'Really informative and spreading a wonderful message.'

Dr Michael Greger, MD,
New York Times bestselling author of *How Not to Die*

'Simon Hill's approach to pl[illegible] with the preachy self-righteousness [illegible]n vegan journey. Accessible withou[illegible] on the shoulders of rigorous resea[illegible] if you'd like to be more aware of wh[illegible] choices do for you and for our world.'

Osher Günsberg, TV host, podcaster and author

'Everyone needs to read this. *The Proof is in the Plants* summarises so eloquently the science of nutrition and what we should be eating more of: plants. Both enjoyable and educational, this book will really inspire you to eat better for your health!'

Ellie Bullen, @elsas_wholesomelife

'Simon Hill has emerged as a leader in the field of evidence-based nutrition because his work is meticulously cited and based on the latest science, and he's not afraid to tackle controversial topics. After reading this book you will feel confident in your food choices and know exactly how to fuel your body for optimal health and athletic performance.'

Robby Barbaro,
New York Times bestselling author of *Mastering Diabetes*

'I highly recommend *The Proof is in the Plants* for anyone seeking practical insight into the power of plant-based nutrition.'

Cyrus Khambatta, PhD,
New York Times bestselling author of *Mastering Diabetes*

'Whether you are already a plant-based foodie, new to the scene, or someone on the fence, *The Proof is in the Plants* will open your mind and fill you up with bountiful new ideas for exploring the next frontiers of health – for you and the planet.'

Dr William Li,
New York Times bestselling author of *Eat to Beat Disease*

'A beautifully written book with a spectacular combination of passion and science, and an absolute page-turner. This book will truly inspire you to think deeply and act differently about health – both your own and that of the planet.'

Jacqueline Alwill, accredited nutritionist,
@brownpapernutrition

'Tired of feeling confused about what to eat? Enter Simon Hill, the nutrition advocate we've all been waiting for. Less about selling absolutes and more about empowering you with scientific truths, Hill delivers with *The Proof is in the Plants*, a rigorously evidence-based primer that will immunise you against diet misinformation and empower you with the tools you need to reclaim your health once and for all.'

Rich Roll, ultra-endurance athlete, top podcast host and
bestselling author of *Finding Ultra* and *The Plantpower Way*

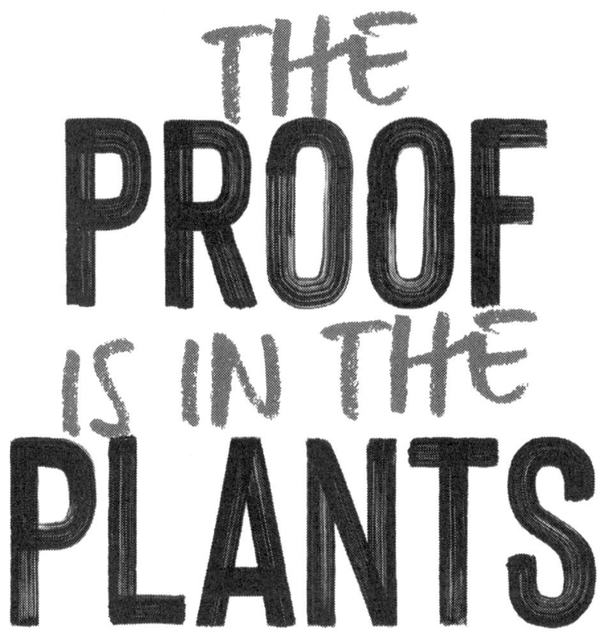

How science shows a plant-based diet could save your life (AND THE PLANET)

SIMON HILL

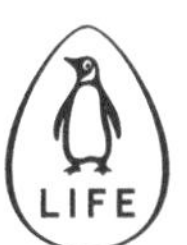

PENGUIN LIFE

AN IMPRINT OF

PENGUIN BOOKS

The information contained in this book is provided for general purposes only. It is not intended for and should not be relied upon as medical advice. The publisher and author are not responsible for any specific health or allergy needs that may require medical supervision. If you have underlying health problems, intend to change your diet or lifestyle, or have any doubts about the advice provided in this book, you should seek the advice of a qualified medical, dietary or other appropriate professional.

PENGUIN LIFE

UK | USA | Canada | Ireland | Australia
India | New Zealand | South Africa | China

Penguin Life is part of the Penguin Random House group of companies whose addresses can be found at global.penguinrandomhouse.com

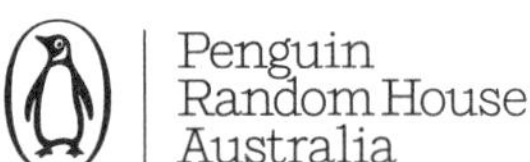

First published by Penguin Life in 2021

The graphic on p. 206 is adapted from the report of the Commission Food in The Anthropocene: the EAT-*Lancet* Commission on Healthy Diets From Sustainable Food Systems. The entire Commission can be found online at eatforum.org/eat-lancet-commission.

Cover photography and styling by Alison Buchanan
Cover design by Adam Laszczuk © Penguin Random House Australia Pty Ltd
Illustrations by Chloe Gordon, madebychloe.com.au
Author photograph by Charles Grant
Index by Puddingburn Publishing Services
Internal design and typesetting by Post Pre-Press, Australia
Set in 12.25/16 pt Minion Pro

Printed and bound in Australia by Griffin Press, part of Ovato, an accredited ISO AS/NZS 14001 Environmental Management Systems printer

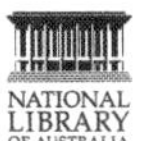

A catalogue record for this book is available from the National Library of Australia

ISBN 978 1 76089 004 9

penguin.com.au

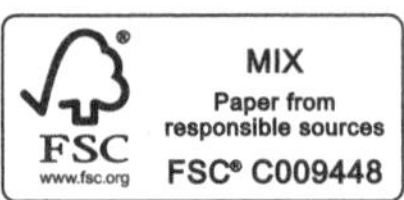

Contents

Foreword

There are certain values that we all hold dear – longevity, prevention of disease and a beautiful, healthy planet. We want a diet that delivers on all these fronts. But how are we to know what to eat to accomplish it? Nutrition feels so confusing these days. Popular diets often conflict with one another, and every click or swipe on the internet reveals a new self-proclaimed expert eager to sell you their agenda. We end up lost in the woods, wandering aimlessly and not getting any closer to the truth. If it's the truth you seek, then it's time we pull out our trusty compass – honest and agenda-free science.

That's exactly what you'll get in this book. Simon combines his expertise as a nutritionist, his insatiable interest in nutritional science and his access to leading experts from across the globe to reveal the scientific truth. Years of research have coalesced around a plant-based diet as the optimal diet for both human and planetary health. So if it's longevity, prevention of disease and a healthy planet that you seek, there is one diet that will deliver it all – a whole-food, plant-based diet. This is where our compass is pointing us.

But to make it happen, you have to be open to the possibility of change. Right now, you may be wondering what you're going to eat. You probably love the food you're currently eating, and may be fearful that your tastebuds aren't going to warm up to this new diet. These are common concerns. In fact, I used to feel the exact same way. Never in a million years did I think that I would give up the foods I love the most – steaks, hot dogs, deli sandwiches – and replace them with fruits, vegetables, whole grains, seeds, nuts and legumes.

But there I was, a shade past thirty years old but feeling at least twenty years older. I was twenty kilos overweight, depressed, anxious and perpetually exhausted. My blood pressure was high and my self-esteem was low. Something had to give. I tried exercising my way out of it, thinking that if I put in enough effort at the gym and in the pool, I could eat whatever I wanted and restore my health. But it didn't work. I had to take a look in the mirror and realize that the food that I was raised on, our family food and the food that I loved, was holding me back.

It all changed for me when I discovered the power of plants. It started small – a smoothie instead of fast food, losing the cream and sweetener from my coffee, adding fibre, fewer French fries and more salads. But these small changes added up to huge results. The weight melted from my body, the anxiety lifted, my blood pressure meds were no longer needed and my self-confidence surged. I was back!

So I brought this approach into my gastroenterology clinic and my patients began having transformative improvements in their health – reversing irritable bowel syndrome, putting their Crohn's disease and ulcerative colitis into remission, and throwing away their acid reflux medications. It was so powerful that I felt compelled to do something completely out of character for me: I started an Instagram account, called @theguthealthmd.

Two years later I connected with an Australian named Simon Hill, who had just started a new podcast called *Plant Proof*. In June 2018 we recorded 'Episode 17: Building a Healthy Gut' and a month later it was released. Over the following weeks we both learned what it meant to go viral. Friends were telling friends that they had to listen to this show, and so it spread across the globe to hundreds of thousands of people. Messages were pouring in from people around the world, sharing how this episode had changed their life.

The overwhelming response to that podcast motivated me to write a book named *Fiber Fueled*, which became an instant *New York Times* bestseller and has sold more than 100,000 copies. *Plant Proof* became one of the most popular podcasts worldwide, with millions and millions of downloads and an avid following. And despite living in different hemispheres, you can see from this book that Simon and I have become close friends.

But it wasn't until reading this book that I understood Simon's own journey to a plant-based diet. Today, he's out there leading the charge to eat more plants, but he wasn't born that way. In fact, plant foods were a total afterthought in the standard Australian diet of his youth. Meat was more than just consumed – it was celebrated. But a series of events in his life challenged him to re-examine his diet. When he started looking at food through the lens of nutritional science, he discovered that simple, sustainable and delicious choices could reduce his risk for disease and supercharge his health for vitality and longevity.

Simon's journey started with a burning desire to understand the optimal diet for human and planetary health. He was confused by all the misinformation out there, and he needed a way to separate fact from fiction. So he turned to science. He obsessively devoured research study after research study searching for answers. He went on to obtain an advanced degree in nutritional science, and he nurtured relationships with leading experts from across the globe. The end result of years of work is this book. It is a triumphant tour de force of modern nutritional science that delivers the knowledge and actionable steps that we all need for human and planetary health. A book I can proudly say that has one hundred per cent of my support. If you're looking for your compass, you are holding it in your hands right now.

Just a few years ago, Simon and I were on opposite sides of the planet consuming a diet that was poisoning our health. We didn't know each other, but we both had our own individual stories that led us to a plant-based diet. Following that path connected us to one another, fuelled by a desire to help others and share what we discovered – that plants heal.

Now here we are to connect with you. You've had your own journey. Maybe your diet hasn't been perfect. Neither was ours! It doesn't matter where you were before, it only matters where you are going. We are inviting you to take the path that heals and invigorates both you and this planet through the power of plants. Join us!

Will Bulsiewicz, MD MSCI
New York Times bestselling author, *Fiber Fueled*

Introduction

Everywhere you turn these days, there are books promising to hack your way to improved health and a better body. Bookshops across the world are lined with diet books that tell you to eliminate sugar, or to eat a high-fat diet rich in animal foods, or that a 100% vegan diet is the *only* way to improve our health, looks and longevity. And I can see why: absolutes and quick fixes are easy to sell. The trouble is, to upgrade our health in the long-term, there are no secret shortcuts or magic pills. The science underlying our wellbeing is much more nuanced than that.

If you're looking for exaggerations, propaganda, questionable science that is bent to fit an agenda or 'hacks' to solve your weight issues in just four weeks, this is not the book for you. What I'm offering is everything you need to know about the optimal way to fuel yourself, based on the best available scientific literature and my unique experience interviewing the world's leading health experts. We'll cover why it's important to consider the health of our planet when making our food choices, too.

I'm not here to sell you anything; I'm here to give you an impartial and agenda-free explanation of how you can enhance your health and wellbeing both today and for decades to come.

Importantly, I'm also not here just to explain *what* we should be eating, but also *why*. Understanding the mechanisms and science behind our food choices offers protection against misinformation and allows us to adapt to a way of eating that works for us. The proof, as you'll see, is in the plants.

Despite the word 'plants' in the title, this book is not about labels and is certainly not just for those interested in veganism. My purpose is to clear the confusion, improve your health and help you understand the impact that your food choices have on the world around you.

The science underpinning nutritional advice is complex, multi-faceted and often convoluted. It makes sense that so many of us are confused about what we should be eating, especially when every year there seems to be yet another fad diet promising weight loss, muscle gain and perfect health. Even most medical professionals receive little training in nutrition. It took me an undergraduate honours degree in physiotherapy, a master's degree in nutrition, a specialised course in plant-based nutrition plus countless hours recording podcast episodes with some of the leading experts in the world to develop the nutritional literacy that I have today. However, we *all* deserve to know how to fuel and look after our bodies. Nobody should be locked out of understanding how to live the longest, healthiest life possible. For this reason, I've done the work for you, sifting through large bodies of evidence-based scientific literature and busting nutrition myths to bring you the agenda-free conclusions to inform the way you feed yourself and your family.

As you'll know if you've ever listened to the *Plant Proof* podcast, I spend countless hours each week breaking down the scientific literature on human nutrition so that we all can make sense of it. It's my passion. I want to help you feel less overwhelmed and confused, and more empowered and optimistic.

My story

I grew up eating a pretty standard Western diet: meat was the star of the plate, whether it was homemade meals or one of our frequent visits to McDonald's or the school 'tuckshop', as we called it, where fried food, meat pies and sausage rolls were always difficult to keep in stock.

When I was fifteen, my dad had a heart attack. We'd spent the day driving around the Yarra Valley, a beautiful wine district about two hours from Melbourne, singing to The Rolling Stones and Cat Stevens. On the way home, Dad felt some pain in his left shoulder but put on a brave face as he always does – he's a doctor – so I thought nothing of it. In the middle of the night, I was woken by a noise and found my dad in the living room, out of breath, in pain and clearly in need of medical assistance.

'I've called an ambulance,' he said, with a worried look in his eyes.

The paramedics arrived shortly after. Within fifteen minutes, he was carried into a helicopter and flown away. Terrified and confused, I followed with paramedics by car to the hospital. Upon arrival, I was told that my dad, who was in his early forties, had suffered a serious heart attack but was fortunately going to survive, thanks to the air transport and emergency medical care that he received. He was extremely lucky – sudden and unexpected cardiac events are the most common cause of death worldwide, often occurring in the prime of a person's life and without any previously identified symptoms of heart disease.[1] Lights out without warning. My dad escaped this and was given a second chance at life, but sadly many do not.

I vividly remember the doctors explaining to me that heart disease runs in families, with no mention of the link to any lifestyle factors such as diet. I assumed that because of our genetics, my brother and I were destined to follow in the footsteps of our dad and our grandfather, who had himself suffered from multiple heart attacks. Since there apparently wasn't anything I could do to prevent cardiovascular disease, I accepted my fate and kept going about my life and eating what I considered to be normal.

The start of my obsession with nutritional science

Seven years later, I had begun working with professional athletes as a sports physiotherapist and was inspired to take greater interest in building strength and muscle. Like many people new to working out, I looked to the major fitness magazines and quickly found myself consuming a diet that was 'cleaner' than before but still extremely animal-focused and with little diversity or appreciation for the power of plants. Chicken breast, lean steak, fish, broccoli, spinach and sweet potato were on heavy rotation. The removal of junk food made me feel much better and, for the first time, I started to draw a connection between what I put into my mouth and my health. At this time I thought I had a good grasp on nutrition from my education and work as a physio, but in retrospect all I really understood was calories, energy balance and macronutrients (proteins, carbohydrates and fats). Thanks to effective marketing, I was protein-obsessed, in terms of how much of it I ate, not in terms of where that protein came from, and had no understanding of the importance of fibre and diversity of plants in my diet.

In 2015, my brother, James, inspired me to take a closer look at the way I was fuelling myself. Given our family history of cardiovascular disease, James had been cutting back on animal products, meat in particular, after hearing about research in this area on various podcasts. He told me there was research showing people who consumed plant-rich diets high in fibre had lower risk of cardiovascular disease. Amazed, I began digging into the science of human nutrition, looking for evidence that dietary changes can promote not only greater longevity (how long you live) but also better health span (how many healthy years you live). Truth be told, I was looking to prove James wrong – I was happy with my diet, and I hoped to find research that supported my continuing to eat a high-protein, meat-heavy diet. I also needed to know if it was possible to change your diet to focus on longevity without sacrificing happiness and physical performance today. Even if science suggested we could live until 140 years old if we ate nothing but kale, there was no way I could do it – food is one of life's greatest pleasures and something to be enjoyed! And as a fitness enthusiast, I didn't want my strength and athletic capability to suffer from changing my diet either.

What followed is probably best described as a healthy obsession with finding out how to make truly healthy food decisions. To dial up my nutritional literacy, I began a master's degree in nutrition, learned how to interpret statistics and critique study methodology, and became fascinated by reading and evaluating scientific literature and commentary surrounding it. Almost immediately, my eyes were opened to the many conflicting interpretations of the science that existed. How could it be that various groups of health professionals, all seemingly legitimate on paper, were giving such contradictory advice? There seemed to be two major camps: those promoting high-fat, animal-focused diets, and those promoting whole-food, plant-focused diets, with each group fervently claiming their diet was the superior way to eat for a long, healthy life. I must admit, initially I felt so bamboozled by all the information that I was tempted to give up and just stick to the diet that I thought had served me well for over two decades of my life.

But the memory of my dad's heart attack compelled me to get to the truth, so I made it my mission to consider not only all the arguments but also to read the science that prominent health professionals used to support their recommendations. In the end, I came to understand that, when interpreted honestly, the research undeniably points to a plant-predominant diet (getting about 85 per cent or more of your total calories from plants) as the *best practice, evidence-based* approach, and probably the single most powerful lifestyle change you can make to better your health. I had my answer. Now I had nothing to lose by giving it a proper go myself.

Feeling the benefits

It took me a few months to transition from that significantly lower meat intake inspired by James to a completely plant-based lifestyle. I'd already stopped consuming dairy as a teenager, as it didn't agree with me, so first I removed all meat from my diet, then fish and lastly eggs. I started eating more whole grains and legumes such as lentils, black beans, tofu and tempeh without even realising then how packed they are with protein, fibre and micronutrients.

What I experienced was nothing short of life-changing. Physically, I immediately felt more energetic and my recovery after workouts was superior. My training intensity and frequency went up, my digestion felt effortless, and my mental clarity improved. I noticed my hair and nails seemed much healthier, and grew faster too! In addition, I felt an overwhelming sense of empowerment: for the first time in my life, I fully understood the power of food and rather than being on autopilot, I was in control of my health. Fast forward six years and I can honestly say that I feel like a new person, mentally and physically. I have a different perspective on food and life, and my body feels better than ever. Since adopting a plant-based lifestyle, I've never compromised on the flavour of my meals and I've become a more conscious person and consumer. By working through this process of questioning the way I had been living for over twenty years, I've learned to separate myself from my thoughts and challenge them. As a result, my actions are now much more aligned with my values and beliefs, which has brought about unexpected inner peace and clarity.

There's no way of knowing for sure what a difference the lifestyle choices we make now will have in ten, twenty or thirty years. However, when I look at the harrowing rates of lifestyle diseases and the totality of the scientific evidence, I am confident that the evidence-based approach that I outline in this book is our best bet for ensuring we are not adding to those statistics. It's like putting on your seat belt while driving: to the best of our knowledge, eating a plant-based diet is a safe and sensible means of protection against unforeseen and potentially avoidable health crises that could otherwise be in our genetic future. It's a precaution that will statistically reduce your chance of developing or dying from a chronic lifestyle disease, and leave you full of energy along the way.[2]

My mission to share the science

In January 2018, after a few years of eating plant-based and feeling more inspired than ever, I started the Plant Proof Instagram account to share my story and, more importantly, the science, with the hope of helping others to experience the same health benefits I had and improve their chances of living a long, healthy life. I wanted to centralise the knowledge I had gained throughout my years at university, in addition to my clinical experience and reviews of scientific literature. Why the name 'Plant Proof'? Well, I was living proof of someone thriving on plants and I was passionate about sharing the scientific proof I was unearthing too.

Initially the account was purely a place to share and store information for my circle of close friends and family who were curious about my lifestyle and routinely asking questions. Before long, people from all over the world were connecting with me – they had an appetite for agenda-free nutritional information that was broken down, non-judgemental, unaffected by dogma and made practical. With this encouragement, I subsequently created plantproof.com and then the *Plant Proof* podcast, which has provided me with the opportunity to connect with some of the world's greatest minds on living a conscious, healthy and active life, including Dr Will Bulsiewicz , Drs Dean and Ayesha Sherzai, Dr David Katz, Dr Emily Manoogian, Dr David Sinclair, Dr Jonathan Foley, Dr Hannah Ritchie and Rich Roll, just to name a few. These information-packed conversations have taught me a huge amount and I have worked hard to sprinkle the wisdom of my incredible guests throughout this book so that we can continue to learn from them.

The three pillars

My interest in human health motivated me to shift to a plant-based diet, but there are two other enormous benefits that come from putting more plants on your plate.

Through some of my podcast interviews and my own reading, I've grown increasingly aware of the destruction of the environment we live in. To feed the billions of people who walk this Earth is no small feat, but doing so with resource-inefficient animal foods has been demonstrated time and again to be one of the main drivers of climate change and the destruction of our ecosystem.[3] Figures vary greatly, but the Food and Agriculture Organization of the United Nations (FAO) cites that animal agriculture alone generates 14.5% of human-induced global greenhouse gases.[4] Beyond emissions, animal agriculture is the main driver behind staggering rates of deforestation and biodiversity loss, and it is the single largest user of freshwater.[5,6] That's why, away from any political agenda, the unified consensus of the leading environmental scientists is that we need to drastically reduce our global consumption of animal foods if we are to limit the devastating impact of climate change.[7] On learning this, it became clear to me that not only is the food we eat contributing to our early deaths – it is killing the planet too. This is the concept of *planetary health.* A thriving natural environment is the necessary foundation upon which we build our societies and without it, we simply cannot exist. With so much at stake, I am convinced more than ever that the only diet that should be promoted on a mass scale is one that benefits our environment too. A plant-based diet does just that: not only is it the diet that most supports *our* optimal health, it is also one that supports optimal *planetary* health.

It almost goes without saying that a diet that removes, or at least significantly reduces, animal products from the plate is a more compassionate choice too. Each day in Australia alone approximately 13.4 million sentient beings are killed for human consumption.[8] Not out of necessity but purely because we like the way they taste and eating them is ingrained into our culture.

Together, these make up the three pillars of my Plant Proof philosophy: human health, planetary health and animal welfare.

If you're reading this and feeling put off by the thought of never again consuming the odd poached egg or piece of fish, I've got good news: the science tells us that it doesn't have to be all or nothing. You can still reap the many health benefits you'll read about in this book with a diet that is about 85% plant-based. This is an important point. The scientific literature that exists today supporting a plant-based diet is very much a combination of studies looking at both plant-predominant diets (that could still include a small amount of meat, fish, eggs and dairy) and plant-exclusive diets. The current science doesn't tell us that a plant-only diet is superior to a diet consisting of about 85% of calories from plants, because separating out these two types of diet to study them thoroughly and conclusively is a near-impossible task. This flexibility between 85–100% plant-based can be really reassuring if you're looking to go plant-based for the first time, and it gives everyone room to find the level of commitment that works for them.

For me, the pillars of planetary health and animal welfare solidified my decision to no longer eat any animal products at all. Once I had gathered the information about how our food choices affect our environment and non-human sentient beings, I knew that as someone fortunate enough to have good food access and the means to change the way I ate, it was something I wanted to commit to. But I want to be really clear from the outset that this book is not about the exact percentage of plant foods in your diet, or what label you might choose – if you want to work towards eating more whole plant foods and fewer animal products, I'm here to help you do that, regardless of the extent of the changes you make.

What to expect from this book

In Part One, we'll unravel the confusion that surrounds what we should be eating in today's world. In Part Two, I'll explain the science that shows how a plant-based diet is the optimal way of eating for your health, the future of our planet and animal welfare. In Part Three, we'll get into the nutrition behind eating plant-based, which foods to eat and why and the practicalities of changing this part of your lifestyle. No matter who you are or what stage of life you're at, you can make big improvements in your energy, health and quality of life with simple dietary changes that will have long-lasting effects. Together, we will tackle common dietary questions, such as where to get protein, whether olive oil is healthy and dairy is essential for strong bones, what type of carbohydrates we should eat and why fibre is important. And you'll feel equipped to take your next steps.

Most of all, I will help you separate fact from fiction so you'll truly understand what a healthy dietary pattern looks like once and for all. I hope to illustrate that what you gain by making small changes in your diet far outweighs what you leave behind. In other words, you have nothing to lose! Join me and let's take a deep dive into how we ended up here and how we can turn things around.

My agenda-free approach

It's important for me to say that, unlike a lot of the 'science' I've come across, my research has no input or funding from any food company, pharmaceutical company or governing body. Nor do I accept any sponsorship for social media posts or feature paid advertising on my podcast. As such, I have been able to interpret the science without any external pressure to bring you unadulterated facts. I've been committed to this approach since the inception of Plant Proof, which is why I have promised to donate 100 per cent of the proceeds I receive from this book to charity.

Our health: What's the problem?

I think it's safe for me to assume that you'd like to add not only more years to your life but also more life to your years: you don't want to die early, nor do you want to be afflicted by chronic health conditions that reduce your quality of life. In Australia, we're not doing too badly on the first point: our average life expectancy is eighty-five for women and eighty-one for men, up from fifty-nine and fifty-five in 1901, and our combined average life expectancy is greater than the OECD average of eighty-one years.[9,10]

However, while we're living longer, we're not necessarily living *better*. Thanks to advances in modern medicine, we've become quite good at keeping people alive through critical high-risk periods of life where they may have otherwise died prematurely, yet we are spending more years of our lives affected by chronic diseases.[11,12] And these diseases that are plaguing us? They're not the infectious diseases that were the main cause of death 100 years ago. They're overwhelmingly diseases impacted by diet and other lifestyle factors: cardiovascular disease, dementia (including Alzheimer's), cancer (lung, breast, prostate and colorectal), chronic obstructive pulmonary disease and type 2 diabetes.[10]

These chronic, non-communicable diseases generally have slow onset and manifest in the form of long-term persistent symptoms, prolonged suffering and disability. They are the leading cause of premature death in Australia, accounting for almost nine in every ten deaths.[13] Globally, they kill 41 million people each year – equivalent to 71% of all deaths.[14]

Sadly, it doesn't stop there. Arthritis, osteoporosis, asthma, non-alcoholic fatty liver disease, chronic kidney disease and inflammatory bowel disease, to name just a few, are also widespread across the nation. Behavioural and metabolic risk factors such as poor nutrition, smoking, physical inactivity, alcohol and drug use, obesity, high blood pressure (hypertension) and high cholesterol (hypercholesterolaemia) are often shared by these chronic diseases, so it's unsurprising that many people who develop chronic disease are affected by more than one. These are called *comorbidities*. In just the past ten years, we have seen the number of Australians with one or more chronic diseases rise from approximately 9.1 million to 11.56 million people.[15] That's almost half of our national population.[10]

Given that around 50% of the Australian population is living with chronic non-communicable diseases, it's highly likely that everyone reading this has been affected by chronic disease either personally or within their family. If you're anything like I was ten years ago, you may be thinking, 'I'm only twenty, this doesn't affect me'. Unfortunately, that's not the case. While it's true these chronic diseases tend to show up when a person is around fifty years of age, or later, the underlying disease pathology often starts during childhood and can even begin in utero depending on the lifestyle of the person carrying the child.[16,17] That means our lifestyle choices, such as diet, can be influencing our disease risk from a young age – which I wish someone had explained to me when I was twenty.

Each day in Australia

- 430 people die, 87% of which are deaths due to chronic disease
- 400 people are diagnosed with some form of cancer
- 250 people develop dementia
- 169 people have a heart attack
- 100 people have a stroke
- 829,000 prescriptions are filled

Sourced from AIHW and Dementia Australia.[10,13,18]

The power is in your hands

Despite the fact we are living longer, more of us are experiencing poorer overall quality of life – more pain, disability, restriction, limitation and psychological distress.[19] But that doesn't have to be your story. Experts now know that the majority of the world's leading chronic diseases are predominantly a result of lifestyle choices rather than a genetic predisposition or inevitability.[20] You could say that genetics load the gun but *lifestyle pulls the trigger*.

A famous study published in 1996, The Danish Twin Study, tracked 2872 sets of identical and non-identical twins from birth for the better part of 100 years, and was able to identify that approximately 20% of someone's long-term health is attributable to their genes, with the other 80% being a result of their lifestyle.[21] A separate study that compared Japanese men living in Japan with Japanese men who immigrated to the United States found much higher rates of heart disease for those who adopted the Western lifestyle.[22]

Together these studies show that we have more control over our health through our daily life choices than what we just have to accept because of our genes – roughly four times more control.[23] This is good news. Every single day, our decisions and behaviours have the power to either feed or prevent disease, and affect not just how *long* we live, but how *well* we live. This interplay between an individual's lifestyle and their genetics, in particular the modifiable factors such as nutrition, can – in simplistic terms – result in genes being turned on or off (something we will discuss in more detail in Chapter 8 – A diet for living longer).

The word 'diet'

Thanks to the generous advertising budgets of weight-loss companies, the word 'diet' is very much seen within the context of 'I'm going on a diet'. As a result, I've always been careful about using it to describe how we eat. But this modern definition is actually far removed from its ancient Greek origins, when *díaita* was used to describe 'a manner of living'.[24] Rather than being a short-term change to food intake in order to lose fat or 'detoxify' the body, it described the habitual foods that people from certain regions ate - for example, the Mediterranean diet or the vegetarian diet. It's with this understanding that I propose we take back the power, remove the stigma, and stand by the more holistic use of the term 'diet' to describe how we eat. It's time to once more think of diet as a noun, not a verb.

Although science has demonstrated this relationship between nature versus nurture, the incidence of chronic disease is so high in the Western world that from an early age many of us start to see these diseases as a routine part of ageing and ultimately our fate. But it shouldn't be considered 'normal', or inevitable, to be dying of a heart attack, living with type 2 diabetes or taking a cocktail of medications just to get through our days. None of us is immortal – we have to die from something – but there's a big difference between experiencing the burden of chronic disease for decades versus spending the majority of your years free from disease.

The reason these chronic conditions are so pervasive, and tend to run in families, could be explained by the fact that family members often adopt the same lifestyle, rather than it being a genetic certainty. Our lifestyle can even affect the disease profile of our pets! A 2020 study out of Sweden, which followed over 200,000 owner–dog pairs for six years, found that owners of a dog with type 2 diabetes were 32% more likely to develop type 2 diabetes themselves.[25] In other words, when we adopt unhealthy lifestyle habits, we are likely to share them with those around us – be it humans or animal family members – and at the same time share the associated risk of developing chronic disease.

The obesity link

Although not everyone who has a chronic disease is overweight, and not all people who are overweight will develop a chronic disease, it is definitely a risk factor.[9,26-33] For example, a large review of eighteen long-term studies, which when combined involved more than half a million subjects, identified that people who were overweight were around three times more likely to develop type 2 diabetes, and people who were obese around seven times more likely.[29] Obesity also increases the risk of developing colorectal cancer by around 30%, postmenopausal breast cancer by around 20–40% and gallbladder cancer by around 60%.[34-36] Carrying excess body fat significantly increases our odds of living a shorter life, too.[37-40]

What's frightening is that since 1975 global obesity, which is described as 'preventable' by the WHO, has tripled to around 2 billion people, or 25% of the global population.[41] While Australia ranks well by many global health measures, we fare pretty poorly when it comes to carrying extra weight and placing ourselves at a higher risk of developing chronic disease. Specifically, one in three Australian adults are obese and two in three Australian adults are either obese or overweight.[42] That's right – being classified as a healthy body weight is actually more uncommon. There are complex reasons behind this that we'll learn more about in the coming chapters.

So while some of us may have genetics that predispose us to certain diseases, like my family and cardiovascular disease, the way we navigate through our lives directly affects what our health and disease span will look like. And when it comes to our lifestyles, and the risk of losing years of good health, poor diet quality tops the list as the most significant contributor.[43,44] Therefore, the food we eat is arguably the single most important thing we should be focusing on to counteract any genetic predispositions to disease that we may have and improve our chances of living a long healthy life. This book will help you do that.

PART ONE

A DIET OF CONFUSION

THE MOST COMPREHENSIVE EPIDEMIOLOGICAL STUDY ever conducted on the causes of premature deaths, the Global Burden of Disease study, found that an unhealthy diet is now responsible for more years of poor health and deaths than any other lifestyle behaviour, having surpassed deaths caused by tobacco, hunger, infections and communicable diseases such as hepatitis and influenza.[1,2] The study, published in 2017, clearly showed that at a global level, we are consuming too much salt, processed meats and red meat, and not enough fibre, omega-3 fats, whole grains, fruits, nuts, seeds, legumes and vegetables, and that these shortcomings in our diet are causing an unprecedented spike in chronic diseases.[3]

Good-quality nutritional research like this study is abundant and available online at the click of a button. It clearly states where we are going wrong and what we should be doing instead, time and again pointing to the undeniable benefits of eating a largely plant-based diet rich in whole foods. But, despite the science being clear, a lot of us are more confused than ever about what we should be eating. It's not uncommon to have friends or family members following completely different diets – with each of them firmly convinced that theirs is the right way! – and to feel bombarded by mixed messages about how the fat you eat is the fat you wear, all carbs are fattening, animal protein is the answer to all your concerns, or the only thing that matters is calories consumed versus calories burned.

How confused are we? Well, the typical Australian currently gets about 42% of their calories from foods that are high in energy, salt, sugar and saturated fats and low in fibre, vitamins, minerals and water[4] – such as sugar-sweetened drinks, processed meats, muffins, cakes, muesli bars, burgers, pizzas and alcohol. These foods, which are not to be confused with minimally processed foods such as brown rice, canned beans and nut butters, add little nutritional value to our diet. It is no wonder then that most of us consume more saturated fats and salt than the national recommendations and 50% of us exceed the World Health Organization's recommendation for added (or 'free') sugars.[5] And it's not just ultra-processed foods where we are getting it wrong: the average Australian consumes approximately 116 kg of meat per year, which is among the highest per capita consumption in the world.[6]

This combination of relatively 'empty' calories from ultra-processed food and excessive meat consumption means we're getting fewer calories from more healthful foods. In fact, very few of us – just over 5% – meet the recommended amount of both daily fruit and vegetables.[7] It makes sense, given our low intake of fruit and veg, that less than 20% of Australian adults reach the suggested daily target of between 28–38 g of fibre, a nutrient only found in plant foods. In fact, the typical fibre intake in Australia is so low (20.7 g per day) that researchers have described it as a 'nutrient of concern'.[8]

Perhaps you're thinking (as I once did), *Shouldn't people show greater willpower, control their cravings and purchase healthier food instead of these ultra-processed foods? Shouldn't the responsibility be on the consumer for buying these products in the first place?* I have learned in my research that over the past seven or so decades, during which chronic diseases have exponentially risen, it is not collective willpower that has changed but rather the environment around us. We cannot underestimate the determination of the industries with vested interests in ultra-processed food and animal products to get their goods in front of our eyes and into our mouths. When you consider the sum of food advertising, social media commentary, industry-funded scientific studies, a healthcare system better equipped to manage disease rather than prevent it, and a nutrition culture that makes huge profits out of our confusion, it's no wonder we struggle to make sense of it all.

I've found that our collective confusion about diet and nutrition comes down to three main areas: our rigged food environment, our hijacked healthcare system and our for-profit nutrition culture. The first and most crucial step in taking control of our health lies in understanding *why* this confusion exists and identifying the many forces at play that have caused it in the first place. If you feel overwhelmed, sceptical or just unclear on what the science says constitutes the optimal diet, you're not alone and it's not your fault. As you'll see, the environment is designed for us to fail. Once we know what we're up against, we can cut through the confusion. ●

CHAPTER 1

A rigged food environment

Eating an evidence-based healthy diet should *not* require obtaining a high degree of nutritional and climate science literacy. Our food environment – the human-built environment in which we buy food (such as supermarkets and cafes) – is influenced by a range of social, cultural, political and economic factors which then have an effect on what we buy and our overall dietary pattern. In a healthy food environment, healthy foods such as fruits and vegetables are easily accessible and affordable. In contrast, in an obesogenic food environment the healthy choices become more difficult to make, often as a result of less healthy products being hard to resist due to their extreme palatability, clever marketing and attractive price points. Thus we are more likely to adopt an unhealthy dietary pattern.

Our food environment *should* favour foods that promote health and reduce the environmental degradation of our planet, yet this couldn't be further from reality. Rather than ensuring that the cheapest and most accessible options are the healthiest, our current food landscape is an out-of-date system that was never intended to prioritise long-term human health.[1] What it does prioritise is industry profit, particularly for Big Food transnational corporations such as Kraft, Unilever, Nestlé and Coca-Cola.[2] The food industry proactively works to create a food environment that makes it incredibly difficult and confusing for us to choose foods that are best for our health. Instead, the most convenient and unhealthful foods are usually those that the industry profits from most.

The food environment in which we live is actually a relatively new development; as recently as the late nineteenth century and early parts of the twentieth century, the majority of the food that Australians consumed did not come sealed in packaging. Rather, people grew and bought vegetables and fruits, and hunted, reared or bought meats and seafood. This was real food – no labels or lengthy ingredient lists. However, after the Great Depression and the two World Wars, countries across the globe, including Australia, implemented policies and incentives to greatly intensify their agricultural production to achieve food security. They introduced government subsidies, new and advanced processing methods, and factory farming; increased the use of pesticides; and sought out ingredients that would be cheap, ample and keep on the shelf for long periods. The aim was to become more self-sufficient, preventing the recurrence of food shortages and nutritional deficiency-related diseases that were prevalent at the time.[3] Governments wanted to protect their people, prevent starvation and support population growth.

While these policies were necessary at the time, they were introduced with a view to increasing *survival* – the top priority – rather than providing *optimal human nutrition*. These new foods were often fortified with major vitamins and minerals, such as the addition of B vitamins to white bread and other refined cereal products. This was successful in reducing rates of malnutrition, but they were still a far cry from whole foods in their natural state.[4–6] At the time we did not possess the scientific knowledge to fully understand the long-term implications of eating such highly processed foods, but now it's clear these new policies came at a cost – the health of generations to come. We created a food environment where people were safe from scurvy and rickets, but at risk of developing heart disease and type 2 diabetes.

Today, we have more than enough resources to feed the global population with foods that are unprocessed or minimally processed (e.g. fruits, vegetables, legumes). In fact, the Food and Agriculture Organization of the United Nations (FAO) estimates that around one-third of all the food that is produced is not even used – it's wasted, costing the world at least US$1 trillion each year.[7]

So why hasn't our food system been adapted to our needs? Unbeknown to most people, a whole range of strategies from the same playbook as that of the alcohol and tobacco industries are used by the food industry[2] – from lobbying to blame-shifting to stressing their importance to the economy – to weaken and block proposed policies aimed at addressing diet-related diseases.[8–10] Devoted to persuading us that its products are central to our health, culture, enjoyment and our overall quality of life, Big Food uses a multi-pronged approach to ensure it stays a part of your life, both here in Australia and in markets around the world. From influencing the scientific literature and dietary guidelines to educating our children about healthy nutrition, these industries, particularly the animal agriculture and ultra-processed food sectors, are one of the greatest contributors to today's dietary confusion.[9,11] Even when there are discussions in Australia around sugar taxes, marketing restrictions for unhealthy foods, subsidisation for fresh produce growers and greater promotion of minimally processed foods, the action that follows is often minimal.[12–15] It's no coincidence that change never seems to get very far.

The revolving door

It's well documented that transnational food companies prefer to operate in less tightly regulated markets. After all, implementation of public health policy tends to conflict with their major goal, maximising shareholder profits.[16,17] In order to influence the development of policies in their favour, a key strategy employed by these companies is establishing relationships with policymakers. This frequently involves personal ties – a mechanism described as the 'revolving door' where senior politicians or government advisers take up jobs in the food industry, no different to what takes place in the mining, gambling and finance industries.[8,9,18,19] This isn't just on the odd occasion – it happens all the time. A 2019 study found that 36% of all registered Australian lobbyists, representing industry, were formerly government representatives.[8] The study noted that the movement from government to industry could be influenced by 'quid pro quo' arrangements, where members of government are motivated to support policy favouring industry interests on the understanding or possibility of a future role in the industry. It works the other way, too, with people from the food industry encouraged to take up political positions while maintaining ties with the industry. This could create the scenario where food industry lobbyists are targeting a government minister they have a personal connection with, which could clearly impact that minister's decision-making.[8,19]

Hyper-palatable processed foods

Using today's advanced technology, food scientists hired by large food companies cleverly formulate products which have undergone significant changes from their natural form, combining them with sugar, salt, fat, preservatives, artificial colours and/or other unnatural additives.[20] These foods have been developed not only to be cheap and durable but also to be addictive – and they are one of the biggest reasons why 95% of Australians are failing to eat enough fruits and vegetables.[21,22] According to research, the average Australian purchases 208 kg of these foods per year![23] This is the equivalent of more than 11,000 Tim Tams – the iconic Aussie chocolate biscuit – per person. More than 30 per day!

What these food scientists look to create is hedonic hunger, an insatiable craving for certain foods without the presence of physical hunger.[24] And it's not just the more obvious senses such as taste, texture and smell that drive these cravings – even the sound of our food can affect how much we enjoy it, making it a commercially valuable area for industry research. When the much-loved Magnum ice cream was reformulated to stop the chocolate coating breaking off and landing on people's clothes, it lost the 'cracking' sound that people found so satisfying when they bit into it, so the company had to quickly revert to the original formulation to rescue their sales.[25] The food industry calls this the *bliss point* – when salt, sugar and fat are combined in the perfect amounts, and are coupled with the perfect texture, to create food that is highly craveable and very difficult to resist.[26]

It is this careful manipulation of food that makes it hard for nature to compete. Would you prefer to bite into a Mars Bar or an apple? For most of us, even though we know it's less healthy, we'd grab the chocolate because we are genetically hardwired to be attracted to energy-dense foods that offer instant gratification. It is widely believed that our ancestors, living in the savannahs of Africa 2 million years ago, evolved in a time when food was scarce, so when they did manage to find energy sources rich in sugar or fat, it made sense to overconsume and put on body fat in preparation for periods without food.[27,28]

Today, we still have a biological affinity for calorie-dense foods yet we live in an enormously different environment. We are constantly surrounded by man-made food options – from 24-hour supermarkets to vending machines to fast food outlets – but the behaviour that once guaranteed our survival is now working against us.[29,30] It's a mismatch that makes us vulnerable to addictive eating patterns, and is the reason why so many of us feel compelled to spend time in the centre aisles of the supermarket, away from the fresh fruit and vegetable section.[31,32] To make matters worse, not only do we have these calorie-dense foods available on tap but, unlike our ancestors, accessing them requires almost no energy expenditure.

More rewarding than cocaine

Studies on mice have shown that the intense sweetness from sugar or calorie-free sweeteners generates a reward signal stronger than the one generated by cocaine.[33] Researchers believe this is because the 'sweetness receptors' in mammals developed in ancestral times, when the sweetest foods available were fruits. Today, hyper-palatable foods, which are far sweeter than fruit, are able to generate supranormal reward signals in the brain that can override our in-built self-control mechanisms. Essentially, they give us a hit so irresistible that we continue to eat in the absence of a physical requirement for calories.[34] The net result? Food addiction.

The impact of these foods in Australia is clear. Research shows that the increasing amount of fat we are carrying is largely a consequence of the fact that the average Australian consumes 826 calories from ultra-processed foods per day.[35,36] And that's just one part of the story. These ultra-processed foods, such as mass-produced packaged breads, breakfast cereals, biscuits, sugar-sweetened beverages, confectionary and ice cream, affect much more than our waistlines. Their consumption has also been implicated in significantly higher risk of developing cardiovascular disease, various cancers, irritable bowel syndrome, inflammation, hypertension and a shortened life span.[37–44] So how do you go about promoting and selling food products with a score sheet that bad?

Establishing credibility

The food industry knows that it needs trust in order to maintain influence. So they employ various strategies to establish a perception of credibility that will keep the faith strong and the sales rolling in. Alignment with health associations and government bodies, including those that create our national dietary guidelines, is one such strategy, which I'll talk about more in the next chapter. But there are plenty of others, including funding their own cleverly designed studies that shift the blame onto a scapegoat, deliberately casting doubt on evidence-based science which suggests their products are harmful, and strategically making their food available in locations of trust.

Shifting the blame

Since as far back as the 1960s, the food industry has been funding and/or sponsoring scientific research in order to boost its credibility and shift the blame for poor health elsewhere.[45] This source of funding is typically welcomed by academics and institutions with open arms – government funding is becoming harder to come by and academics, under unprecedented pressure to publish studies, are commonly expected to raise their own salaries. However, this funding does not come without limitations. Analysis shows that industry-funded research almost always finds benefit or lack of harm to support the funding companies' products, and thus needs to be treated with scepticism.[46] An investigation by a team of American researchers into industry-funded science and outcomes looked at 206 studies, 54% of which received industry funding. It identified that industry-funded studies were 400% to 800% more likely to find a favourable outcome in support of the funding company's product/s compared with non-industry-funded research. Of the intervention trials included, not a single industry-funded study published unfavourable results.[47] Similarly, in 2015, Marion Nestle PhD, professor of nutrition, food studies and public health at New York University, identified seventy-six industry-funded studies that were published over an eight-month period, of which seventy showed results that were favourable to the sponsor's interests.[46]

Is the food industry truly motivated to add to our understanding of human nutrition? Coca-Cola, for example, has publicly pledged to do research honestly yet still reserves the right to terminate studies if the findings are not in its interests.[47,48] This way, it can be lauded for its corporate responsibility initiatives while still protecting its profits. Big Food corporations are funding studies purposefully designed to produce favourable outcomes and/or are not publishing studies that go against their interests. We will never get the full picture if only the 'successful' studies ever make it out into the public domain. The issue with withholding this information is that although it may not be beneficial from a commercial perspective, it's important for adding to the totality of evidence and giving us a more complete picture. If all we are seeing are the studies that show lack of harm, or benefit, for a particular product (a phenomenon known as *positive publication bias*), how can we make an informed decision? If we are going to allow industry to work with academics and fund nutrition science, then we really do need more transparency. Researchers should maintain academic freedom and have full control of the study design and methodology, and all results – whether favourable or unfavourable for the brand – should be made available.

There are many studies out there that are industry-funded and are at odds with the totality of scientific evidence, illustrating the extent to which members of the food industry will go to in order to have published research supporting the consumption of their products. Here are a few examples.

In 1965, the Sugar Research Foundation (SRF), known today as the Sugar Association, secretly funded a literature review published in the *New England Journal of Medicine* which, against all the evidence at the time, exonerated sucrose (table sugar) consumption from increasing the risk of heart disease and instead shifted the blame to dietary cholesterol and saturated fats.[49,50] It is now known, as a result of historical documents made public, that the SRF not only set the objective of the literature review, but also provided studies for the scientists to include and reviewed the draft before it could be published. On top of that, the SRF paid the three scientists the equivalent of US$50,000 to publish the paper, which failed to disclose any conflicts of interest.[49,51] From the documents obtained, it's quite clear that these scientists knew exactly what the SRF wanted and then delivered on it.

More recently, it's become public knowledge that Mars, Pepsi, Nestlé, McDonald's and Coca-Cola have been funding studies to take the focus off their products and instead shift the blame for rising rates of obesity and type 2 diabetes from sugar to lack of exercise.[52–56] Coca-Cola even gifted US$100,000 to a Queensland professor to help fund research looking at the benefit of exercise in treating obesity.[57] In other words, they are trying to protect their profits by sending the message that people are unhealthy because they aren't moving enough, and a diet high in sugar can simply be offset by more exercise. I'm not convinced: the 210 calories in a 500 ml bottle of regular Coca-Cola would take me personally about 2.5–3 km of moderate jogging to burn off. This idea that it's not the food, or drink, but the consumer that is responsible for their behaviour and subsequent health status is regularly used by these companies to position proposed government policies, such as a sugar tax, as irrational and oppressive.[58,59] This in turn may give the public the impression that the likes of Coca-Cola and McDonald's will fight for the right of 'freedom of choice'. But, let's not kid ourselves, these studies on the role of physical activity in obesity are nothing more than marketing – deliberate diversions to turn our attention away from the harm these products are doing to our bodies. These corporations care little about our wellbeing and a lot about their profits.

Planting seeds of doubt

The food industry is well aware that changing our habits is harder than just sticking with what we know, and they use this to their advantage by funding scientific studies that cast doubt on the findings from non-industry-funded science. Because the consumption of animal products and ultra-processed food is deeply ingrained in our culture, all the food industry has to do to protect its market share is to create enough confusion that it's hard for the average person to know how and why to make healthy changes to their plate.

One example of this is eggs, which have been the subject of decades-long debate around their effect on cholesterol levels. Over the years, high-quality studies have identified that it's probably best to minimise our consumption of eggs because they are a rich source of dietary cholesterol, which is well established to increase blood cholesterol levels, an independent risk factor for cardiovascular disease.[60–63] Yet other studies, mostly funded by the egg industry, with rather 'creative' study methodologies, have concluded that the effect of dietary cholesterol, and thus of eggs, is harmless. In fact, a recent review of studies on eggs and cholesterol levels found that significant amounts of industry research conducted since the 1950s have been tactically used to water down the results of non-industry-funded studies.[64]

FIGURE 1.1:
EGG-INDUSTRY-FUNDED CHOLESTEROL STUDIES OVER TIME[64]

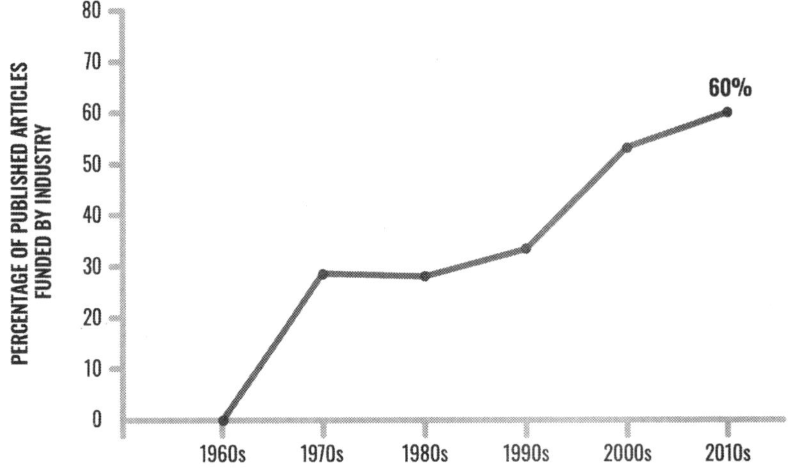

The result? Enough confusion for many people to throw their hands up in the air and point to the studies that support their desire to continue consuming eggs unhindered.

Another recent example is the series of systematic reviews and meta-analyses, published along with a 'Dietary Guideline Recommendations' paper, in the *Annals of Internal Medicine* in 2019 by a group of researchers known as NutriRECS. The study exonerated red and processed meats, claiming most people do not need to reduce their consumption of either in order to maintain good health.[65] Their recommendations – which caused a media frenzy – directly challenged the findings from decades of high-quality science linking red meat and processed meat consumption to cancer, other chronic diseases and premature death. This is science so consistent that the World Health Organization (WHO) in 2015 declared processed meats as *carcinogenic* (cancer-causing) and red meat as *probably carcinogenic.*[66]

There were several problems with the NutriRECS research and the way it was interpreted. First, none of this was new science. They had crunched old data in a way typically assigned to drug research, not nutrition science, which watered down the associations. Second, even with their novel way of reviewing this data, positive associations were still observed between cancer and consumption of unprocessed red meat and processed meats, meaning they still found evidence of harm. To get around this, the researchers also decided to take into consideration personal preferences and health-related views related to meat consumption.[67] In other words, their recommendations considered the fact that people *like the taste* of meat. Since when has nutrition science been about personal preference?

A month after these articles were published, the lead author, Bradley Johnston, was linked with industry funding that he had failed to disclose for the second time in his career.[68–70] The first time was in 2016, when his published research contradicted the American Dietary Guidelines on restricting added sugars. That study was financed by a sugar industry lobby group called the International Life Sciences Institute, which receives funding from the beef industry and companies such as Coca-Cola, McDonald's and PepsiCo.[71–73] This same organisation was engaged by the tobacco industry back in the 1980s to challenge WHO's tobacco control efforts.[74] This time around for the *Annals of Internal Medicine* paper, Johnston had an undeclared conflict of interest because he had received over US$75,000 funding for separate research on saturated fats from the industry group AgriLife Research, which is partly funded by the Texas beef industry. This conflict of interest was only later added as a correction when leading nutrition scientists and policymakers brought the researchers' ties to the beef industry to light, a correction that was all too easy to miss.[68,69] When it comes to grabbing consumer attention with headlines about 'new' advice on eating meat, these mixed messages can create a sense of fatigue with nutritional advice altogether and undermine public perception of *all* the science, regardless of its validity. The net effect? We stick to eating what we always have, a diet we've been conditioned to see as *balanced and healthy*.

To be clear, just because a study is industry-funded does not mean its results should be immediately thrown out. In fact, without funding from the food industry, many academics would find it hard to conduct research and the overall body of literature would be much smaller. We'll clear up what exactly the science says about red meat and eggs in Part Two. The point I'm making here is that we need to approach industry-funded studies with a level of scepticism and ask ourselves each time, 'Is this science or marketing?'

Opportunistic touchpoints

Another element to building credibility is the strategic placement of food products in key social environments to win public favour and be seen as a positive contributor to the community. I'm sure you will be familiar with the types of food found in kiosks, canteens and vending machines at schools and hospitals – highly refined packaged foods, fried foods and processed meats. Not only is this highly opportunistic, given these environments usually offer very limited choice, it's also worrying when you consider that school students and people in hospital are some of the people who most need to be nourished with healthy food. Yet the food industry deliberately targets its products and marketing towards these environments that are associated with trust, sending a mixed message about whether they're the kinds of things we should be eating.

The food industry in Australia also directly influences what ends up in our schools, more than you might realise. For example, the Healthy Kids Association, a not-for-profit charity that aims 'to educate and empower families, children and school canteens to make the healthiest choices possible', appears to receive financial support from Dairy Australia.[75]

It's not just the physical food at schools where industry has a touchpoint with our children. In Australia, it is not uncommon for industry associations to develop information with teachers for the curriculum. They position this as providing 'free education' on schools' behalf, just like the pharmaceutical industry 'educating' our doctors, and the Commonwealth Bank kindly taking on the task of teaching our kids about money with their Dollarmites scheme! Dairy Australia have created a specific website targeting school kids which states, 'All the tools and curriculum linked resources needed to bring the Australian dairy industry into the classroom'.[76] Similarly, Meat and Livestock Australia has also developed its own curriculum, 'Good Meat', for Australian children from kindergarten to Year 10.[77] The aim of the program is to educate children about the healthfulness of red meat and how the industry cares for its animals and the environment. It's clever, but we have to realise that it's marketing and if there wasn't a commercial agenda, they wouldn't do it. I'm not saying that this tactic in itself suggests dairy or red meat is unhealthy – we'll get into the specifics of that later on – but surely the food industry, which obviously has vested commercial interests, shouldn't be educating our children on food choices for human health, planetary health and animal welfare?

Conditioning by the food industry also occurs in hospitals – shockingly, there are even paediatric hospitals in Australia with a McDonald's restaurant on site![78,79] This sends the message to the broader community that fast food is endorsed, or at least considered acceptable, by children's healthcare services – especially worrying given one in four Australian children are considered to be either overweight or obese.[80]

Then there's the strategic alignment with professional athletes and sporting leagues. At the time of writing Australia's largest sport, the Australian Football League (AFL), receives money from McDonald's, Coca-Cola and Milo in exchange for exposure.[81] What sort of exposure? In 2019 alone, there were over 103 million TV viewers of AFL, and it's not uncommon for games to fill a stadium with over 50,000 patrons.[82] Safe to say, many of the kids watching will assume that their idols running around on the field, who are incredibly fit and healthy, also eat and drink these foods – after all, that's the implicit association these industry corporations are paying for, right? At the very least, it's going to stop the kids questioning the healthfulness of these foods at their school kiosk.

Big Food's self-regulation

One of the primary strategies used by transnational food corporations to keep markets open and profits high is that of self-regulation.[83] Essentially, this means introducing their own industry-developed regulations so they can be seen to commit to a set of rules and practise corporate responsibility while avoiding more stringent public health regulations from being put in place that would hurt their bottom line and disgruntle their shareholders. The problem with self-regulation from a public health perspective is that ultra-processed foods are a huge driver of the obesity and chronic disease affecting our population, but success for these companies is not realised through a reduction in sales of these foods.[83] So what we end up seeing is self-regulation initiatives that look like they are responsible on the surface, such as the 'Responsible Children's Marketing Initiative' code in Australia, but in reality do little to promote health.[84,85] Despite this particular self-regulated code, and others existing in Australia, multiple studies have identified that marketing to children on TV remains largely unchanged.[14,86]

These touchpoints all act to create an environment where the consumption of these products is considered a normal part of life. This is no doubt why as a young teenager I would regularly polish off ten chicken nuggets and a McFlurry after a game of football. By targeting kids from a young age, businesses acquire lifelong customers who are conditioned to consume with no questions asked. The ironic part? When these kids become adults and bad eating habits begin to catch up with them, many inevitably wind up in hospital with chronic disease . . . only to be again surrounded by industry-driven foods and marketing.[87,88] This is akin to selling cigarettes to patients hospitalised with lung cancer. These foods are positioned as being good for our sports stars, our youth and those with illness; surely, then, they're healthy? You'd be forgiven for thinking so.

How to deal with a system that is set up for us to fail

Despite all of the science that we have, hyper-palatable ultra-processed foods loaded with sugar, salt and fat continue to stare you in the face each time you go to the local supermarket, and now you know why. We don't have much control over this; government decisions affecting industrial agriculture are complex and updating policies is much harder and slower than we might imagine.

In a healthy food environment, foods such as fruits and vegetables are easily accessible and affordable. We live in an unhealthy food environment, where less healthy products are hard to resist because of their extreme palatability, pretty packaging and attractive price points. This makes healthy choices more difficult and we are therefore more likely to adopt an unhealthy dietary pattern.

While eating these foods every now and then is not going to be the end of the world, you certainly don't want to be consistently getting a substantial amount of your calories from them. And, ideally, they should come with a disclaimer about the real effect they have on your body, not the false pretence that they are healthy and part of a balanced diet. By delving into *why* we eat the way we do – including the mistruths and confusion that have circulated, often intentionally – we can safeguard ourselves against this rigged food environment and make positive changes to our diets based on science, not marketing.

CHAPTER 2

Our hijacked healthcare system

Australia certainly has one of the better healthcare systems in the world, a hybrid of free public health care and the option to purchase private health insurance if desired. Unfortunately, while our access to basic medical care is great, the system itself contributes to our not-so-healthy food habits in several ways.[1] From the influence of the food and pharmaceutical industries to insufficient funding for preventative care and a lack of nutrition training for medical professionals, our healthcare system often adds to our confusion about what we should eat.

Sick care over health care

While over one-third of the country's health burden is attributed to conditions and diseases caused by lifestyle, public spending focused on preventing illness through lifestyle changes does not reflect that reality.[2] Just 1.7% of Australia's national health expenditure goes towards public health services targeting prevention, and that is then split up across activities focused on physical activity, road safety, smoking, skin cancer, nutrition, etc. This figure pales in comparison to what Canada (5.9%) and New Zealand (7%) are spending on disease prevention, and sees us ranked in the lowest third of OECD countries.[3]

You may be wondering why such a small percentage of the overall healthcare budget is being spent on preventing the most expensive diseases.[2,4] Surely Australia's economy would benefit from a healthier, more productive population? The reality is that government campaigns and policies targeting chronic disease prevention would drastically reduce sales for the food and pharmaceutical industries, affecting their bottom lines.[5,6] These industries therefore have a vested interest in maintaining the status quo.

In Australia, it's well documented that pharmaceutical companies, food giants and industry representatives such as Coca-Cola, Woolworths and the Australian Food and Grocery Council collectively donate millions to political parties to influence policymaking.[7,8] However, there's a loophole that allows these donations to fly under the radar. As it stands, any donation to an Australian political party under AU$13,800 does not need to be declared to the public. This means it is possible for a company or individual to donate a huge sum of money to a political party and keep it a secret, as long as each individual payment remains under the $13,800 threshold. There's a name for these donations – 'dark money' – which in the 2018–2019 election year was calculated to amount to over $100 million dollars in donations to the two major Australian political parties.[9] Of course, these donations lead to alliances being drawn and promises being made for the next term of government – it's just another way that the food industry is able to buy influence. In addition to financially supporting political campaigns, it's undeniable that the food and pharmaceutical sectors stimulate the economy, boost the national GDP and generate an enormous amount of tax revenue. To give a sense of scale, every single day around 829,000 prescriptions are filled across Australia. The Australian red meat industry (the third largest beef exporter in the world) generates over $30 billion in revenue per year and employs 450,000 people.[10–12] It would take a brave political party to enact significant policy changes that prioritise health over profits and disrupt the contribution of these sectors to our economy.

This is how the interests of big business indirectly set the agenda for our public health programs. Lower rates of disease would mean fewer jobs in these industries, lower sales of junk food, less reason to buy insurance, less revenue for the government and a financial hit to the economy. Improving our health and reducing preventable deaths starts to look less financially attractive for the powerful players – no wonder large-scale prevention campaigns and new health-focused policies never seem to materialise. A prime example of this is the National Partnership Agreement on Preventative Health – Australia's single largest investment ever into tackling these chronic lifestyle diseases. Sadly, despite those involved setting the optimistic goal of being 'the healthiest country by 2020', the campaign was abolished after a change in government following the 2013 federal election.[13] Other government prevention campaigns, such as the Australian Dietary Guidelines and the Health Star Rating front-of-pack labelling system, have lasted longer but are not without their own issues.

Food industry influencing health recommendations

Our national dietary guidelines should be working for us, but these recommendations tend to be ambiguous at best and industry-influenced at worst. Every decade since 1980, Australia has released national guidelines aimed at providing the public with up-to-date, evidence-based advice on how to eat in order to stay healthy and vital. Over the years, the guidelines have been gradually modified, shifting from a nutrient focus to more of a food group focus that today includes grains, fruits, vegetables, milk and milk alternatives, and a protein group which includes red meat, poultry, fish, eggs, nuts, seeds and legumes.

Despite these improvements, there are a few standout problems with the 2013 Australian Dietary Guidelines. Rather than clearly recommending people consume more sources of plant-based protein, and fewer sources of animal protein, which was definitely shown to be beneficial by the science of the day,[14–21] foods such as red meat, chicken, eggs and dairy are featured prominently. Curiously, the guidelines also advocate eating whole grain cereals *or* cereals with high fibre – the latter claim essentially endorsing the consumption of highly processed cereals as long as they are advertised as 'high fibre'. But there's a stark difference between consuming whole grain cereals that naturally contain fibre, such as steel-cut oats, and consuming fibre-enriched heavily processed and sugar-packed cereals with a 'high-fibre' claim on its colourful box. The science supporting grain consumption to reduce the risk of chronic disease is very clear and is based on the consumption of grains in their whole form, *not* in a refined form.[22]

Unless the consumer or health professional reads 210 pages of guidelines or a 45-page summary, it's likely they will just look at the image of the dietary guidelines 'plate', a bird's-eye view of the various food groups we should stick to. That leaves us with an oversimplified graphic of a plate with a clear emphasis on animal protein and foods in wrappers, and mild, ambiguous language such as *sometimes* and *small amounts* that will mean something different to everyone. This plate essentially promotes the ideas of 'everything in balance' and 'moderation', ideas that junk-food companies such as Nestlé and McDonald's wholeheartedly support and regularly use when campaigning against the introduction of policies that would negatively affect their sales.[8]

How can we be recommending people consume ultra-processed foods, such as soft drinks, hamburgers, potato chips and ice cream, 'sometimes' or in 'small amounts' when we know these foods are designed to be insatiable, addictive and to promote weight gain?[23] Why haven't we taken a hard line, like Brazil, whose latest dietary guidelines emphasise the consumption of fresh foods and specifically advise people to 'Avoid consumption of ultra-processed foods'?[24] Or like Canada, whose dietary guidelines make it clear that such foods 'undermine healthy eating'?[25] At least with messaging like this, if we do choose to eat these foods, we are making an informed decision.

The organisation that provided the recommendations to the government is the Dietitians Association of Australia (DAA), which was paid $522,221 in 2009 to perform a systematic literature review that could be used to draft the dietary guidelines.[26] As the major dietetic association in Australia, representing over 7000 health professionals whose stated mission is to 'build healthier communities', it would be reasonable to assume that the DAA would be a trustworthy candidate to perform this task.[27] Yet, due to the guidelines' failure to clearly recommend evidence-based eating, I was sceptical and decided to investigate further. What I found was shocking but illuminating. During the DAA's review and recommendations period, the organisation had a long list of 'corporate partners' including Dairy Australia, the Meat and Livestock Association, Nestlé, the Egg Nutrition Council and Unilever, to name a few.[28] With such clear affiliations, it is no surprise that the recommendations were based on a huge amount of industry-funded research – happy corporate partners means more sponsorship dollars. It's a recurring theme – keep large food corporations on side because they keep the lights on.

Lack of nutrition training for our doctors

If you were to assume your doctor is well versed in nutritional science, you wouldn't be alone. Sadly, this is not the case. On average, medical students undertake less than twenty-four hours of nutrition study during their four-year degree and most graduate with little understanding of what lifestyle modification means in practical terms for patients.[29–32] In fact, at many universities across the world, including in Australia, taking nutrition classes is not even a mandatory part of a medical degree.[33] That means it's possible for medical students to graduate without undertaking *any* specific nutrition classes. Even if students do take units about nutrition, these are mostly spent learning about specific nutrients (e.g. vitamin absorption or fat metabolism) rather than the science studying food choices and disease prevention.[34] Furthermore, if these students choose to become specialist doctors, there are no fields of specialty practice focused on nutrition that they can pursue.[35] So, where then *do* doctors get their dietary information? A recent survey of more than one thousand first- to fourth-year medical students in Australia identified that just 16% of students read published studies in nutrition journals. Instead, the majority of these students reported getting their nutrition knowledge from consumer websites.[36] This doesn't sound like the best path to truly understanding how food affects our health. It's no wonder that a systematic review looking at sixty-six studies across the world on the nutrition education provided to medical students found that insufficient training leaves doctors lacking the confidence to talk to their patients about nutrition.[37,38]

Clearly, this glaring lack of formal nutritional education is not the fault of individual doctors – they get into this field because they genuinely want to improve the health of patients. Nor is it the first time in history that our doctors have not been informed about the impact of lifestyle behaviours on disease risk. It took multiple decades and more than seven thousand scientific studies before the landmark 1964 US Surgeon General's Report, which linked smoking cigarettes with significantly increased chances of cancer and early death, made its way into medical practice.[39] This was due to a multitude of reasons – one notable one being that tobacco companies did everything they could to discredit the research and cause confusion about the lethality of their products, knowing full well that people – doctors included, many of whom were addicted to smoking themselves – love to hear good things about their bad habits.[40,41] Since 1964, more than 20 million Americans have died from conditions attributable to smoking. How many of these people would have lived longer healthier lives if our medical system was quicker to act?[39]

Thankfully, today it is now generally accepted that smoking causes cancer, but there is a new blind spot. Food is *not* medicine, but science clearly demonstrates that it is an important predictor of your health and longevity.[42] Specifically, the research shows that eating more whole grains, fruits, legumes, vegetables, nuts and seeds and eating less animal protein and highly processed foods is associated with lower risk of developing chronic diseases, such as cardiovascular disease, type 2 diabetes and colorectal cancer, and is a clear commonality among people who live long, healthy, relatively disease-free lives.[43–45] But, as we've seen, the food industry is fighting tooth and nail to deter governments from modifying the food environment, and has strategies to sprinkle just enough confusion throughout the literature to give people (doctors included) a reason to stick with what they know.[8,42] My point here is not to blame doctors but rather to illustrate that, while I believe in time this will change, it's perhaps not your best bet to wait for this to happen.

Big Pharma and the appeal of medications

The standard consultation time of fifteen minutes restricts doctors' capacity to educate patients about diet and promote behaviour change. What's easier, quicker, and typically more commercially attractive to healthcare organisations is prescribing medications – often those promoted to them by pharmaceutical representatives. At its heart, the way the pharma industry operates is informed by the economic theory that *curing* someone is not a sustainable business model but *managing disease* will create returning customers for decades. And that philosophy has had a flow-on effect on how our healthcare system deals with sick people.

During a four-year period from 2011 to 2015, there were over 116,000 'educational events' funded by the pharmaceutical industry in Australia alone. These events saw over 3.5 million attendances from Australian health professionals, mostly doctors, and cost the pharmaceutical industry over $286 million to host.[46] While the pharmaceutical industry will argue that professional education is important for improving patient care, being educated by a company that wants you to prescribe more of their products surely poses a huge conflict of interest. Despite an industry code of conduct supposedly preventing it, speakers at these events often have financial ties with the pharmaceutical company putting on the event, creating an implicit understanding of favourable coverage.[47] To illustrate just how effective this strategy is, it's been shown that simply paying for a doctor's meal, valued on average at US$20 or less, results in a significant increase in prescriptions for the company's brand-name medication.[48]

Yes, doctors need regular updates about which drugs work for certain conditions as new developments are made. This is an important part of medicine. But research shows generic drugs offer the same results as brand-name equivalents, are equally safe and, in specific cases, have been shown to result in even better patient outcomes because their affordability results in better patient adherence.[48,49] So while these events are promoted as educational, they are far better described as marketing for what is a $25 billion market in Australia alone.[50] Meanwhile, there is no financial incentive or wining-and-dining culture encouraging doctors to give their patients information about diet modifications such as eating more beans and broccoli, which could reduce their need to come back for a subsequent consultation and help others, like members of their family, avoid disease in the first place.

Of course, there are layers of complexity beyond what I have described above. In a subset of the population who simply cannot access fresh, healthy food, these medications are the only, or most important, solution that can offer an improved quality of life. Even for people of higher socio-economic class whose diets are less restricted by their financial means, pharmaceutical medications are often life-saving – for example, for my dad. Medications are also particularly important for acute conditions. My focus here on Big Pharma is not about demonising Western medicine or shaming doctors or those who take medications. It's about addressing the elephant in the room. If we truly want our doctors to be able to provide the greatest service and value to our community, they need to be part of a system that values prevention ahead of profits. Today, this is not the case. Through no fault of their own, our doctors are part of a system built to manage and cure, which sadly means that something has to go wrong before medical interventions take place.[10] All of this is a distraction from the most powerful prescription of all – a healthier lifestyle.

The rise of 'medfluencers'

There has also been a huge push from the food industry, particularly the dairy sector, to conduct influencer campaigns on social media, in which they team up with qualified health professionals and pay them to endorse the consumption of their products. To see this for yourself, search #dairyaustralia #dairymatters. Yet another way for big business to feed their messaging to us.

No one is safeguarding *your* health except *you*

So, we have little public health funding going towards preventative care, the food industry using their power to influence public health recommendations, and a healthcare system that has little to no nutrition training but lots of influence from Big Pharma. It's easy to see why many of us feel confused about what to eat and leave doctors' appointments with pills in hand, none the wiser that the food we're putting into our mouths multiple times a day feeds the very diseases that our medications are helping to manage. Even if you're fortunate enough that your doctor is well versed in lifestyle medicine and nutrition, in the short time you have together they can really only scratch the surface of what a healthy dietary pattern looks like. On top of that, the moment you step out of the clinic, you're back in a food environment that makes it incredibly challenging for you to act on any advice.

You only have to look at the success that tobacco control measures have had on smoking – even if it took decades after the first studies linking smoking with lung cancer to have them implemented – to see the good that can be done if our healthcare system aligns to support our optimal health. Through a combination of policies affecting the smoking environment – including taxes, advertising bans, smoking restrictions at venues and graphic warnings on packs – as well as a change in attitude towards smoking by doctors, the number of daily smokers in Australia has more than halved, falling from 25% of the population in 1991 to 12% in 2019.[10] Unsurprisingly, during this period, deaths caused by lung cancer per 100,000 persons have dropped by around 25%.[51]

When it comes to nutrition, there's a lot that could be done: tax unhealthy foods, subsidise healthier foods, improve food labelling requirements, restrict the marketing of unhealthy foods and beverages to children, develop nutrition standards for schools and hospitals, and introduce other government policies that specifically act to make it easier for people to choose the healthy option. This is working well in the Philippines, where they introduced a sugar-sweetened beverage tax to reduce obesity. A single month after introducing the tax in January 2018, the shelf price of such beverages had increased by 16–20%, and sales had fallen by 8%.[52] Similarly, when a Melbourne hospital convenience store trialled a 20% price increase on sugar-sweetened beverages over a seventeen-week period, sales of soft drinks dropped by 27.6% and sales of bottled water increased by the same amount.[53]

We need to acknowledge that there are fundamental flaws with the way our healthcare system operates, which make it easy for healthy people to become sick and difficult for sick people to become healthy. If Australia truly wanted doctors to be up-to-date with the evidence, the government would introduce policies that regulate contact between the pharmaceutical industry and our health professionals and would create an environment that first and foremost sells health rather than medicines. This is not exactly a new idea –Thomas Edison predicted exactly this in 1903, when he wrote, 'The doctor of the future will give no medicine, but will instruct his patient in the care of the human frame, in diet and in the cause and prevention of disease.'[54] Unfortunately, we're not there yet, and I won't hold my breath. I don't recommend you do either. However, with awareness of these influences and an understanding of how the system works, you're in a much better position to take control of your food choices *now*, rather than waiting for our healthcare system to catch up with science.

CHAPTER 3

A for-profit nutrition culture

It's common to hear people describing their diet by the very nutrients it contains: 'high-fat, low-carb', for example, or 'high-protein'. This way of thinking about food, which reduces it down to its key nutrients and assesses its value simplistically based on those, is called *nutritionism*.

Nutrients are the compounds in foods that are essential for growth and life. The six we need to function properly are carbohydrates, lipids (fats), proteins, vitamins, minerals and water. Historically, the focus on nutrients has been on identifying and curing diet-related diseases that are caused by nutritional deficiency, such as treating scurvy with vitamin C, or beriberi with vitamin B_1. Even though widespread deficiencies and malnourishment are rare in Australia and most developed countries, this link between disease and nutrients still shapes our way of thinking. According to the Australian Institute of Health and Welfare, despite not eating anywhere near enough fruits and vegetables, and far too much ultra-processed foods, 'Australians generally get enough key nutrients in their diet', namely carbohydrates, fats, protein, vitamins and minerals.[1] But how can we be getting our nutrients right when our diet has such severe shortcomings?

The nutrient approach actually says very little about the healthfulness of what goes into our mouths and through our digestive tracts. In order to eat, you have to consume macronutrients – that's a given. But we don't eat nutrients, we eat *food*. The somewhat unexciting truth is that it's not helpful to look at one or two nutrients in isolation – we also need to consider how we get them and what comes along for the ride. This means the source of your nutrients is what determines the quality of your overall dietary pattern. It's not just a case of ticking a few boxes of key nutrients and therefore you're 'eating well'.[2] All macronutrients are not created equal. For example, when it comes to their effect on our bodies and health outcomes, plant protein differs from animal protein, unrefined carbohydrates differ from refined carbohydrates and saturated fats differ from unsaturated fats. We'll discuss this in more detail in Part Two.

The Health Star loophole

Australia's answer to the World Health Organization's recommendation to introduce front-of-pack labelling is the Health Star Rating (HSR) system. Launched in 2014, the HSR system rates a food product from 0.5 to 5 stars, with 0.5 being the least healthy and 5 being the healthiest food in its category, with the goal being to help consumers make healthier food choices.

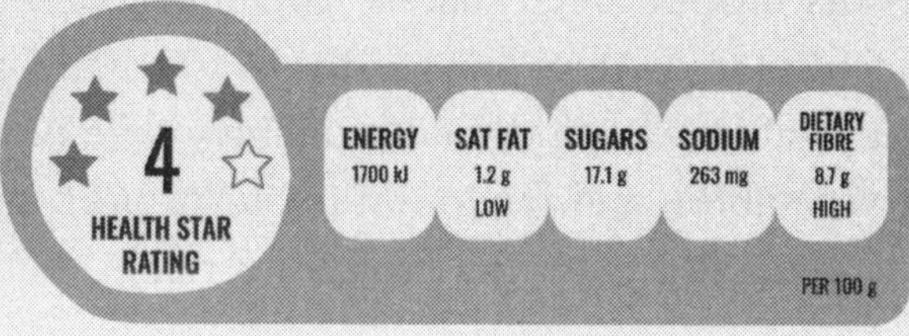

While the HSR system has many issues, arguably the greatest is its focus on nutrient type and quantity without consideration for the source of those nutrients. The rating is calculated using what is called a *compensatory system*. If a product contains negative attributes, such as sugar, sodium, saturated fats, etc., the effect of these can be neutralised through the addition of positive attributes such as protein and fibre. Unfortunately, clever food manufacturers have taken advantage of this system: for example, if they know they need X grams of sugar added to their product to make it hyper-palatable, they can add the necessary amount of fibre to offset the sugar and maintain an attractive star rating.[3] As a result, many energy-dense ultra-processed foods such as biscuits, cakes and icy poles receive a rating of 3 to 5 stars.[4] No wonder almost half of the average Australian's calories come from ultra-processed foods![5] To add insult to injury, the HSR system doesn't differentiate between natural sugars found in fruits and vegetables, and added sugars found in ultra-processed foods. As a result, under the HSR system, not all whole fruits and vegetables – foods consistently shown to reduce chronic disease risk, and which the Australian Dietary Guidelines say Australians need to eat more of – would receive 5 stars.[6-8] Talk about confusing.

Manufacturers of ultra-processed foods in the food industry worked in collaboration with the Australian government in the development of the HSR system, and lobbied against certain features that would affect their profits.[7,9,10] So the fact the HSR system reduces the healthfulness of food down to a handful of nutrients without consideration of their source, and that it is not mandatory, isn't really all that surprising.

This raises the question: how has the nutrient approach and all the trendy diets that stem from it become so popular – and who's benefiting from it?

The food industry loves nutritionism. Defining our diets by its macronutrients creates an environment where we forget the importance of the source of our food, opening the door for processed food companies to put unhealthful products in front of us under the guise of providing us with the nutrients we 'need'. In the 1980s, for example, the prevailing recommendation from national dietary guidelines was to reduce consumption of saturated fats. The intention was to encourage consumers to eat more fruits, vegetables, whole grains, etc. – foods naturally low in saturated fats. However, manufacturers took advantage of this by reformulating industrially processed foods, such as Oreos and Snackwell cookies, creating new versions that were now lower in saturated fats, but higher in refined carbohydrates (e.g. added sugars and white flour). The public could continue to enjoy their cookies, now with a 'reduced fat' claim emblazoned across the front. Unfortunately, this tactic still gets a lot of use today. Food manufacturers spend millions of dollars innovating to create on-trend ultra-processed foods in response to the latest dietary craze, like the plethora of ultra-processed 'vegan' and 'gluten-free' products that have hit the shelves in the past few years, often loaded with added fats, sugar and salt. They make appealing health claims on pretty packaging and in clever advertising campaigns, promoting key nutrients such as 'source of fibre' or 'high-protein'. If we take these marketing messages at face value, we can easily mistake an ultra-processed blueberry muffin emblazoned with a 'real fruit' claim for an actual serving of fruit, while a bar packed with sugar, fats, fillers and additives seems like a good choice because it is 'low-carb' and 'high-protein'. With our busy lives, we rarely have the time to stop and critically analyse the healthfulness of food and are driven by buzzwords emblazoned on the packaging, and by price. In fact, along with the United States, New Zealand, Italy and the United Kingdom, Australian consumers are the most price sensitive in the world, buying roughly 40% of their food on sale.[10] Of course, food manufacturers are well aware of this data and use it to their advantage.A 2019 study that looked at price promotions on 1579 products over a one-year period in Australia's largest supermarket corporation identified that ultra-processed or 'junk' food is on sale almost twice as often as healthy foods.[11]

The ever-changing media narrative

The media, too, has a lot to answer for when it comes to our nutrition confusion. Consider how traditional media companies function and what drives them: their profits are generally built on the number of eyeballs they can attract.[12] To draw people to their content, they need to be constantly offering something new and surprising. Feeding you a consistent message and truly informing you would go against this – the more nutritional literacy you have, the less thirsty you are for further information, making you progressively less valuable to them.

It's in the media's commercial interests to keep the narrative around health and nutrition constantly changing. How do they do this? They employ an endless rotation of sensationalised headlines, industry-funded science and the latest fads to keep you grasping for clear and solid information you can confidently hold on to. Nutrition becomes a more fluid and exciting topic for them to cover if there are seemingly constant 'breakthroughs' updating our knowledge at a rapid pace, and it begins to feel as though whatever new dietary habit you take up today for your good health is only going to be superseded by something new and better in a month's or a year's time. While it's true that what we know about diet is evolving, the scientific consensus doesn't rapidly change from day to day based on a single experiment. It is carved out over decades. And despite how it is often portrayed, new science is not by default better than old science. What's most important is how a study was conducted, the reliability of its findings and how it fits within our existing understanding of nutrition for optimal human health. Without context, all science should be taken with a grain of salt!

The gluten-free trend is a prime example. Thanks in part to mainstream media inaccurately touting this diet as great for gut health, energy levels and weight loss, the global gluten-free product market is currently worth approximately US$22 billion and projected to double by 2027.[13] Yet, beyond the small percentage of people who the science shows clearly do benefit from avoiding gluten (those with coeliac disease or gluten ataxia), the majority of people following a gluten-free diet are actually likely to be doing more harm than good. Removing gluten-containing grains, such as wheat, makes it harder for people to reach their daily fibre target, increases the chance of nutritional deficiency and is likely to result in lower consumption of whole grains – all of which can increase the risk of developing chronic disease and living a shorter life.[14,15]

The media also know how much we love to hear that our 'bad' habits are – hang on a second – actually healthy! It's this type of news that drives clicks and shares. Who doesn't want to read that red wine and chocolate are heart-healthy?[16,17] Mars and Hershey's are aware of that – it's why they have poured millions and millions of dollars into scientific studies showing the benefits of cocoa. Of course, when the results of these studies are hyped by the media, what is left out is that any potential benefit is likely offset by cocoa's delivery vehicle – a combination of sugar, salt and fat.[18] When something confirms our beliefs and justifies our behaviours, we accept it on face value and often feel compelled to share it with our friends and families. In contrast, when something challenges our beliefs, we either work out a way to make it fit our pre-existing beliefs, demand more evidence or tune out entirely and pretend we didn't see it. This is *confirmation bias*, and it is to the detriment of our health as it stops us from being able to objectively evaluate new information and moves us further from where the science truly lies.

So what should we do in the face of the media confusion? One solution could be inspired by areas of the world where people are eating well according to traditional diets and living long healthy lives (which we'll learn more about in Chapter 8). I think it's safe to say that 'diet news' does not form a part of the culture in these places. There is no jumping from diet to diet based on a new headline, they aren't waiting to hear about the latest 'superfood' and their diets are not informed by what's on TV. They eat real food, predominantly or entirely plants, in their whole or minimally processed form and drink mainly water.[19–21] Although news can be exciting, and certainly grab our attention, we don't need to overcomplicate things.

Social media and the allure of anecdotes

Diet culture runs rampant on the internet, particularly on social networks such as Facebook, Twitter and Instagram, where pseudo-experts speak passionately and compellingly about their individual health experiences such as curing gut health issues with a Paleo diet or reversing diabetes with a ketogenic diet.

These anecdotes are interesting and can be incredibly persuasive, especially when told as stories, which as humans we are so receptive to. But no matter what diet these individuals advocate for, their testimony is not reliable evidence. Anecdotes are usually very short-term, telling us nothing about the long-term risks associated with a certain diet or supplement. Someone on YouTube who is thirty days or even two years into a meat-only diet, for example, cannot reliably tell us the long-term pros and cons. Chronic diseases have very long latency periods. That person advocating for a meat-only diet can be both feeling great *and* building up plaque in their arteries, and setting themselves up for a heart attack or stroke in the future, at the same time.

There are many things we can do in the short-term to feel better that are not conducive to long-term health. For example, substituting food with cocaine will of course result in weight loss, and could even lead to improvements in insulin resistance and other biomarkers in subjects with disease, but I'm sure we can all agree it wouldn't be a good idea long-term!

Health is a spectrum

Any move away from a standard Western diet is generally a healthy one and will typically leave people feeling better. This is no doubt why we all know people who swear by their dietary framework based on the fact it improved their personal health. However, the only thing these anecdotes tell us is that relative to the person's previous diet, they feel better. It doesn't tell us if their new dietary pattern is the optimal diet for human health.

We also have no way of validating that the information shared in anecdotal stories is accurate. Even if we could, it would be incredibly risky to extrapolate information from these individual experiences to create recommendations for the general population. That's what long-term epidemiological studies involving thousands of people from various populations are helpful for – they show us far more reliably how dietary patterns among large groups of people play out over decades. That's not to say that someone who has first-hand experience cannot share their stories and information about what they eat. But when anecdotal information that goes against the scientific consensus is spread as fact, and referenced as if it has equal weight to decades of consistent science, it simply adds to the confusion. Anecdotes and opinions sit at the bottom of the evidence hierarchy (see page 70), and that's worth remembering when we find ourselves getting too carried away, no matter if said anecdotes support your preferred diet or not.

There are also more purposeful misrepresentations of science prevalent in the media. It's called 'cherrypicking'. Think of it as a game of abstract hunting, where one searches for 'science' that fits a predetermined narrative, finding studies with conclusions that support pre-existing beliefs without critically evaluating the methodology, while turning a blind eye to any studies that challenge those beliefs. An example of this is someone who rejects the findings of a study that disagrees with their position because it's 'observational', not a 'clinical intervention', but uses the findings of observational research elsewhere when it fits their narrative. Cherrypicking studies reassures us about the foods we like to consume and provides further justification for our chosen behaviours. Social media influencers regularly use this strategy to provide credibility for their e-books, meal plans and products. I'm sure you've seen this. Perhaps you've come across someone who believes the dietary framework they advocate is a panacea and has no weaknesses. Someone who doesn't critically analyse even the science that supports their beliefs. Someone who will find any reason *not* to believe science that challenges their chosen dietary pattern. This is not evidence-based practice, this is confirmation bias.

It's very difficult for most of us to understand who on social media is cherrypicking from the science and who is actually objectively evaluating the literature. We end up with lots of 'experts' with very different opinions and another reason for people to lose trust in nutrition science. When there is enough disagreement within the science – or apparent disagreement – we tend to resort to familiar patterns and choices based on things like our upbringing and beliefs. And that's understandable – there is an agenda-driven minefield out there and it can feel exhausting trying to keep up.

Resisting the allure of quick fixes and fads

Whether it's weight management, addressing nutritional deficiencies, building muscle or improving our cholesterol, nothing beats lifestyle changes that we can adhere to in the long-term.

The problem is that even though most of us understand this, we crave overnight results – and we are bombarded with diets promoting quick fixes that are far sexier and more appealing to implement than sustained lifestyle changes that require discipline and focus. Why make long-term dietary changes, or perform regular physical exercise, if you can lose ten kilos simply by drinking juice for four weeks?

Businesses know this. They develop commercially appealing products and services, often backed by self-funded scientific studies or anecdotes, that promise the world and target our thirst for instant gratification, such as bone broth for digestion and exogenous ketones for fat burning.[22] Sometimes we do notice benefits from these products, though that can come down to other factors. One of these is the placebo effect – because we expect to feel improvements, we do feel them. Another is the fact that we commonly try these quick fixes in conjunction with making other small lifestyle changes, such as going for morning walks or drinking more water. This means we can't get an accurate measure of the effect of the new product independently from our other improved habits.

Why do these distractions, advertisements, media narratives and social media 'experts' promising the world work on us? Why is it that even when we know something may not be great for us, such as extremely low-calorie 'detox' programs, we often succumb to the instant results it can provide? The simple answer is that bypassing immediate pleasure to instead work hard for something that is ultimately more gratifying is an adaptive skill called *delayed gratification*. It's a skill we must actively build throughout our lives to overcome the evolutionary wiring that would have us believe that we need everything immediately for survival. As we get better at delayed gratification, we can more easily resist sources of immediate fulfilment with an understanding that it will be a worthwhile 'sacrifice'. However, in a world where the average person spends 144 minutes on social media per day,[23] constantly performing actions that create micro hits of feel-good neurotransmitters such as dopamine, our craving for instant gratification is arguably at an all-time high. We have become more and more conditioned to experience pleasure and gratification with minimal effort, and that's what we expect when it comes to improving our health too.

There's a behavioural economics model that's been well studied by neuro-economic researchers called *hyperbolic discounting* that helps explain this cognitive bias (*an error in thinking*) that so often prevents us from achieving our long-term goals. If I were to offer you $50 today versus $100 tomorrow most people would take the $100. Why? Because it's double the money, and the time, the delay period, is minimal. However, if I were to offer you $50 today versus $100 in a year's time, most people would opt for the $50. Why? Because even though the difference in value is the same, we discount the future satisfaction we will derive from the $100 reward because of the delay to receive it. This is like staying in to watch more Netflix rather than doing the workout you had planned. Avoiding chronic disease and maintaining your health in decades to come seems so far away, so the immediacy of the pleasure from Netflix wins.

So, how can we improve our ability to practice delayed gratification and resist the temptation of quick fixes or the latest diet craze? Behavioural neuroscience research suggests that trust is at the heart of this ability. In the famous 1972 Stanford marshmallow experiment by Professor Walter Mischel, some of the children studied were able to wait for fifteen minutes to receive two marshmallows rather than one, whereas others opted to eat the single marshmallow they were offered straight away.[24] Researchers then followed these children for more than forty years and were able to identify that those who demonstrated the ability to delay gratification in the original experiment went on to have fewer problems with managing their weight, fewer issues with substance abuse and ultimately became more socially and cognitively competent.[25–27]

So does this study indicate that some of us are just inherently better at self-control? In 2012, researchers from Rochester University replicated the marshmallow experiment with a new set of children, making a small tweak to the experiment to introduce an element of trust.[28] At the beginning of this experiment, children were given a set of used crayons in a closed jar and told by the researcher that if they could wait a few minutes, they would be given a brand-new set. All the children were able to wait. When the researcher returned, they broke the promise for 50% of the children (an unreliable experience) and gave the other 50% the new set of crayons (a reliable experience). They then carried out the marshmallow experiment. The kids who'd had an unreliable experience had no reason to trust the researcher and thus chose the single marshmallow. In contrast, the kids who'd had a reliable experience realised that waiting for a bigger reward was worthwhile and were able to wait on average up to four times longer.

So in order to get better at delaying gratification, we need to build trust with ourselves. Set goals that require us to resist immediate pleasure (e.g. a morning jog for thirty minutes three times per week instead of sleeping in) but are still achievable so we are able to experience delayed gratification. If it's unrealistic, it's likely to create an unreliable experience (failure to achieve the goal) and send us back to craving instant gratification. Each time we are successful, we are strengthening the delayed gratification part of our brain, just as a bodybuilder strengthens their muscles with each rep. With practice, you'll become more disciplined and find it easier to resist the urge to give in to instant gratification. Instead of grabbing the chocolate bar on your way home from work, you'll wait until you get home and cook the healthy dinner you had planned. And you'll be able to sustainably build a dietary pattern that will allow you to live more years in good health.

In the same way that modifiable risk factors for chronic disease, such as obesity and high cholesterol, develop and play out over years, the lifestyle changes targeted at combating them need to be equally sustainable and long-lasting. While we may wish that science could deliver us a magic pill, there really is no shortcut to long-term health – but the rewards to be gained from being patient and consistent are truly enormous.

A way out of the maze

When you combine all of these sources of confusion, it's pretty clear why most people want to just throw their hands up in the air and continue on eating as they always have. While I wholeheartedly believe that the information in this book will free you of this confusion and put you and anyone you share it with on the path to a long and healthy life, making the monumental shift required to fix the chronic disease pandemic isn't as simple as education. We also need significant changes in the way our governments think about nutrition and disease, and the way the food industry is regulated. It should be made easier for everyone to follow a dietary framework that's known to prevent and fight disease, and harder to follow one that feeds disease.

Until that happens, the good news is that while there are many powerful players who would like you to think no one knows what is best for humans to eat, the science is not confused. There really is a lot that we can do as individuals to upgrade our diet and lead a lifestyle that is known to promote good long-term health. When we understand what the science truly shows, we can quiet these voices of confusion and build the confidence required to make long-lasting changes to our plate.

PART TWO

A DIET OF SCIENCE

WITH ALL THE CONFUSING, MISLEADING SCIENCE – THE pseudo-experts, industry-funded studies and media frenzy – and all the distractions of the ads, shiny products and prominently placed ultra-processed foods, it's easy to think there is no consensus when it comes to the optimal diet. But the best science is actually quite clear, and it all points to the protective power of plants.

The three primary sources of confusion we explored previously – the food and healthcare industries, and for-profit nutrition culture – can make us feel a bit scattered when we choose what to put on our plates, as if we've got nothing concrete on which to base our decisions. My deep dive into the research has shown me that there is, in fact, a very solid foundation for adopting a diet centred on plants. The three pillars supporting that foundation are human health, planetary health and animal welfare. In other words, what's good for us is also really good for all life and the planet itself.

When it comes to human health, the scientific literature makes it stunningly clear that the best diet for us is one in which about 85% or more of our calories come from whole plant foods. I call this a *plant-predominant* diet, or sometimes *plant-based* for short. Any variation of this theme – Paleo, keto, vegetarian or vegan – can deliver good health, as long as it's plant-predominant. As you'll see in the chapters in this section, a plant-predominant diet is a way of eating that improves your health span and life span – a diet that adds more years to your life and more life to your years – while also providing benefits to your short-term health and wellness goals.

Although we tend to categorise chronic diseases by their unique properties and treat them as individual diseases, they are largely manifestations of the same underlying cause and lifestyle risk factors. We can eat in such a way that feeds disease or we can eat in order to fight disease. Regardless of which disease we are talking about (and the list in this book is not exhaustive), the same overarching diet principles apply: a heart-healthy diet is also a kidney-healthy and liver-healthy diet. Just one dietary pattern can protect you from all of them – talk about efficient!

You'll soon see how plants can prevent, slow or stop the progression of, and in some cases even reverse, chronic disease: obesity, type 2 diabetes, heart disease, cancer and dementia. The science supports plant-based foods for living longer too.

When we look at our food choices through the lenses of planetary health and animal welfare, the case for adopting a diet that is as plant-exclusive as possible solidifies. Thus, we'll move from human health to the second and third pillars that support a plant-exclusive diet in the last chapter of this section, taking a close look at the impact of animal consumption on the health of the planet and animals' lives. While I am by no means asking anyone to be perfect, I think it's important we are aware of how the way we choose to eat affects the world around us. We can then use this information to make the best choices possible within the context of our personal circumstances.

The science in this section and throughout this book is the strongest, most evidence-supported and up-to-date data available, all brought together in one place. I have avoided drawing conclusions from anecdotes, case studies (reports of a single person's experience), expert opinions and/or laboratory studies (e.g. animal studies are great for generating hypotheses but the findings often do not play out in humans) – all of which are levels of evidence that are considered weak and unreliable for making public health recommendations. Instead, I've primarily used a mixture of findings from observational research, which shows us health outcomes for people in the general public who eat a certain way, clinical trials or randomised controlled trials (RCTs), which show us what happens in a clinical setting if person A adopts a certain diet compared with person B who adopts a different diet, and systematic reviews and meta-analyses, which are reviews that synthesise and evaluate findings from similar studies to determine the combined effect. As I walk you through the many ways a plant-predominant diet is good for our health and the health of the planet, you'll notice I'm always mindful of the hierarchy of evidence (see Figure 2.1). To inform our food choices, it's important to look for consistent patterns that emerge not only from the lab, but play out in well-designed observational studies of health outcomes of people in our populations today, and in tightly controlled clinical trial interventions and meta-analyses as well.* While there are no absolutes in science, when you understand the ins and outs of the different forms of scientific investigation and are able to interpret their findings in an unbiased fashion, there are clear patterns that emerge, shining light on how we should eat for optimal health. It's these patterns that I've dedicated my time to uncovering. At every level, it all points in the direction of a diet with great emphasis on whole plant foods.

---

* A common retort is that RCTs are the gold-standard and observational research is crummy. While it would be great to always be able to use RCTs to prove causation, they do have their limitations. They can't be used to answer certain questions, such as what diet is best for longevity? It would be near impossible to control compliance, a huge number of subjects would be required to show a significant difference, and it would cost a significant amount of money. The findings from observational research, often called 'correlations', can still be meaningful and illuminating. Did you know that smoking has never been definitively proven to cause cancer? Over 7000 studies link the two, but they are all observational (also known as 'epidemiological', epidemiology being the branch of science that deals with the incidence, distribution and causes of a disease within a population). When RCTs cannot be performed, remarkably consistent patterns on a large scale cannot be ignored.[1]

FIGURE 2.1:

THE HIERARCHY OF EVIDENCE IN NUTRITIONAL SCIENCE

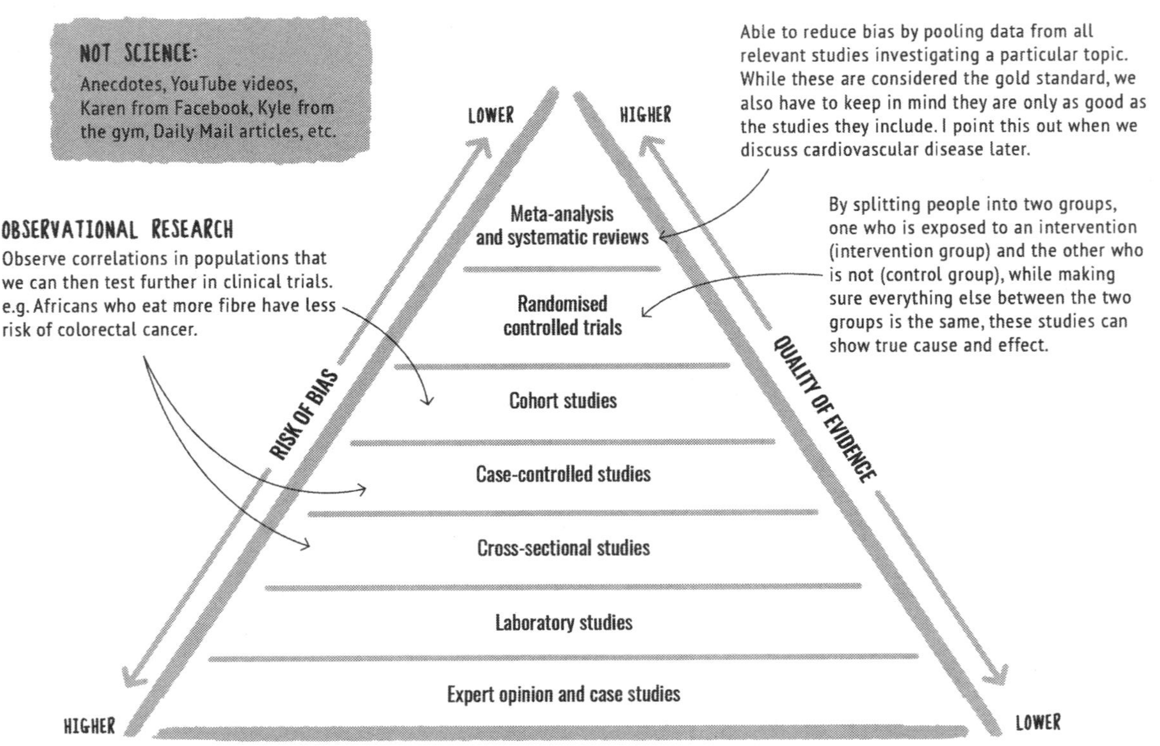
NOT SCIENCE:
Anecdotes, YouTube videos, Karen from Facebook, Kyle from the gym, Daily Mail articles, etc.
OBSERVATIONAL RESEARCH
Observe correlations in populations that we can then test further in clinical trials. e.g. Africans who eat more fibre have less risk of colorectal cancer.
Able to reduce bias by pooling data from all relevant studies investigating a particular topic. While these are considered the gold standard, we also have to keep in mind they are only as good as the studies they include. I point this out when we discuss cardiovascular disease later.
By splitting people into two groups, one who is exposed to an intervention (intervention group) and the other who is not (control group), while making sure everything else between the two groups is the same, these studies can show true cause and effect.
LOWER
HIGHER
RISK OF BIAS
HIGHER
QUALITY OF EVIDENCE
LOWER
Meta-analysis and systematic reviews
Randomised controlled trials
Cohort studies
Case-controlled studies
Cross-sectional studies
Laboratory studies
Expert opinion and case studies

Dietary labels and what they mean

There are a lot of dietary labels in use today and sometimes their meanings are pretty subjective. So to make sure we're on the same page, here are some quick definitions of terms I use frequently. These definitions are not my own, nor are they labels that I'm asking you to use for your own diet. They reflect what's used within the scientific literature, and as such might be a bit different from what you're familiar with from social media and the news.

PLANT-BASED

A diet that maximises calories from whole, or minimally processed, plants. In scientific research, the term *plant-based* can be used to refer both to diets that consist of 100% of calories from plants *and* to diets in which most, but not all, calories come from plants. Not so helpful! To make things a bit clearer, where possible I use the terms *plant-exclusive* (meaning 100% of calories from plants) and *plant-predominant* (it's impossible to give an absolute, but I use it to mean around 85% or more calories from plants) to help differentiate between the two. Roughly speaking, this works out to two plant-based meals per day and one meal that contains animal products. Plant-predominant diets include dietary patterns such as the vegetarian, pescetarian, Mediterranean and DASH diets (see Chapter 5). A whole-food plant-based diet (WFPBD) is a plant-exclusive diet.

VEGAN

A diet that excludes all animal products, including meat, fish, eggs, dairy and even honey. A vegan diet is a type of plant-exclusive diet, but since this can mean anything from fried potato chips to steamed sweet potato, it's important to recognise that the label 'vegan' does not automatically mean healthy. It is an ethical term, not one used to designate the healthfulness of a diet. A WFPBD, on the other hand, is a healthy vegan diet based on whole plant foods.

VEGETARIAN

A diet without meat but that may contain eggs and/or dairy. Like a vegan diet, the label 'vegetarian' doesn't speak to how healthy the diet is.

SEMI-VEGETARIAN/FLEXITARIAN

A mostly vegetarian diet that contains red meat (beef, lamb, pork, veal, goat, etc.), poultry, fish or shellfish occasionally (i.e. less than once per week).

PESCETARIAN

A diet that includes fish and shellfish, eggs and milk but not red meat or poultry.

NON-VEGETARIAN/OMNIVOROUS

A diet including both animal and plant products with no focus on maximising calories from plants. Depending on the study, this can be anything from the standard Western diet (which is rich in animal products and ultra-processed foods and low in whole plant foods) to the American Heart Association diet (a diet with a focus on lean meat, fish, low-fat dairy, fruits, vegetables and whole grains).

PALEO

A low-carbohydrate, whole-food diet that includes meat, fish, eggs, nuts, seeds and most vegetables but excludes dairy, grains, legumes and highly processed foods. While these days the typical Paleo diet prominently features animal products, it doesn't have to, and can be done in a plant-predominant manner.

KETOGENIC

Rather than being defined by the source of its nutrients, the ketogenic (or 'keto') diet is very low in carbohydrates, moderate in protein and high in fat. It can therefore be omnivorous or plant-based.

When we are no longer influenced by industry or media hype and look at the science objectively, a plant-predominant diet becomes the obvious answer. Consider Canada's recent dietary guidelines. In 2019, Health Canada took a hard stance and publicly stated they would no longer use research funded 'by industry or an organization with a business interest' in the creation of their national food recommendations.[2,3] This move created headlines globally – finally, a government body was able to review the totality of the evidence *without influence from the food industry*.[4]

The result? Canada's new guidelines promote a plant-predominant diet. They recommend eating plenty of vegetables, fruits and whole grain foods, and to 'choose protein foods that come from plants more often'.[5] They also suggest eating nuts, seeds, avocado and/or fatty fish (good sources of unsaturated fats) instead of fatty cuts of red meat, processed meats, full-fat dairy, coconut milk and deep-fried foods (sources of saturated fats). They even removed dairy as a necessary food group for the first time. And, importantly, they explicitly make clear that plant-based foods have less environmental impact compared with animal-based foods – a message to Canadians to consider the environmental footprint of their diet too.[2]

This is what I call a diet of science. Science doesn't care about labels: its goal is simply to uncover the truth. When we look at what it has to teach us, we come up with the power of plants. We can let go of the narrative that sells us one fad diet after another and the uncomfortable feeling that human health comes at the expense of the environment. When we choose to eat what most nourishes our health, we are also choosing what's best for the health of the Earth and the animals who live here too. ●

A quick note

It is very important to note that the evidence-based recommendations put forward here are specific to the Western world and do not always apply to developing countries, where food security and disease prevalence – and thus their prioritisation within public health – are often completely different.

CHAPTER 4

Eating for a healthy body weight

Carrying excess body fat, whether being overweight or obese, is a major risk factor for many of the leading chronic diseases reaching epidemic proportions in modern society.[1–10] For example, studies suggest that being overweight in our forties, fifties and sixties may well increase our risk of developing Alzheimer's disease by 35%.[10] Being obese is likely to place us at around seven times the risk of developing type 2 diabetes and at up to two to three times the risk of developing cardiovascular disease, our top killer.[6,11] This extra body fat is also a recipe for a shorter life.[1,5,12,13] Importantly, a 2016 meta-analysis of 239 studies involving over 10 million people identified that this risk of living fewer years isn't exclusive to people who are obese – even those who were classified as overweight were significantly more likely to die during the study observation periods than matched individuals of a healthy body weight.[13] While society certainly assigns undue value to our size and the way we look, and I have no desire to compound that, the statistics around disease and mortality show that there are indisputable advantages to maintaining a healthy body weight. Yet body fat is incredibly easy to gain and very difficult to get rid of because we live in an obesogenic environment, which promotes the overconsumption of calories while discouraging physical activity. It's this that separates the human species from wild animals, none of whom have the food availability that we do, nor the sedentary habits, and thus they rarely have excess body fat.

When the societal pressures to be thin are coupled with an environment that promotes the exact opposite, it's no wonder weight is a topic that arguably receives far more air-time than any other health issue. Even if you are not currently on a diet aimed at weight loss yourself, I'm sure you can recall a recent conversation with a friend or family member who is. While 821 million people across the world are starving, there is a global US$200-billion-dollar (and growing!) weight-loss industry built predominantly on supplying products promising quick fixes that fail to deliver long-term results.[14] We are not very good at losing weight and keeping it off. In fact, only around 20% of people who lose weight are able to keep it off in the long-term.[15] Of course, this leaves many of us frustrated and confused about why we were unable to maintain the results we had experienced.

Weight loss is mainly a product of energy balance – a calculation of the amount of energy we consume in the form of calories or kilojoules from fat, alcohol, protein and carbohydrates versus how much energy we utilise in basic life-sustaining functions (e.g. breathing, digesting food and moving our bodies throughout the day). We gain weight when we 'overfill our tanks' because our bodies have evolved to store almost unlimited amounts of fat. Historically, this feature helped our species survive during times of food scarcity – our ancestors could gain a lot of fat and then draw on that fat as energy at a later time when food wasn't available. Today, however, food scarcity is not an issue for the majority of people living in the Western world, so we are far less likely to draw down on the excess fat we deposit. The truth is, because of this energy balance equation, it's possible to lose weight with many different diets. Any diet that helps you consume fewer calories than you expend will promote weight loss, but not all diets are necessarily health-promoting or sustainable in the long term.

You may be wondering if, rather than changing the foods you eat, you can exercise your way to weight loss (just as Coca-Cola would like us to believe). It's true that exercise can help make a weight-loss journey successful as well as improve our fitness levels and increase our chances of living a long life.[16] However, research shows that, when it comes to our weight, no amount of exercise can counteract an unhealthy diet. The typical number of calories burned during exercise is far less than the calorie content of our favourite foods. For example, a person who weighs 70 kg jogging at a moderate intensity for thirty minutes burns around 298 calories.[17] This figure includes the fifty-five or so calories that they burn at rest over half an hour, meaning that the exercise itself was responsible for burning 243 extra calories beyond what this person would have expended just by being alive. A single chocolate bar or a couple of 'bliss balls' – either of which would be easy to eat without much thought – would pretty much exactly offset these calories burned! This is not to say that either of these foods should be off limits; I'm simply pointing out why positioning exercise as the key to healthy body weight is misguided. Physical activity is a much smaller contributor to body weight than the food you consume multiple times a day, hence the saying, 'You can't outrun a bad diet.'

While the basic principles of energy balance tell us that it's possible to lose weight on any diet, even an ultra-processed junk food one – such as the Twinkie diet, on which Professor Mark Haub famously lost 12 kg in 2010[18] – we aren't likely to sustain that long-term, or even feel great doing it. In order to nourish your body in such a way that lends itself to a healthy body weight over the long-term, you need to know which foods make you more and less likely to fall into a calorie surplus, and which foods will make you feel satisfied while consuming fewer calories. Once you know this, you are looking for a dietary pattern that is naturally rich in these foods that promote a calorie deficit or equilibrium, so you can avoid counting calories, constantly craving food or beating yourself up for hours on the treadmill.

If weight loss or maintenance is your goal, the evidence across all levels of science supports a diet rich in whole plant foods that minimises calories from ultra-processed foods, alcohol and animal foods, as you'll see in this chapter.

BMI

In order to make sense of findings from observational studies looking at body weight, we first need to understand Body Mass Index (BMI), which is a helpful indicator of the link between body mass and health at a population level. BMI is calculated by dividing a person's weight (in kilos) by their height (in metres, squared).

FIGURE 4.1:
BMI CLASSIFICATION[19]

BMI (kg/m²)	CLASSIFICATION
Below 18.5	Underweight
18.5–24.9	Normal weight
25.0–29.9	Pre-obesity
30.0–34.9	Obesity class I
35.0–39.9	Obesity class II
Above 40	Obesity class III

In observational studies, BMI gives us a good idea as to whether people within a certain population (e.g. vegetarians from California) are generally underweight, a healthy weight or overweight. While it is certainly not a perfect measurement - particularly for people who are significantly taller or shorter than average, people who have a physical disability, people who are pregnant or are elderly, and for athletes or bodybuilders, as muscle mass reduces its reliability - it is considered by the World Health Organization (WHO) as a reasonable proxy for determining body fat percentage and subsequent risk of developing weight-related health issues.[19,20] Indeed, a 2016 systematic review and meta-analysis looking at BMI and risk of premature death among more than thirty million people, from 230 cohorts that were followed for around fourteen years, found that those at lowest risk had a BMI between 20-24 kg/m^2.[1]

Why a plant-based diet works

The primary mechanism behind how a plant-based diet works for weight loss is increased satisfaction with fewer calories. Plant foods in their whole form are much less calorie-dense than animal and ultra-processed foods, which means fewer calories per bite. They also contain a lot of water and fibre, which fills our stomach and feeds our good gut bacteria, resulting in the production of these incredible compounds called short-chain fatty acids (SCFAs) which then stimulate the production of specific appetite-suppressing hormones, such as GLP-1, PYY and leptin.[21–24] At the same time, a high-fibre meal decreases ghrelin, an appetite-stimulating hormone. The end result? Feeling full while consuming less.[25]

In contrast, one of the major reasons why the typical Western diet leads to weight gain is because we don't experience the same level of appetite suppression (or feel as full) when eating fibre-poor ultra-processed foods, which make up 42–58% of our total calories (see Figure 4.2). As a result, we end up consuming more calories than we actually require.[26]

FIGURE 4.2:

PERCENTAGE OF CALORIES THE AVERAGE PERSON GETS FROM ULTRA-PROCESSED FOODS PER DAY IN FOUR WESTERN COUNTRIES[27-30]

COUNTRY	DAILY CALORIES FROM ULTRA-PROCESSED FOODS
United States	58%
United Kingdom	57%
Canada	46%
Australia	42%

It's long been thought that the reason ultra-processed foods are inherently unhealthy is because they contain more salt, sugar and fat and less fibre than whole foods. Given what we just learned about fibre in particular, that would make sense! However, while this is no doubt a major contributing factor, there may be more to it than that. In 2019, a brilliant study by Kevin Hall PhD, a researcher of body weight and metabolism, investigated the effects of ultra-processed foods (e.g. French toast or a plain bagel with cream cheese) versus whole foods (e.g. a berry and walnut quinoa breakfast cereal) on energy consumption and weight gain.[26] In this tightly controlled metabolic ward crossover study, twenty subjects ate the ultra-processed diet for two weeks followed by the unprocessed diet matched for macronutrients (fat, protein and carbohydrates), sugar, salt and fibre for two weeks, in a random order. Subjects were given food with a surplus of calories beyond their energy requirements (around 5500 calories) and told to eat as much (or as little) as they wanted, essentially until satisfied. On average, subjects consumed about 500 calories more per day on the ultra-processed diet, which resulted in weight gain of approximately 1 kg over the fourteen days. On the unprocessed diet, meanwhile, they *lost* an average of 1 kg over the fourteen days. In other words, consuming ultra-processed foods is a great way to gain weight! Even when matching protein, fat, carbohydrates, salt, sugar and fibre, it took fewer calories from the unprocessed foods to satisfy the subjects.

Researchers believe this can be attributed to two things: first, even though fibre was matched, they observed that the unprocessed foods resulted in an increase in the production of the appetite-suppressing hormone PYY, whereas the ultra-processed foods resulted in decreased production of this hormone. Put another way, when it comes to feeling full, eating ultra-processed foods that contain added fibre isn't the same as consuming the fibre that's naturally found in whole plant foods. Second, the subjects ate the ultra-processed meals faster, potentially resulting in a delayed sense of fullness and therefore a greater number of calories consumed per sitting. This study underscores that even if we have the very best of intentions, ultra-processed foods have been cleverly designed to exploit our biology, making them very easy to overconsume.

FIGURE 4.3:

KEVIN HALL'S METABOLIC WARD STUDY COMPARING THE EFFECTS OF AN ULTRA-PROCESSED DIET VERSUS AN UNPROCESSED DIET ON APPETITE AND WEIGHT

Diets were matched for protein, fat, carbohydrates, salt, sugar and fibre.
Subjects were given an excess of calories and were told to eat until satisfied

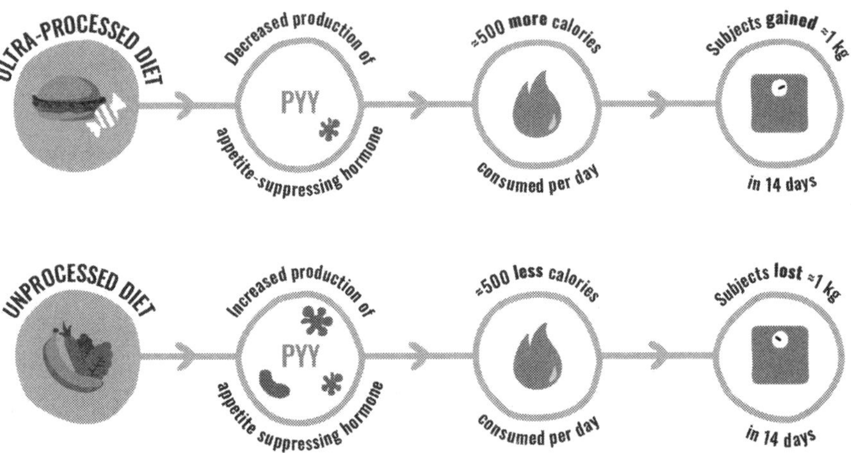

It's not just ultra-processed foods that are problematic for our waistlines, but also the amount of animal products in our diet. Whether you look at people from North America, Canada, United Kingdom, Germany or Belgium, you see a consistent reduction in BMI as they remove more animal products from their diet, with omnivores consistently having the highest BMI and vegetarians/vegans the lowest, as shown in Figure 4.4.

FIGURE 4.4:

AVERAGE BMI OF NON-VEGETARIANS AND VEGETARIANS IN MAJOR OBSERVATIONAL STUDIES ACROSS THE WORLD[31-35]

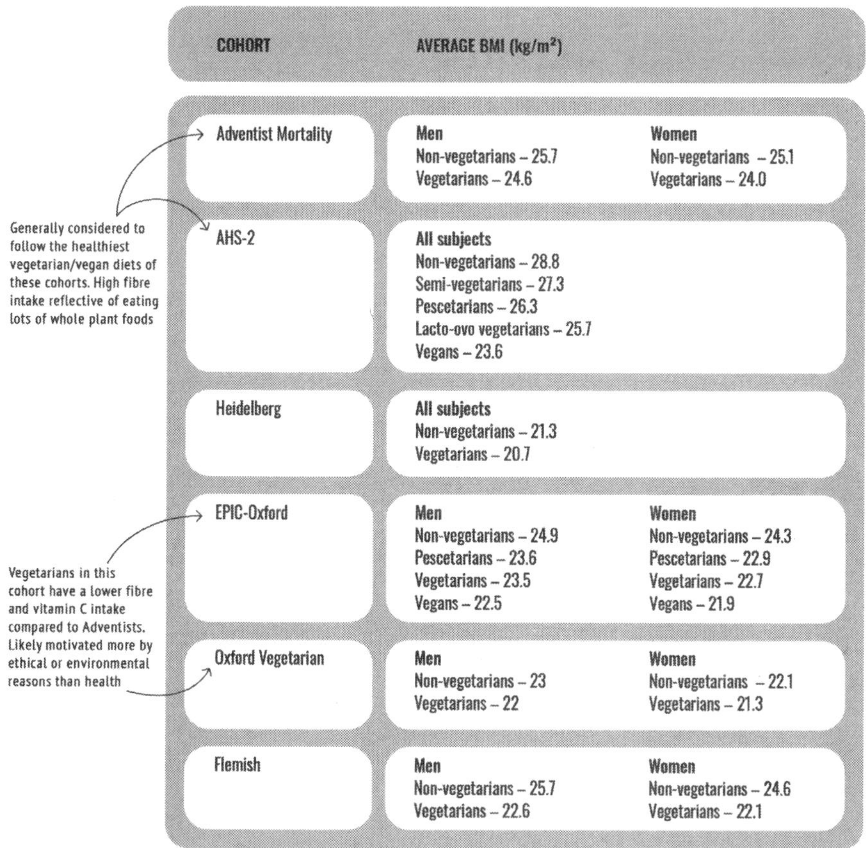

COHORT	AVERAGE BMI (kg/m²)	
Adventist Mortality	**Men** Non-vegetarians – 25.7 Vegetarians – 24.6	**Women** Non-vegetarians – 25.1 Vegetarians – 24.0
AHS-2	**All subjects** Non-vegetarians – 28.8 Semi-vegetarians – 27.3 Pescetarians – 26.3 Lacto-ovo vegetarians – 25.7 Vegans – 23.6	
Heidelberg	**All subjects** Non-vegetarians – 21.3 Vegetarians – 20.7	
EPIC-Oxford	**Men** Non-vegetarians – 24.9 Pescetarians – 23.6 Vegetarians – 23.5 Vegans – 22.5	**Women** Non-vegetarians – 24.3 Pescetarians – 22.9 Vegetarians – 22.7 Vegans – 21.9
Oxford Vegetarian	**Men** Non-vegetarians – 23 Vegetarians – 22	**Women** Non-vegetarians – 22.1 Vegetarians – 21.3
Flemish	**Men** Non-vegetarians – 25.7 Vegetarians – 22.6	**Women** Non-vegetarians – 24.6 Vegetarians – 22.1

Generally considered to follow the healthiest vegetarian/vegan diets of these cohorts. High fibre intake reflective of eating lots of whole plant foods
Vegetarians in this cohort have a lower fibre and vitamin C intake compared to Adventists. Likely motivated more by ethical or environmental reasons than health

When researchers looking at various populations around the world have measured waist circumference, considered a more accurate marker of body fat percentage and risk of chronic disease than BMI in certain populations, the results are the same – a lower waist circumference as one eats fewer animal products.[36–38] The most likely explanation for this is that by maximising the amount of whole plant foods in their diet, vegans and vegetarians are displacing more calorie-dense animal foods and feeling satisfied while consuming fewer calories thanks to the extra fibre and higher overall volume of their food.[39] This is the protective benefit of eating more plants.[40]

The fat versus carbs debate

There's a school of thought that exists in certain diet circles that since we were told to eat less fat in the 1980s and we have since become increasingly fatter and more likely to develop chronic disease, the guidelines must have got it wrong. While on face value this might seem like a logical conclusion, the data says otherwise. The 1980 US dietary guidelines (which were largely used to inform the rest of the Western world) encouraged people to lower their intake of foods high in fat, such as meat and dairy, with good reason – it was hoped this would lead to people lowering their saturated fat intake and increase their consumption of health-promoting low-fat foods such as fruits, vegetables, whole grains and legumes in order to lower their risk of chronic disease.[41,42] Unfortunately, humans do not always do what they are advised to! Today it's clear that our fat intake, in terms of grams per day, has stayed at essentially the same level while we have simultaneously increased our total energy intake by between 200–450 calories per day.[43,44] The higher end of this, 450 calories, is almost equivalent to consuming a can of Coca-Cola and a McDonald's cheeseburger on top of a typical day's eating. It's foods like these, along with others rich in heavily refined carbohydrates, such as desserts, pasta, tacos and alcohol – foods that we know do not adequately satisfy our hunger – that make up these increased calories.[43-46] Unfortunately, the reality of our increasing waistlines has been used to demonise carbohydrates as a macronutrient group. The problem with this is that not all carbohydrates are created equal.[47] Rather than blaming black beans for the problems caused by jellybeans, we need to consider the differing health effects that refined and unrefined carbohydrates have on our health. While it's clear that we should be limiting foods that are high in refined carbohydrates, unrefined carbohydrates, found in whole or minimally processed plant foods such as fruits, vegetables, whole grains and legumes, come packed with fibre, vitamins, minerals, phytonutrients and water, which are all incredible for promoting a healthy body weight and reducing the risk of chronic disease and premature death.[40,48,49]

It's not carbohydrates making people sick; it's the foods those carbohydrates are coming in.

These population studies, taken together, include data from hundreds of thousands of people, and the results are consistent: people who eat fewer animal products and more whole plant foods have lower BMIs. But this is only *part* of the overall evidence in support of a diet that gets most, or all, calories from whole plants. A 2016 review of twelve clinical intervention trials comparing vegetarian (including vegan) and non-vegetarian diets for weight loss concluded that significant benefit is associated with adopting a vegetarian diet compared with a diet that includes meat, with the greatest benefit seen by those adopting a vegan diet.[39] Although only twelve trials were included in this study, it does support the idea that vegetarian and vegan diets are generally better for promoting healthier body weight than diets that include meat.

The most compelling trial included within this meta-analysis compared a vegan diet with a low-fat non-vegetarian diet (taken from the US National Cholesterol Education Program) and found greater weight loss for subjects who followed a vegan diet at both one year (4.9 vs 1.8 kg) and two years (3.1 vs 0.8 kg).[50] I find this to be compelling for a few reasons. First, it was the longest of the included trials, following subjects for up to two years. Given we know all sorts of diets can result in short-term benefits, the longer we can follow subjects, the more confident we can be that the diet is sustainable. Two years is hardly a lifetime, but it's more than many studies which look at weight loss. Second, the control diet used is generally recognised as a healthy omnivorous diet (one low in saturated fats, cholesterol and refined grains), so we know control subjects were not eating a standard Western diet. Finally, unlike many studies that use calorie restriction (e.g. a 1500 kcal per day diet), subjects from both groups were simply told to eat until they were satisfied, which better reflects how we eat in real life.

Alcohol and weight gain

While ultra-processed foods no doubt play a huge role in weight gain, another source of calories that is often overlooked is alcohol. According to a 2018 WHO global report, Aussies guzzle down 40% more alcohol than the global average, and almost half of us are classified as binge drinkers.[51,52] Specifically, the average Australian aged over fifteen drinks 2.72 standard drinks a day while the US Centers for Disease Control and Prevention (CDC) recommends a maximum of one drink per day for women and two drinks per day for men (zero alcoholic drinks being the healthiest option).[53,54]

While there are many health reasons to avoid or minimise alcohol consumption, there are a few specific reasons why anyone aiming to lose weight should watch their alcohol intake:

1. The calories in alcoholic drinks don't come purely from the sugar in them. The compound ethyl alcohol, or 'ethanol', contains seven calories per gram, so even a shot of vodka contains around 100 calories. The higher a drink's alcohol percentage, the more calories it contains from ethanol. This is why most dry red wines tend to be slightly higher in calories than dry white wines, despite containing less sugar.

2. The human body cannot store alcohol. Upon consumption, it gets prioritised above all other nutrients (fat, protein and carbohydrates) for metabolism because it's a toxin and the body wants to remove it.[55] The extra calories from alcohol are therefore utilised before calories from food.

3. It's not just the calories in your cocktail that are promoting weight gain. Research shows when people drink, they usually eat more calories and move less – the former attributed to alcohol's ability to stimulate appetite and inhibit mechanisms that under unintoxicated conditions would allow you to control food intake.[56,57] This results in three factors working together against weight loss: more calories from alcohol, more calories from food and less energy expended through movement, making it more likely you fall into a calorie surplus. If there is any day to be extra focused on the food you eat and how much you move, it's the days you drink alcohol, and the few days after.

If you want to be more in control of your weight for any health-related reasons, alcohol intake is one of the biggest factors to be mindful of.

Another study from this meta-analysis was a 2015 trial that randomised sixty-three overweight subjects to one of five diets: vegan, vegetarian, pescetarian, semi-vegetarian or non-vegetarian. Over a six-month period, without restricting calories, vegan subjects lost significantly more weight (-7.5% of body weight) than pescetarians (-3.2%), semi-vegetarians (-3.2%) and non-vegetarians (-3.1%).[58]

Since this meta-analysis, an interesting RCT out of New Zealand was published called the BROAD study, which investigated the benefits of a low-fat WFPBD for weight loss without calorie restriction with sixty-five subjects diagnosed as obese or overweight and living with chronic disease.[59] Subjects randomised to the WFPBD were compared with a control group receiving standard advice from their doctors. In both groups, subjects were advised to focus their efforts on diet, not exercise. At six months, the control subjects averaged 1.6 kg of weight loss and the WFPBD subjects averaged 12.1 kg! The researchers concluded: 'To the best of our knowledge, there are no [other] randomised controlled trials that have achieved a greater average weight loss over a six-month or twelve-month period, without mandating regular exercise or restricting total caloric intake.'[59]

Unfortunately, there was no data specifying what the control diet was like, so it's hard to know what the plant-based diet was really up against. Were they following a specific diet? Were they told to eat whatever they wanted? We don't know, which makes the 'compared with what' principle tough to evaluate here. Nonetheless, because the differences between groups were so significant, the researchers ended the control group at six months so the control subjects could also benefit from the WFPBD intervention. At twelve months, the WFPBD subjects were able to maintain 95% of their weight loss.

Despite its limitations, the BROAD study does show a low-fat WFPBD, with food education and social support, is a great option for those wanting to adopt a dietary pattern that promotes weight loss in the medium-term without having to count calories and without an emphasis on exercise. What it can't tell us is whether such a diet is superior to, say, a diet with mostly plants and a small amount of animal products, or a higher fat WFPBD.

The other dietary pattern that is known for promoting a healthy body weight is the Mediterranean diet. However, up until very recently there were no clinical trials directly comparing the effectiveness of this dietary pattern with a completely plant-exclusive diet. In 2021, researchers from the United States published a study that randomised 62 overweight adults into a Mediterranean or a low-fat vegan diet group for a sixteen-week period. It was a crossover trial, so each subject got to experience both diets – one diet for sixteen weeks and then, after a one-month break, the other diet for sixteen weeks. The participants were told to eat without restriction, simply until they were satisfied. Over the study period, subjects lost 3.4 kg more fat on the vegan diet.[60]

What's clear is that a diet centred on plant-based foods in their whole or minimally processed form is one that lends itself to a healthy body weight. As the observational studies show us, it can be plant-exclusive or it can equally include modest amounts of animal products. And while vegan diets tend to produce greater weight loss in clinical trials, interventions with small amounts of animal products, such as vegetarian diets, were also better than non-vegetarian diets.[39] When it comes to animal products and weight, it seems that some is okay and less is better.

Should I count calories?

We can easily be led to believe that the answer to our growing waistlines is calorie-counting, slaving away at the gym and/or buying gimmick products. Yes, calories matter, but with good food selection, they need not be obsessed over. In other words, calories count, but we don't need to count them!

A hundred years or so ago, when our not-too-distant ancestors ate whole foods until they were satiated, they weren't plugging their food intake into calorie calculators, taking fat-burner supplements or doing 'cardio' at the gym. Put simply, they weren't subject to the same environment we are today, and just like all other mammals living in the wild, the way they naturally ate and moved was far more likely to result in a healthy body weight.[61]

Today, as a result of being genetically wired to source and feast on calorie-dense foods, combined with living in an environment that provides these foods in abundance without us having to burn much energy to access them, we have a lifestyle that lends itself to an unhealthy body weight. We've been conditioned to believe the only way to combat that is to 'diet'. Why? Because being overweight makes us vulnerable to the billion-dollar food and supplement industries while keeping us at a distance from understanding how to truly address our body weight.

This is why I am not an advocate for 'dieting' or 'counting calories'. As I said earlier, I think we should see our diet as a noun, not a verb.

It's not an issue if you want to count calories – for some people, it can be a helpful tool, particularly if you have a very specific body composition goal (such as bodybuilding). But for most people looking for optimal health, the answer does not lie in calorie-counting but in shifting our focus to an eating pattern rich in whole, or minimally processed, fruits, vegetables, grains, legumes, nuts and seeds.

Can this be done in our obesogenic environment? Absolutely. If you look at Table 4.4, you'll see the AHS-2 population, which includes over 96,000 subjects from North America.[62] Despite living in a similar environment to ours, their healthy lifestyle is protective against obesity. While 40% of Americans are obese, only around 9% of the vegans in the AHS-2 population are obese.[48,63] This shows that it is possible to live in an obesogenic environment and not be affected by it. By focusing on a new way to see the foods we do and do not eat, or eat in abundance versus minimising, we are describing a permanent shift in our lifestyle that allows us to better navigate today's food environment, rather than the temporary restrictions and inevitable rebound that comes with a 'diet'.

What about low-fat, low-carb and high-protein diets?

Most of us have likely either tried a low-fat or low-carb diet, or know somebody who has – both diets have been popular for a few decades. Among experts and in the media, there are two camps, each arguing that one is better than the other. But what does the science show? If calories are equal, is there a particular fat-burning advantage to consuming fat in preference to carbohydrates, or vice versa?

The most compelling evidence looking at exactly this is a 2017 meta-analysis that pooled the results from thirty-two metabolic ward studies, meaning subjects eat the food given to them in a closely monitored hospital setting, the restrictions of which make it the gold standard for RCTs.[64] These studies fed subjects two different diets (low-fat versus low-carb) that provided the same amount of total calories and protein, the idea being that if one group lost more weight, you could attribute that to the low amount of fat or carbohydrates that they were eating. While there was slightly more fat loss during the low-fat high-carbohydrate diet (16 g per day), the findings were considered clinically meaningless, confirming the conventional theory that, when it comes to weight loss, 'a calorie is a calorie' – and that, unlike what some may claim, carbohydrates are no more fattening than fat.[64]

These feeding trials are calorie-controlled, though, and while they can accurately convey what subjects ate and how much weight they lost, they can't tell us whether one dietary pattern was more satiating, an important factor when considering how sustainable those diets will be when transferred to the real world. After all, a diet that provides greater satisfaction on fewer calories would presumably be better at promoting weight loss in everyday life. So what do we see when comparing low-fat to low-carbohydrate diets outside of a metabolic ward? Trial after trial shows us that neither a low-carb nor a low-fat diet is *clinically superior* with regard to weight loss.[65–69]

It's hard to really control how subjects eat outside of a metabolic ward though. Wouldn't it be nice if we could compare a fairly healthy low-carb diet with a fairly healthy low-fat diet, without calorie restriction, while ensuring that people don't deviate from the foods they're allowed to eat? Enter Kevin Hall (again), who, in early 2021, published the highly anticipated results from an extremely cleverly designed RCT. In a four-week metabolic ward trial, he compared a very low-carb or ketogenic omnivorous diet with a low-fat, high-carbohydrate WFPBD.[70] Subjects completed each diet for two weeks, were given their meals with an excess of calories beyond their normal requirements and told to simply eat until satisfied. They could eat as much as they wanted – just like we can in our everyday lives. When subjects were eating the high-carbohydrate, high-fibre WFPBD, they consumed about 700 fewer calories per day and burned more body fat, despite being just as satisfied! Here, finally, is an RCT that explains the power of whole plant foods for promoting a healthy body weight, and further disproves the notion that 'carbs make us fat'. While I could easily go as far as saying the results of this study were mind-blowing, they really are just confirming what we've known for a long time – carbohydrate-rich plant foods, such as sweet potato, black beans, brown rice and bananas, are not to blame for the rates of obesity we see today. Whole plant foods rich in unrefined carbohydrates help people eat fewer calories, not more.

What about protein? Is protein the secret to losing weight? Protein does have a higher thermic effect than both carbohydrates and fat, which means that our bodies burn more energy to process it.[71] But while higher protein diets can result in modest increases in fat loss, it's not the silver bullet that it's often made out to be. If it were as simple as eating a high-protein diet, very few of us in Western populations, where we are protein-obsessed and eat more meat per capita than most, would struggle with weight gain.[72]

Sometimes it pays to step outside the lab and see what happens in the real world. The populations that naturally achieve healthy body weight around the world are not obsessing over protein – with most consuming around 70 g per day.[33,48] While this meets the dietary recommendations for protein, it is by no means a crazy high amount. In fact, we know that as populations become more Westernised and increase their protein intake, their BMI tends to increase. Take Okinawa, Japan, for example. Okinawans eating the traditional diet of the region are known for being some of the longest-living and healthiest people in the world, with a remarkable number of people reaching 100 years of age. In just two generations, as younger Okinawans have moved to a more Western diet that has almost double the protein, their BMI has gone from the lowest among Japanese populations to the highest.[73]

So protein isn't the be-all and end-all for weight loss – it can't save us from a poor diet – and as we continue to look at the relationship between the foods we eat and chronic disease in the following chapters, it will become increasingly obvious that obsessing over protein, particularly animal protein, is detrimental to our health and longevity.

Diabetes and weight

Type 2 diabetes used to be something of a marginal disease, but today affects approximately one million Australians and over 30 million Americans, and is one of the leading causes of death in Western countries.[74,75] It is said to be the fastest-growing chronic disease in Australia, growing at a rate faster than heart disease and cancer.[76] For the majority of people, type 2 diabetes is a lifestyle disease, with 80–85% of the risk of developing type 2 diabetes believed to be driven by unhealthy body weight.[77] As a result, in most cases, type 2 diabetes is a disease that we can prevent or even put into remission by adopting a lifestyle that promotes a healthy body weight.

We know that you can lose weight on any diet, but a plant-based diet is particularly helpful for people living with type 2 diabetes – and for anyone who wants to prevent type 2 diabetes – for three main reasons. First, as we've seen throughout this chapter, a plant-based diet is great for weight loss without having to count calories. Second, a plant-based diet is protective against major complications of type 2 diabetes, including cardiovascular disease, chronic kidney disease and dementia.[78-81] And third, a plant-based diet addresses the root cause of type 2 diabetes.[81] Let me explain.

Both type 1 and type 2 diabetes are characterised by *impaired blood glucose control* due to problems with a hormone called insulin. Under normal conditions, insulin, produced by our pancreas, triggers the flow of glucose (a single unit of sugar) from the blood into muscle cells for energy production and thousands of critical cellular functions. Think of this like a lock and key relationship: insulin is the key that unlocks the front door of the muscle cells, allowing glucose to enter. When a person has diabetes, glucose cannot enter the muscle cells and thus glucose levels become elevated in the blood, which can have serious health implications, including cardiovascular disease, kidney disease, poor psychological wellbeing and blindness. In fact, cardiovascular disease is the number one cause of premature death among people with diabetes.[81]

While type 1 diabetes is an autoimmune condition in which the body mistakenly activates its immune system to destroy cells in the pancreas and is not linked with lifestyle factors, type 2 diabetes is a progressive condition in which the body fails to produce enough insulin, and that insulin is ineffective due to a physiological state called *insulin resistance*.[82] * To return to our lock and key metaphor, insulin resistance means that despite the presence of the key, the gate does not open – like a jammed lock. With that, you get a build-up of sugar in the blood much like a traffic jam on a highway. In the early stages of this disease, the pancreas compensates

* Diabetes is not the only condition related to insulin resistance. Another one you may have heard of is polycystic ovary syndrome (or PCOS), which insulin resistance is believed to play a key role in the development of. This is a condition that can cause difficulties falling pregnant, menstrual cycle irregularities, skin conditions, weight gain and a heightened risk of developing cardiovascular disease during the reproductive years of a woman's life.[83]

for this by working harder to produce more insulin to combat insulin resistance and bring down blood sugar levels.[84,85] This is like your body creating stronger keys that, for a time, are able to turn the jammed locks and open the cellular gates. This stage is what we call pre-diabetes, a condition that affects at least 2 million Australians and over 84 million Americans.[86,87] The CDC estimates over 90% of those with pre-diabetes do not know they have it, which means that most of these people are walking around with underlying insulin resistance but no noticeable symptoms.[88] Over time, the pancreas may begin to wear out, and when 50–70% of the insulin-producing cells have shut down, the person has type 2 diabetes.[82]

I am sure you are wondering, just what is it that jams up the lock? If you think maybe sugar has something to do with it, you would not be alone. Impaired blood glucose control is a characteristic of both type 1 and type 2 diabetes, so people have long blamed sugars for playing a role in insulin resistance. And I get it: if someone who is insulin-resistant tries to eat a banana, which contains 14 g of sugar, they'll notice a spike in their blood sugar. However, that idea that the sugar found in whole foods is to blame is one of the biggest misconceptions about diabetes, and one that is now widely refuted by diabetes associations and scientists around the world.[89] It's clear from observational studies of vegetarians and vegans, and of the longest-living people in the world, that people who regularly consume large quantities of fruit, vegetables, whole grains and legumes (which are all sources of sugars and/or carbohydrates that break down into sugars) are protected from developing type 2 diabetes.[90,91] Blaming the natural sugars found in whole plant foods for diabetes is akin to blaming firefighters for fires because they are first on the scene. Both are just trying to get to where they are supposed to be in order to do their jobs. Elevated blood sugar is merely a symptom of insulin resistance, not the cause.

So, if it's not unrefined sugar, what are we eating that is causing insulin resistance and the skyrocketing rates of type 2 diabetes? Research indicates that a significant part of the answer is fat. More precisely, microscopic fat particles building up in muscle and liver cells – not where they are supposed to be.[92-94] Saturated fats in particular appear to be the type of fat that overwhelms the muscle and liver cells and really jams up the lock. A 2016 meta-analysis of 102 randomised controlled feeding trials showed that replacing an equivalent number of calories from saturated fats with calories from polyunsaturated fats reduced insulin resistance.[95] That means when we reduce foods like meat and dairy in our diet, in favour of foods like tofu, nuts and seeds, our bodies become better at moving glucose into our cells.

Various studies have also implicated animal protein, heme iron (top sources in a typical Western diet include red meat and poultry), advanced glycation end products (AGEs, which occur in high levels in cooked meat), isolated fructose and sucrose (table sugar) in the development of insulin resistance and type 2 diabetes.[96-104] Isolated fructose and sucrose are refined sugars that are mainly found consumed in sugar-sweetened beverages and desserts, and increase the chances of developing type 2 diabetes by contributing to weight gain and increasing insulin resistance in the liver. In simple terms, unlike the sugars in whole fruit, when you consume an excess of these refined sugars, your liver converts them into fats that are then stored in your liver cells, which is bad news if you want to reduce your risk of developing fatty liver disease and type 2 diabetes.[105-108]

On the flip side, plant-based dietary patterns and the nutrients they provide in abundance (unsaturated fats, plant protein, unrefined carbohydrates, dietary fibre, magnesium and antioxidants) have proved effective not only in reducing the risk of developing type 2 diabetes in the first place, but also for restoring normal biology, or 'unjamming the lock', in those who suffer from existing insulin resistance and/or type 2 diabetes.[77,95,109-117]

This is where a plant-based dietary pattern differs from a low-carbohydrate diet for managing type 2 diabetes. While it's true that you can lose weight on very low-carb diets, such as the ketogenic diet, and improve blood sugar levels, there are a few things that need to be considered. First, the ketogenic diet does not offer a magic fat-burning advantage over any other dietary pattern.[70] It's true that when someone removes carbohydrates from their diet, their body switches to utilising fat for energy but unless that person is in a calorie deficit, they are simply burning dietary fat, not mobilising stored body fat. Second, when it comes to insulin resistance and type 2 diabetes, the approach of removing carbohydrates from your diet is really only a band-aid. Of course removing carbohydrates means you will have improved blood sugar. When you're not eating carbohydrates, your body doesn't have to worry about getting glucose from the blood into the cells. By default, such exclusion means that ultra-processed foods with added sugars are off the menu (a good thing). Along with a loss in water weight, this is one of the major reasons people adopting a ketogenic diet lose a good amount of weight in the first few weeks. The problem is that these diets are usually rich in saturated fats from the animal products they contain, and while on the surface things seem to improve, the underlying cause of insulin resistance is not addressed.

If someone is prepared to limit themselves to 25–50 g of carbohydrate per day for the rest of their life (the limit when following a ketogenic diet), and is able to keep the excess weight from returning, this could be an option for them. Practically, though, this means avoiding whole grains, potatoes, most legumes and most fruit. Unfortunately, clinical trials tell us that by one year, most people struggle to adhere to this extreme restriction,[118] and as carbohydrates are reintroduced, their body is extraordinarily lousy at handling them.[70,119,120]

That doesn't mean there aren't exceptions. A small minority of people can stick to a very low-carbohydrate diet long-term and lose a significant amount of weight, so if it works for you, all power to you. However, I would strongly encourage anyone who goes down this path to source most of the fats in their diet from unsaturated fats found in plant-based foods. Why? Well, other than the fact that consuming foods rich in unsaturated fats instead of saturated fats helps to decrease insulin resistance, numerous studies, including a 2018 meta-analysis of eight observational studies involving over 400,000 subjects from all over the globe, have identified that people following low-carbohydrate diets made up of animal-based foods tend to live shorter lives than people following low-carbohydrate diets rich in plant-based sources of protein and fat.[121] Practically, this would mean dialling down your consumption of foods like meat, eggs and dairy while at the same time placing greater emphasis on foods like tofu, nuts, seeds and avocado (and even modest amounts of fish, for those who eat animal products). This is in line with the 2020 American College of Endocrinology guidelines – which clearly recommend plant-based dietary patterns as the preferred way of eating for people living with type 2 diabetes.[122]

Plant-based nutrition beyond weight

Data from long-term weight-loss studies shows that the benefits of most diets are somewhat short lived. Typically, more than 50% of the weight lost has been regained at the two-year mark, and by five years, about 80% has been regained.[122] While these results are certainly better than no progress towards a healthier body weight, it does underscore the fact that even though energy balance is a simple concept, sustained weight loss is highly complex – particularly when you factor in the obesogenic environment that most of us live in. If you've struggled with weight and had someone tell you 'eat less and move more', I empathise with you. This is hard stuff. I commend anyone who has lost weight on any diet. Simply being proactive with your health is something I admire.

Ultimately, if we want to lose weight it's clear there is a powerful advantage to eating more whole plants – they keep us full with fewer calories – but if we want to keep the weight off long-term, our rationale to choose kale over potato chips is going to need to be based on something more meaningful than a number on the scales. For the best results, research shows that it helps to choose a dietary pattern and lifestyle that prescribes greater purpose and meaning to our food choices – a manner of living that becomes an important part of who we are.[123] As we'll see in the coming chapters, as we continue to look at our health and the health of all life on the planet, a plant-based diet can offer exactly that.

Podcast highlight: Episode 91, 'Healthy weight loss is not a diet'

In this solo episode, I expand on a number of principles touched on here, including energy balance and high- versus low-carbohydrate diets for weight loss, and cover many practical tips for achieving a healthy body weight.

CHAPTER 5

Eating to prevent cardiovascular disease

Globally, cardiovascular disease (CVD) is both the leading cause of death and of years lost due to ill health.[1,2] It's responsible for one in four deaths in Australia.[3] Due to this prevalence, many people have come to accept heart attacks and strokes as a normal part of ageing or the result of bad genes, yet the American Heart Association estimates that *80% of all cardiovascular disease is preventable.*[4] To a large degree, we have the power to do something about it.

Although the rate of deaths from cardiovascular events in most developed countries has actually declined steadily since the 1980s, this is primarily a result of a reduction in smoking and better pharmaceutical management for risk factors such as high blood pressure and high cholesterol.[5] But we can only rely on Western medicine so much – if we want to really squeeze cardiovascular disease out of our society, we have to address it at the root cause: diet and lifestyle.

Since both my father and grandfather had heart attacks, understanding this area of research was particularly important to me.

I wanted to know if my dad could prevent further damage to his heart, and whether I could avoid what I had reluctantly accepted as my fate.

Cardiovascular disease is a group of disorders primarily affecting the blood vessels that supply the heart and brain. The two most common forms are coronary heart disease leading to a heart attack (which I will call just heart disease from here on in) and cerebrovascular disease (*cerebro* meaning relating to the brain, the most common form of which is stroke).[1] While a heart attack or stroke is the *acute* manifestation of vascular blockage preventing blood flow to the heart or brain, there is an abundance of science that tells us the underlying disease process typically starts decades earlier.[6–10] The acute event is just the result of years of compounding damage. In fact, the narrowing of our arteries, described as atherosclerosis in the medical world, can actually begin in utero, particularly if the person carrying the child has high cholesterol.[11] This means that even if you are young and for all intents and purposes a healthy person, you could still have asymptomatic cardiovascular disease, depending on your lifestyle and what foods you've been eating.

Atherosclerosis explained

The most common underlying cause of stroke and heart disease is the presence of *atherosclerosis*,[12] or chronic hardening, inflammation and narrowing of the arteries that supply blood to the heart and brain.[13] The narrowing begins with damage to the inside of the artery wall, which is typically caused by a combination of factors. The most studied and well understood of these is elevated LDL-cholesterol, elevated blood sugar levels and high blood pressure.

When the artery wall is damaged, the body issues an anti-inflammatory response and sends a type of white blood cell called macrophages to protect the blood vessel and clean up anything that doesn't belong there.[14] Unfortunately, they go about their business somewhat indiscriminately and end up engulfing LDL-cholesterol particles,[13] which results in cholesterol and protein becoming trapped in the artery wall and hardening into crystal-like molecules.[13,15] Over time, more and more LDL-cholesterol particles build up, creating a plaque. This process, depicted in Figure 5.1, is something we want to avoid!

FIGURE 5.1:

THE ATHEROSCLEROSIS PROCESS

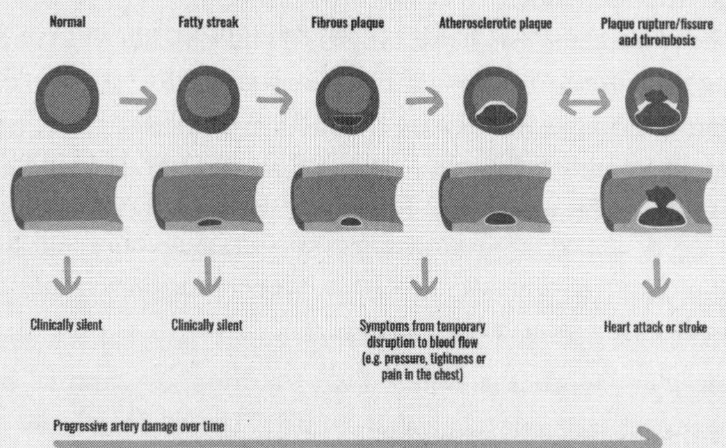

In cases of coronary artery disease, it is the arteries supplying the heart with oxygenated blood that develop atherosclerosis. In minor cases, this results in shortness of breath and chest pain, or 'angina'. In more serious cases, where the plaque build-up is larger and less stable, it can rupture, causing blockage of the artery and a heart attack. In cases of ischaemic stroke (the most common form of stroke), it is blood vessels supplying the brain tissue that are affected – usually the carotid arteries in the neck.

Something that caught my attention when I started reading the literature in this area was the dietary habits of various populations around the world that have extraordinarily low levels of cardiovascular disease. For example, it is normal for traditional populations such as the Okinawans in Japan, people in rural China, the Tarahumara Indians of Mexico and the Tsimane people in Bolivia to live into old age with little to no risk of having a heart attack. Other than the fact that people in these populations tend to be active and non-smokers, the commonality between them is that they share a diet that is made up of predominantly whole plant foods with minimal calories derived from animals or ultra-processed foods.[16–20]

The research, as you'll see, is clear: if you want to avoid developing this disease in the first place or you want to stop or slow the progression of the disease if you have it already, you'll want to adopt an anti-inflammatory diet that's low in saturated and trans fats, cholesterol, refined carbohydrates, salt and heme iron, and rich in unrefined carbohydrates, fibre, unsaturated fats, plant protein and antioxidants. In other words, a plant-predominant or plant-exclusive diet based on whole foods. So what is it about whole plant foods that offer this protection? Or animal and ultra-processed foods that inflict damage? Let's dig a little deeper.

The dietary causes of high cholesterol and high blood pressure, two of CVD's biggest risk factors

When we think of cardiovascular disease, most of us think of cholesterol and high blood pressure, and for good reason. The link between elevated LDL-cholesterol (or LDL-C for short) – what we often hear described as the 'bad' cholesterol – and increased risk of cardiovascular disease is one of the most studied relationships in medical science.[12,21,22] And it's thought that around 50% of all deaths caused by cardiovascular disease are due to high blood pressure (hypertension) – more than any other risk factor.[23] As of 2015, the global prevalence of hypertension was around 1.13 billion people, or 30–45% of all adults.

So why are high LDL-C and elevated blood pressure not so great for the health of our arteries? And how can we use our lifestyle, particularly our diet, to promote healthier levels of these biomarkers of cardiovascular disease?

LDL-cholesterol

Data from more than two million subjects across a broad and diverse range of studies has unequivocally and consistently shown that the more a person's LDL-C is elevated above normal, and the longer the period of elevation, the greater the risk that person will develop atherosclerosis.[12,21,24,25] The evidence is clear: elevated LDL-C *causes* CVD.[21] To lower your risk of having a heart attack or stroke, you want normal LDL-C levels for as many years as possible, as we can see from Figure 5.2.

FIGURE 5.2:

RESULTS OF STUDIES LOOKING AT HOW THE RISK OF DEVELOPING CORONARY HEART DISEASE IS AFFECTED BY LDL-C LEVELS[21]

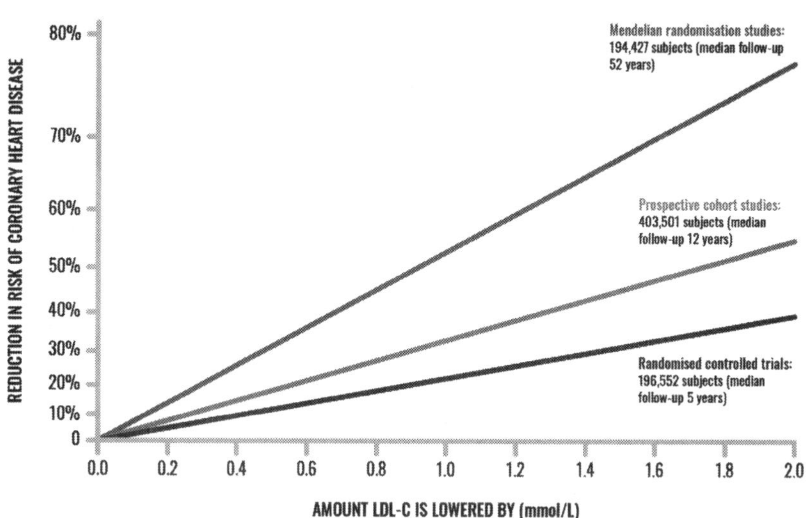

Here's what we're looking at in this graph. Each line represents a different type of study examining how the risk of developing coronary heart disease is affected by LDL-C levels. Across the three study types, this graph comprises data from nearly one million subjects across more than thirty studies.

The top line shows the results of Mendelian randomisation studies. These studies take advantage of genetic variations that result in a person naturally having higher or lower LDL-C levels. These genetic mutations take place at conception, and so they allow us to look at the effect of LDL-C levels independent of other lifestyle variables, just like an RCT. Nature's RCT, you could say. Regardless of the genetic variation someone has, out of more than fifty different genetic variations that lead to lower LDL-C, these studies have shown that lower LDL-C levels decrease the risk of developing heart disease. And vice versa – genetic mutations that cause higher LDL-C increase the person's risk of developing heart disease.

The middle line shows the results from large observational studies of people living in the real world – such as the cohorts we've discussed elsewhere. These observational studies consistently show that people living with lower LDL-C levels have lower risk of developing heart disease.

The bottom line represents RCTs. Many RCTs involving cholesterol-lowering medications have shown that the greater the reduction in LDL-C, the lower a person's risk of developing heart disease. Importantly, several different types of cholesterol-lowering medications have shown the same result, indicating that it is the absolute reduction in LDL-C that matters most, not the pathway by which it is lowered.

Lipids 101

Lipids are fat-like substances that circulate in your blood. Two lipids you may have heard of are triglycerides and cholesterol. Triglycerides come mainly from the fat in foods you eat, but your liver can also produce triglycerides from excess protein and carbohydrates in your diet. Once digested, triglycerides circulate in the bloodstream to be used as energy by your cells. Cholesterol, on the other hand, is produced by your body – mostly by the liver, but also to a lesser extent by other cells throughout the body. Where triglycerides are a type of fuel, cholesterol is needed for various metabolic processes, such as making hormones and building cells.

Lipids aren't able to dissolve in water (the technical term for this is hydrophobic) so they are unable to flow through your blood by themselves – but they need something to sit on. What do they sit on? On proteins known as *lipoproteins*. You can think of lipoproteins as cargo ships and lipids like cholesterol and triglycerides as the shipping containers. The cargo ships (lipoproteins) cruise through your blood carrying shipping containers (lipids) where they need to go, from one port to the next.

There are a handful of different lipoproteins, but the two that are most important when it comes to CVD are low density lipoproteins (LDL) and high density lipoproteins (HDL). When we have elevated levels of LDL particles, they can penetrate artery walls and cause plaque build-up, like if the cargo ship were to get to port and, instead of docking, it crashes through and causes damage to the dock. This is why LDL-C is called 'bad' cholesterol.

HDL particles are more like cargo ships that are covered in rubber – the particles are soft at the edges, and this stops them from crashing in and lodging in the artery wall. Unable to penetrate the artery wall (or get stuck in the dock), they instead take the cholesterol along with them, helping to clear it from the blood and take it back to the liver. Hence HDL-C is called 'good' cholesterol.

A normal LDL-C level, according to the US Centers for Disease Control and Prevention (CDC), is 100 mg/dL (2.59 mmol/L) or lower (cholesterol levels are measured in milligrams of cholesterol per decilitre of blood (mg/dL) or millimoles per litre of blood (mmol/L), depending on where you are in the world).[26] However, we should probably be aiming for an even lower level – two studies have shown that targeting a range of 50–75 mg/dL is actually more optimal to avoid clogging our arteries and reduce our risk of developing CVD.[27,28] Both the average Australian's and American's LDL-C is approximately 120–130 mg/dL (3.1–3.3 mmol/L) which is *twice* the level shown to be associated with no atherosclerosis.[29,30]

The good news is that if you can reduce your LDL-C from these average levels to below 100mg/dL, you will reduce your risk of developing and dying from cardiovascular disease. Dramatically, in fact. In 2018, results from one of the most eloquently designed observational studies investigating LDL-C and cardiovascular disease were published. The Cooper Center Longitudinal Study took 36,375 healthy subjects who were in their late thirties and early forties, without a history of cardiovascular disease or type 2 diabetes, and followed them for 27 years![22] They found that those whose LDL-C was below 100 mg/dL were 30–40% less likely to die from cardiovascular disease than those whose LDL-C was between 100 and 129 mg/dL (2.59 and 3.33 mmol/L).

Our diet significantly affects our LDL-C levels – and the fewer animal foods, the better. This has been seen in observational studies, such as a 2007 study in Brazil which found a stepwise reduction in LDL-C as a person's diet consisted of fewer animal products (see Figure 5.3), with vegans being the only group to have a cholesterol level below 70 mg/dL (1.81 mmol/L) – the level where studies show people have zero, or very little, atherosclerotic plaque.[31] This makes sense given that vegans are the only people who have cholesterol-free diets and typically consume less saturated fats and more dietary fibre than vegetarians and omnivores – key aspects of our diet that affect our LDL-C levels.[32–34]

FIGURE 5.3:

LDL-C LEVELS OF BRAZILIAN SUBJECTS WHO ADOPT DIFFERENT DIETARY PATTERNS[31]

CHOLESTEROL	OMNIVORES	LACTO-OVO VEGETARIANS	LACTO VEGETARIANS	VEGANS
LDL-C mg/dL (mmol/L)	123 (3.2)	101 (2.6)	88 (2.3)	69 (1.8)

While not as significant as the Brazil cohort, a 2018 meta-analysis that included over forty observational studies with 12,619 vegans and 179,630 omnivores identified that among Western populations, the average LDL-C level for vegans is 23.2 mg/dL (0.6 mmol/L) lower than non-vegetarians.[35] Based on clinical trials investigating the efficacy of statins (cholesterol-lowering drugs), this difference in cholesterol still equates to a roughly 14% lower risk of having a major cardiovascular event.[25]

In fact, clinical trials directly comparing dietary interventions with cholesterol-lowering drugs have shown that the adoption of plant-based dietary patterns can in certain circumstances be just as effective in lowering LDL-C as using medications. A prime example of this is the Portfolio diet, which is a plant-based diet known to dramatically lower LDL-C levels to a similar degree to that achieved by low-intensity statins.[36,37] Researchers specifically credit the success of this dietary pattern to its inclusion of plant sterols (derived from margarine and supplements), dietary fibre (mainly from oats, barley, psyllium, legumes, fruits and vegetables), nuts and plant protein (e.g. soy), all known to significantly reduce cholesterol. This being said, in many circumstances, statins and other cholesterol-lowering drugs are necessary and life-saving. You should discuss any possible changes to medications and your dietary pattern with your doctor.

What about HDL-C, or 'good cholesterol', levels?

HDL-C is often labelled the 'good cholesterol' and for decades has been thought of as protective for cardiovascular disease risk, and thus something we want to elevate in our blood.[38] However, vegan and vegetarian populations have been shown to have a lower risk of cardiovascular disease compared with omnivores, despite often having lower HDL-C levels.[39-41] How can vegetarians and vegans have lower risk of cardiovascular disease but also lower amounts of 'good cholesterol'? It seems paradoxical.

In recent years, as science has advanced, it's become widely accepted that the actual quantity of HDL-C is less important than how well your HDL-C is functioning - specifically, its capacity to remove cholesterol from the blood to the liver for excretion.[12,42] Unsurprisingly, diets high in saturated fats have been implicated in reducing the beneficial functions of HDL-C,[43] which could explain why vegetarians and vegans consuming less saturated fats have lower risk of cardiovascular disease despite having lower HDL-C levels.

So what is it about the standard Western diet that drives up our LDL-C? The main culprits are foods high in saturated fats, trans fats and dietary cholesterol.

Saturated fats

Many studies have shown that saturated fat consumption increases blood cholesterol (both total and LDL). The most compelling summary of this was a meta-analysis of 395 metabolic ward studies which clearly showed that within just a few weeks of reducing saturated fat intake, both total and LDL-C were also reduced.[44] The evidence is compelling – feed people less saturated fats and their LDL-C goes down, which in turn decreases their risk of cardiovascular disease. Feed them more, and it goes up.

To paint a picture of the severity of the impact that saturated fats and the associated rise in LDL-C has on cardiovascular disease, data from the Nurses' Health Study involving over 80,000 American women showed that by replacing just 5% of calories from saturated fats with polyunsaturated fats, people lowered their risk of heart disease by 42%.[45] Another study, which included data from over 120,000 subjects from two different populations, found that replacing just 5% of calories from saturated fats with whole grains also reduced the risk of heart disease – this time by 9%.[46] These findings are consistent with multiple meta-analyses of RCTs that clearly show benefit in reducing saturated fats, particularly in exchange for foods rich in polyunsaturated fats.[47–49] The most recent of these is a 2020 Cochrane Review, which identified that replacing saturated fats with polyunsaturated fats lowers the risk of having a cardiac event by 27%.[47]

We've known this since the 1970s. In the late 1960s, men in North Karelia, a town in Finland, had the highest incidence of death from heart disease in the world.[50] In addition to being regular smokers, these men had very high LDL-C, high blood pressure and were consuming more than twice the WHO recommended intake of saturated fats (22% of total calories), mostly from cheese, milk and butter.[50–52] Following implementation of a community prevention program in the 1970s, which emphasised a reduction in saturated fats (cut by almost half to 13% of total calories), rates of death from heart disease in Finnish men reduced by 80%, more than any other population in the world. Importantly, most of this reduction was explained by dietary changes, not other lifestyle changes.[50]

How to clog arteries from birth

In 1994, researchers randomised 108 West African green monkeys, both male and female, into two groups eating different diets from birth – a study which would never get approved for human subjects. Both diets were rich in dietary cholesterol, but where one was high in saturated fats, the other was low in saturated fats and instead high in polyunsaturated fats. After five years, the average amount of plaque that had developed in the arteries of the monkeys eating the diet high in saturated fats was five times that of the monkeys eating the diet low in saturated fats.[53] While I am the first person to acknowledge that we shouldn't draw firm conclusions from animal studies alone, these results are a good example of all levels of science pointing in the same direction – whether it's studies looking at non-human primates that are genetically similar to us, human populations living in the real world, or clinical interventions in human adults, they all show the same thing. It's simply not in our best interests to make friends with foods rich in saturated fats.

Although we use the umbrella term 'saturated fats', there are actually a number of different types of saturated fats, and they have different effects on cholesterol and CVD risk.[54] The most common sources of saturated fats that increase LDL-C in the standard Western diet are animal products – cheese, beef, milk, butter and so on – and ultra-processed foods.[55]

FIGURE 5.4:

TOP SOURCES OF SATURATED FATS IN A TYPICAL WESTERN DIET[55]

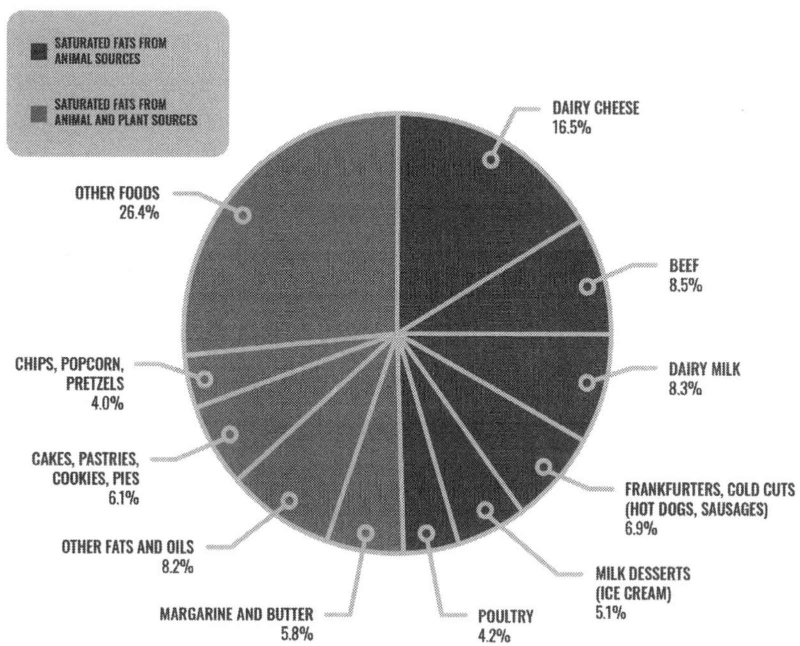

There's one important detail to note: if you replace saturated fats with refined carbohydrates low in fibre (e.g. chocolate bars, cookies, cakes, white flour products, sugar-sweetened drinks, highly refined cereals and candy), rather than whole plant foods, it may actually *increase* your risk of cardiovascular disease, or at best it's a lateral move.[56–59]

This caveat is why certain people claim there is no need to reduce saturated fats – they are usually forming that opinion based on studies that fail to factor in the foods and nutrients that saturated-fat-rich foods are either displacing or being replaced by.[57]

For example, if I want to make red meat look good, I could cite studies that compare red meat consumption against the consumption of low-quality carbohydrate sources such as white bread, pasta, white rice, cookies and biscuits rather than whole plant foods.[57] Alternatively, if I want to make dairy look good, I could cite studies comparing dairy with red meat or refined carbohydrates. Replacing 2% of energy from saturated fats found in red meat with 2% of energy from saturated fats in dairy was found to lower the risk of cardiovascular disease by 25%, a benefit attributed to the calcium found in dairy.[60] Does that mean dairy is healthy? Well, yes, in the context of risk of cardiovascular disease and compared with red meat or refined carbohydrates. However, there are options other than replacing red meat with dairy that have more favourable outcomes. For example, we know that replacing calories from dairy (butter and cheese) with calories from foods rich in polyunsaturated fats, monounsaturated fats or unrefined carbohydrates significantly reduces LDL-C and the risk of developing cardiovascular disease.[61–64] One set of researchers determined to investigate the 'compared with what' question combined three cohorts from the United States, which contained more than 200,000 subjects, and identified that replacing just 5% of calories from dairy fat with the same amount of calories from whole grains led to a 28% reduction in cardiovascular disease risk.[63]

FIGURE 5.5:

CHANGE IN CARDIOVASCULAR DISEASE RISK WHEN YOU REPLACE 5% OF CALORIES IN YOUR DIET FROM DAIRY FAT WITH 5% OF CALORIES FROM OTHER NUTRIENTS[63]

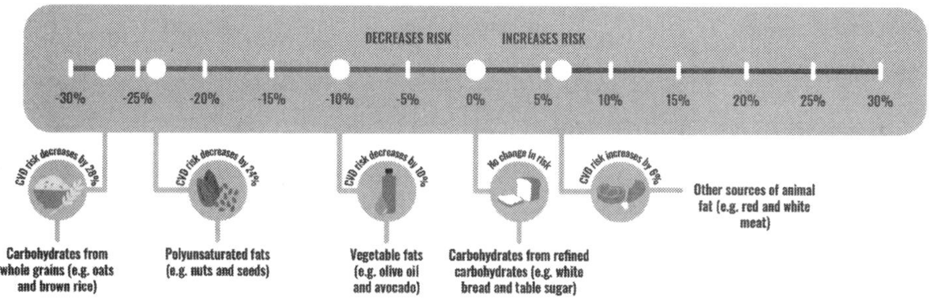

Why replace red meat with dairy when you can get an even better benefit by consuming foods such as nuts, seeds, legumes and whole grains instead? The key takeaway here is that if you want to prevent your arteries from becoming clogged, it's best to replace the calories from saturated fats in your diet with foods rich in polyunsaturated fats (e.g. flaxseeds, chia seeds, walnuts and fish), monounsaturated fats (e.g. avocados and olive oil), unrefined carbohydrates (e.g. whole grains such as oats and brown rice) and/or plant protein (e.g. lentils or black beans).

FIGURE 5.6:

THE EFFECT OF REPLACING SATURATED FATS WITH OTHER NUTRIENTS[46-48,57-59,65]

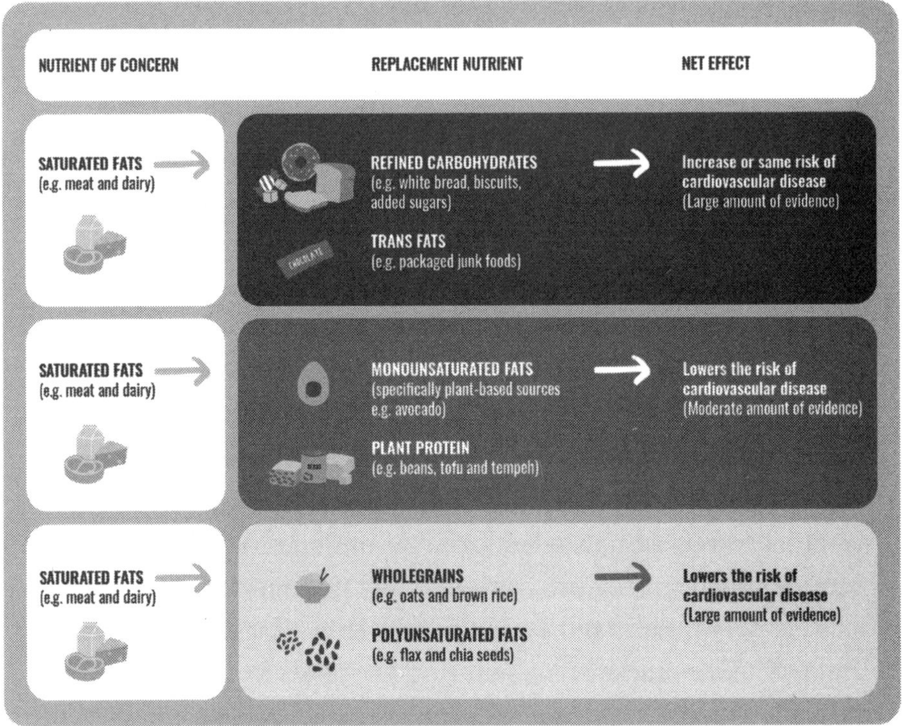

What is it specifically about refined carbohydrates such as white bread that are so bad for our cardiovascular health? There seem to be a few major mechanisms at play. First, refined carbohydrates raise our triglyceride levels, which, just like high LDL-C, increases our risk of atherosclerosis.[12,46] Second, unlike when we eat whole unrefined carbohydrates packed with fibre, water and phytonutrients, when we consume refined carbohydrates, we get a much larger spike in blood sugar.[66] Essentially, without the fibre, the sugars from our food rapidly enter our blood. This elevation in blood sugar above a healthy level makes LDL particles more likely to damage our arteries and build up as plaque.[67,68]

So, while a diet that is rich in both saturated fats and refined carbohydrates (such as the standard Western diet) will create the perfect conditions for clogged arteries, any diet that is rich in either saturated fats or refined carbohydrates can be bad news. This has played out in clinical trials, which show us that there are multiple ways of achieving good outcomes as long as you get a predominance of calories from a diet low in saturated fats and refined carbohydrates, and high in whole plant foods.

But hasn't the connection between saturated fats and CVD risk been debunked?

There have been a handful of studies, including three meta-analyses, looking at saturated fats and cardiovascular disease that are often cited to 'prove' that saturated fats are not a problem.[49,58,69-72] However, while the conclusions of these studies may be welcomed by those who consume copious amounts of meat and wish to justify their diet, the data within is less convincing.[73] One of the major ways these studies make saturated fats look good is by failing to consider what they are being compared with.[57,58,74,75] If you compare people eating lots of saturated fats from foods such as meat and butter with people consuming less saturated fats who are instead getting more calories from ultra-processed foods rich in refined carbohydrates, you wouldn't see any real difference in cardiovascular disease risk. Swapping saturated fats for refined carbs doesn't give you the heart protection that whole plant foods do![58] All these studies really tell us is that, when it comes to the health of our heart, fatty cuts of meat and butter are no worse than (ultra-processed) cookies and cakes. This is what their conclusions should have made clear.

There are six clinical trials that are regularly cited as evidence that dietary changes can help reduce the risk of developing cardiovascular disease and reduce the risk of subsequent events for those with existing cardiovascular disease. It's important to understand the differences between these trials and what they can and cannot tell us, as often this is lost in communication.

The first four trials are commonly cited as evidence that a plant-based diet can truly reverse cardiovascular disease. These are two studies by Dr Caldwell Esselstyn Jr, as well as the Lifestyle Heart Trial and the Mount Abu Trial, all of which looked at the ability of certain interventions to reduce atherosclerosis and prevent further cardiac events in subjects with existing cardiovascular disease.

First, I want to clear up the claims of 'disease reversal' that stem from these studies. While it's certainly possible that we can reverse cardiovascular disease through lifestyle changes including diet, more recent science suggests the imaging methods used to detect the amount of plaque in the arteries of subjects in these studies are not very reliable.[76,77] So, whether there was truly any disease reversal is up for debate. However, what's of more relevance to us, more than what happened to this plaque, is the hard outcomes – did these subjects experience improvements in their health (e.g. lower risk of having a heart attack)?

In 1985 Dr Esselstyn Jr used a low-fat, 100% whole-food, plant-based diet in twenty-four patients with severe coronary artery disease.[78] After observing significant benefits, he was inspired to do a larger study in 2014 with 198 subjects who had severe coronary artery disease.[79] During a four-year follow-up, only 0.6% of the subjects who adhered to the diet had further cardiac events, compared with 62% of those who failed to adhere to the diet. The major limitation of Esselstyn's studies is that there were no formal control groups, and subjects were taking medications, as prescribed by their doctors, which have since been shown to effectively reduce the progression of cardiovascular disease.[80,81]

This means we cannot attribute the benefits observed in these studies to the dietary intervention alone.

Dr Dean Ornish produced similar results with his Lifestyle Heart Trial in 1990.[82] His five-year trial randomised forty-eight patients with existing cardiovascular disease into two groups: a usual care group (standard doctor advice) and a lifestyle intervention group that involved a low-fat (around 8% of total calories) whole-food vegetarian diet. Importantly, whereas control subjects were taking cardiac medications, the subjects in the lifestyle intervention group were not. After one year, the intervention group had a 37.2% reduction in LDL-C versus a 6% reduction in the control group and a 91% reduction in frequency of angina versus a 165% *increase* in the control group. After five years, there was an average of 0.89 cardiac events per subject in the intervention group versus 2.25 per subject in the control group.[83] However, even with the inclusion of a control group, we cannot attribute the benefits purely to dietary intervention because diet was not the only difference between the groups. The intervention group was also doing substantially more exercise and stress management, were encouraged to discontinue smoking and were attending group support sessions, and no analysis was done to tease out the individual effects of each of these components. What this study *does* tell us is that a total lifestyle intervention that involves a plant-based diet can be more effective for preventing future cardiac events for people with existing cardiovascular disease compared with the 'usual care' approach, which usually involves multiple medications and little to no dietary change.

The 2011 Mount Abu Trial is somewhat similar to the Lifestyle Heart Trial in that it investigated the effectiveness of an intervention which in addition to including a low-fat vegetarian diet, involved daily exercise and stress management through Raja yoga meditation, for subjects with existing cardiovascular disease.[84]

The most notable finding was that compared with subjects who least adhered to the lifestyle intervention, the subjects who best adhered had about 40% lower risk of having a cardiac event over the 6.5 years that the study was conducted. However, just like the Lifestyle Heart Trial, while this shows the value of adopting a holistic lifestyle approach to treating cardiovascular disease, it is impossible for us to conclude that these benefits are produced solely by the low-fat vegetarian diet. In order to determine that we would need another trial that looks at a control group versus a group who adopts a low-fat vegetarian diet, with no other lifestyle changes.

Fortunately, we do have evidence from two long-term (for an RCT, that is) studies, where diet was the only difference between control and intervention subjects, that clearly show that dietary change can significantly improve cardiovascular health. These are the Lyon Diet Heart Study and the PREDIMED trial.[85,86] Together these two studies show that whether you are trying to prevent heart disease in the first place, or prevent subsequent events for those who already have cardiovascular disease, the adoption of a Mediterranean diet that's low in saturated fats and primarily vegetarian is an option worthy of consideration.

The Lyon Diet Heart Study was similar to the previous four studies in that it evaluated a dietary intervention for secondary prevention of cardiovascular events – that is, how well dietary changes can affect a person's risk of a subsequent event.[86] The researchers randomised over 400 subjects to either a low-saturated-fat (8% of calories) Mediterranean diet rich in polyunsaturated omega-3s or a control diet that contained more than 11% of calories from saturated fats, more dietary cholesterol, more meat and more refined cereals, and less fruits, vegetables, legumes and omega-3 polyunsaturated fats. Over 27 months, the group consuming the Mediterranean diet experienced 70% fewer cardiac events.

The Mediterranean diet

A traditional Mediterranean diet is characterised by:[87]

- A predominantly vegetarian diet based on the consumption of fresh whole foods.
- A great diversity of whole plant foods including fruits, vegetables, whole grains, legumes, nuts and seeds.
- Virtually non-existent amounts of ultra-processed food, including processed meats and sweets.
- No more than moderate consumption of fish.
- Low consumption of meat, eggs and dairy.
- Low consumption of alcohol (mainly red wine, a glass or two with dinner).
- Low consumption of saturated and trans fats while being rich in unsaturated fats, predominantly from olive oil.

While the actual foods may differ from country to country across the Mediterranean Basin (i.e. Spain to Italy), the overall dietary pattern is consistent with the above characteristics. This traditional non-Westernised Mediterranean diet is associated with health benefits, and is not to be confused with the Western take on Mediterranean cuisine, which can include pepperoni pizza, pasta and lamb chops with a Greek-style dressing.

Over the course of five years, the PREDIMED trial, which involved more than 7000 subjects, compared two versions of a healthful whole-food Mediterranean diet (one with added nuts, the other with added olive oil) rich in polyunsaturated fats, and low in saturated fats, to a 'low-fat' control diet in people without cardiovascular disease but with a high risk of developing it.[85] I put 'low-fat' in quotation marks because despite the advice from researchers, the control subjects barely reduced their fat (39% of calories down to 37%) intake and all three groups ended up consuming the same amount of saturated fats. The major difference between the two groups was that the Mediterranean diet groups consumed slightly more unsaturated fats and fewer refined carbohydrates. Furthermore, the control diet was lower in fruits, vegetables, legumes, nuts and fish. Subjects in both of the Mediterranean diet groups had around 30% fewer cardiac events over the five-year period. Most of this benefit was due to a lower risk of stroke rather than heart-related cardiac events, and there was no difference between the groups when it came to risk of dying during the trial. This is likely explained by the fact all groups were consuming the same amount of saturated fats. Interestingly, when researchers doubled back to look at the PREDIMED data and focused only on subjects consuming what they called a 'pro-vegetarian' Mediterranean diet (a truly low-saturated-fat version of the Mediterranean diet that included less fish, red meat, dairy and eggs, and more whole plants), these subjects were 41% less likely to die during the five-year trial.[88] So, even when it comes to a generally healthy Mediterranean diet, people seem to do better when reducing calories from animal products – or, in other words, what makes the Mediterranean diet healthy is not the selection of the animal products included but that, when done well, it emphasises calories from whole plant foods and heart-healthy unsaturated fats while being low in saturated fats.

FIGURE 5.7:

ADHERENCE TO A PRO-VEGETARIAN MEDITERRANEAN DIET AND ITS EFFECT ON RISK OF DYING DURING THE FIVE-YEAR PREDIMED TRIAL[88]

	VERY LOW ADHERENCE	HIGH TO VERY HIGH ADHERENCE
Subjects' diet	More meat, fish, eggs and dairy	More fruits, vegetables, legumes, nuts and olive oil
% of calories from saturated fat	11.7	8.1
% of calories from polyunsaturated fat	5.8	6.8
Fibre (per day)	19 g	36 g

41% lower risk of dying during the 5 year trial

Olive oil and heart health

It's probably clear by now that a Mediterranean diet is certainly heart-healthy, but perhaps you have come across information suggesting that olive oil is not! Some people argue that, yes, compared with butter, olive oil is healthy, but compared with no oil it is not and we would be better off eating whole olives. However, to date there is no compelling evidence comparing olive oil with oil-free diets that suggests harm, so this is purely speculation.[89] This message about totally avoiding oils, including olive oil, for cardiovascular health is based on the findings of limited mechanistic studies (zooming in at a microscopic level and seeing how arteries function after consuming olive oil). Not only are there conflicting studies at this level of science, the limited findings that suggest we should be worried don't play out when we look at the actual health outcomes of humans consuming olive oil over the long-term.[89] If anything, current evidence suggests olive oil improves artery function and can be enjoyed in modest amounts within the context of a dietary pattern that places a strong emphasis on total calories from whole plant foods.[89-91] It's the antioxidant activity of the polyphenols that olive oil contains that is thought to be responsible for the cardiovascular benefits it offers. For further exploration into cooking oils, see Part Three.

So what can we make of all of these trials in addition to the rest of the evidence available to us? First, although I realise an absolute answer is often easiest to run with, we need more research looking at the independent effects of dietary intervention on the prevention and reversal of cardiovascular disease in order to categorically say what is the single best diet for a healthy heart. It would be nice to one day see an RCT comparing a Mediterranean diet with a WFPBD while ensuring there are no other differences between groups. Until then, the science that we do have, including clinical trials that show what happens to cardiovascular risk factors when we substitute nutrients (e.g. swapping saturated fats for polyunsaturated fats as discussed earlier), and large observational studies looking at dietary patterns and cardiovascular health, indicates that what matters most is not the dietary label, but the overall theme.[48,57,92] Dietary patterns that consist of an abundance of fibre-rich whole plant foods, are low in saturated fats and place significantly less emphasis on animal-based and ultra-processed foods are good for cardiovascular health.[93] A traditional Mediterranean diet is a good example of this, as is the DASH diet, a pescetarian diet and a well-planned WFPBD. Furthermore, in addition to adopting a diet with these characteristics, it's clear that while diet is arguably the biggest lever we can pull, we cannot discount the effect of other aspects of our lifestyle – particularly exercise, stress management and cessation of smoking, all of which appear to have a cumulative effect on our risk of developing this disease.

Trans fats

In 1901 Wilhelm Normann, a German chemist, successfully converted liquid fat (vegetable oil) into a semi-solid using a process called hydrogenation.[94] Following this scientific discovery, it wasn't long until food manufacturers began using hydrogenation to convert vegetable oils that are otherwise highly susceptible to rancidity into semi-solid fats (trans fats) to improve the shelf life of food products (e.g. margarine). Fast forward some eighty years and researchers had clearly identified that high saturated fat intake increases the risk of cardiovascular disease. The response from the food industry was reformulation of products, and a surge of industrially produced trans fats entered the food system. Despite the best of intentions, what was not known at the time was that these industrially produced trans fats are arguably just as bad as saturated fats when it comes to cardiovascular disease, if not worse.[95,96] Several studies have shown that consumption of hydrogenated oils significantly increases total cholesterol and LDL-C, and thus increases the risk of developing cardiovascular disease.[97-102] In fact, data from the Nurses' Health Study found that replacing 2% of energy from trans fats with unsaturated fats reduced the risk of developing heart disease by 53%.[45]

Because the links between trans fats and cardiovascular disease are so strong, and trans fats are not essential for human health, the WHO and the Food and Agriculture Organization of the United Nations recommend trans fats should be limited to 1% of total dietary energy, with the goal of completely eliminating them.[103] Denmark was the first country to take a hard stance on trans fats, banning the sale of any fats or oils containing more than 2 g of trans fats per 100 g of fat.[104]

In Australia, and many other countries around the world, trans fats are yet to be banned. Until this takes place, the best advice I can give is to steer clear of deep-fried or packaged 'junk' food altogether, and if an ultra-packaged food does not say 'No' or 'Free from' trans fats or partially hydrogenated oils, assume that it contains them. And, of course, you should absolutely avoid any foods that voluntarily mention trans fats and/or hydrogenated oils in their ingredients. Minimising or removing animal fats from your diet may also be helpful, as they too contain a small amount of trans fats, though the jury is out as to whether these naturally produced trans fats are harmful, due to insufficient studies focusing on their effect on cholesterol.[105]

FIGURE 5.8:

TOP SOURCES OF TRANS FATS IN AUSTRALIA

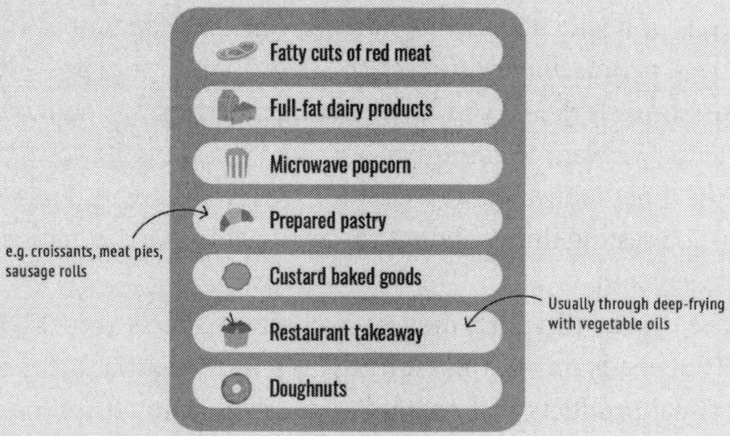

Adapted from The Heart Foundation[106]

Dietary cholesterol

When it comes to cardiovascular disease, dietary cholesterol is one of the most misunderstood and heavily debated dietary risk factors. One day we hear eggs (a top source of dietary cholesterol in Western diets) are heart-healthy and the next they are off the menu! Despite the confusion, the science is clear.

Dietary cholesterol does negatively affect blood cholesterol, but context is key.[107,108] Most of the confusion stems from the fact that 60% of all studies looking at eggs and their effect on cholesterol levels have been funded by the egg industry, with one primary objective: to convince us that eggs are completely harmless when it comes to plaque building up in our arteries, despite each egg yolk containing about 186 mg of cholesterol. On close inspection, however, despite the way the industry wishes to position eggs, more than 85% of the industry-funded studies suggest that eggs do have unfavourable effects on blood cholesterol, although these findings are often downplayed or dismissed when the studies then go on to be reported by the media.[109]

The strongest science we have that tests the relationship between dietary cholesterol and blood cholesterol – a meta-analysis of nearly 400 metabolic ward studies – found that when you feed people dietary cholesterol, their LDL-C goes up – albeit more modestly than if you fed them saturated fats.[44] As we learned earlier, if we want to minimise our risk of atherosclerosis this is not the direction we want to see our LDL levels moving. There are a few interesting things about this relationship that are important to understand.

The degree to which dietary cholesterol affects your LDL-C levels depends on your baseline diet. If your routine diet is rich in animal products that contain appreciable amounts of dietary cholesterol (e.g. red meat, poultry, eggs and shellfish), the addition of more dietary cholesterol (e.g. a few extra eggs) has less of an effect on your cholesterol levels compared with someone who adds the same amount of dietary cholesterol to a baseline diet that is either low in, or excludes, animal products.[110] This is one of the tactics the egg industry has used – adding eggs to a typical Western diet that's already rich in foods that contain dietary cholesterol to prove it has minimal effect on LDL-C levels. But the bottom line is that when you add dietary cholesterol to a heart-healthy dietary pattern, it does raise cholesterol before its effect begins to plateau (see Figure 5.9). And if the egg-industry-funded studies looked at this relationship in reverse, and instead observed what happens when dietary cholesterol is removed, they would see that cholesterol decreases to a more favourable level.

FIGURE 5.9:

EFFECT OF DIETARY CHOLESTEROL ON BLOOD CHOLESTEROL[110]

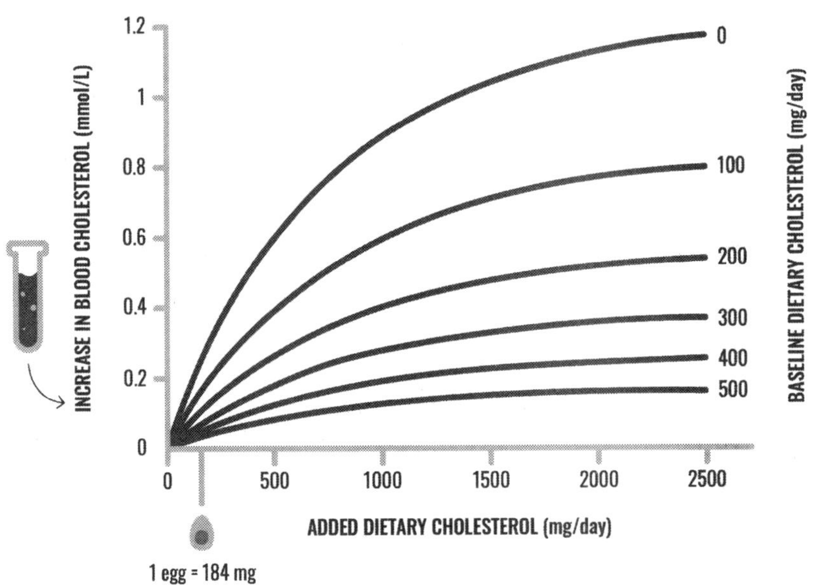

While we have understood this relationship since the early 1990s, a 2020 meta-analysis of 66 RCTs provides more recent evidence that the consumption of dietary cholesterol (in this case from eggs) significantly raises LDL-C levels. Specifically, the researchers identified that this significant increase in LDL-C was produced by the consumption of more than one egg per day.[111]

Also, in the presence of dietary cholesterol, saturated fats' ability to raise LDL-C is considerably more pronounced. Dietary cholesterol's presence has an additive effect, worsening the effect that saturated fats have on LDL-C.[112] In other words, if you're eating bacon and eggs, the high amounts of dietary cholesterol from the eggs will worsen the effect that the saturated fats from the bacon has on your cholesterol levels.

So what does this mean for our food choices? We need to zoom back out and think about the context of our overall diet. When it comes to the foods we eat and lowering our risk of cardiovascular disease, our number one priority should be reducing foods rich in saturated fats – as these have the greatest effect on our LDL-C levels.[44,113] This means considerably reducing, or eliminating, foods such as meat and full-fat dairy, in favour of whole plant foods. For example, swapping red meat for lentils. In doing this, we will be inadvertently lowering our dietary cholesterol intake at the same time because around 55% of all dietary cholesterol in a typical Western diet comes from red meat, poultry, processed meat, seafood and milk products.[114]

What about eating lean meat – for example, chicken breast instead of thigh? A 2019 RCT looked at exactly this and found that even though there were benefits to consuming lean meat, a diet where plants were the major protein source still resulted in significantly lower LDL-C.[115] Despite having their fat trimmed, both lean red and white meats still contain more saturated fats than sources of plant protein, and still contain dietary cholesterol. So while choosing lean red or white meat is certainly a step in the right direction, you can go one step better by choosing to opt for beans or lentils – which are both cholesterol-free and contain almost zero grams of saturated fats per serve.

It's a similar story for eggs. It really depends on what they are displacing. If you choose to eat eggs instead of meat or fruit loops, that's a healthy step in the right direction.[116] But if you choose to swap eggs for whole plants, such as a bowl of porridge, blueberries and ground flaxseeds, the science suggests you are upgrading your diet considerably more.[89] Of course, this isn't black and white, as it does appear to get to a point where the foundation of your diet is so health-promoting that you can afford to include some of these foods in modest amounts without it dramatically affecting disease risk – which is why I have defined a plant-predominant diet as one that provides around 85% of calories from whole plants. Are a few eggs a week within the context of such a diet going to significantly increase the risk of cardiovascular disease? I'm not convinced of that. This is in line with the latest guidelines from the American Heart Association, and the 2020 meta-analysis mentioned earlier, which state that individuals with normal cholesterol can include up to one egg per day (seven per week) in a heart-healthy dietary pattern that emphasises plant protein over animal protein.[111,113] This recommendation is for people who are free from cardiovascular disease who also consume meat. For vegetarians who are free from cardiovascular disease and have normal cholesterol levels, this could be slightly higher (around two eggs per day).

The bottom line here is that, regardless of the nuance, if you want to get your LDL-C down to an optimal level, reducing sources of dietary cholesterol (see Figure 5.10) can be a useful strategy to adopt in addition to minimising the consumption of saturated and trans fats. And if you choose not to completely exclude them, their inclusion should be in modest amounts within the context of a heart-healthy plant-predominant dietary pattern. A stronger case can be made for complete elimination of dietary cholesterol if you are wanting to stop or slow the progression of underlying disease from years of poor diet, smoking, drinking, sedentary living, etc. and/or have high cholesterol. Which is no doubt why the 2020 US dietary guidelines state that dietary cholesterol should be kept 'as low as possible without compromising the nutritional adequacy of the diet' – about half of all adults in the United States (and Australia) have borderline-high or high cholesterol.[117–119] While it's not overtly clear in the US guidelines, this statement is a clue as to how to eat for optimal health. Remember, cholesterol is found in just about every animal product, other than egg whites and honey, and is not present in plants. Make of that what you will.

FIGURE 5.10:

FOODS RICH IN CHOLESTEROL

FOOD*	SERVING SIZE	CHOLESTEROL	SATURATED FAT
Liver (chicken, veal, lamb), raw	150 g	594 mg	4.4 g
Squid	150 g	349.5 mg	0.5 g
Prawn (shrimp)	150 g	241.5 mg	0.2 g
Eggs	1 large	186 mg	1.6 g
Chicken breast, raw	150 g	127.5 mg	1.9 g
Steak (lean cut), raw	150 g	115.5 mg	2.5 g
Salmon, raw	150 g	96 mg	1.5 g
Oysters (Pacific)	6 oysters	92.2 mg	1 g
Butter	2 tbsp	61 mg	14.6 g
Mussels (blue)	12 mussels	53.8 mg	0.8 g
Cheddar cheese	50 g	49.5 mg	9.4 g
Bacon	4 pieces	47.5 mg	5.7 g
Milk	1 cup	24.4 mg	4.6 g
Prosciutto	4 thin slices	21.7 mg	1.1 g

* Weights based on raw weight

This may leave you wondering, 'Isn't some cholesterol in our diet essential for optimal health?' While it's true cholesterol is important for the production of various hormones, and the health of almost every cell in our bodies, this shouldn't be confused with a requirement to include it in our diet. This simply is not the case. Rest assured, we will clear this up in Chapter 7.

Does having low cholesterol increase the risk of stroke?

From time to time, I hear it suggested that it's a bad idea to have low cholesterol because it increases the risk of stroke. There are a few things about this claim to clear up. First up, we know from mountains of data, including a 2010 meta-analysis of 20 RCTs containing 170,000 subjects, that the benefits associated with having low cholesterol far exceed the risks.[120] Around fifty times greater, to be precise! Which means that if you have low cholesterol you are likely to live more years in good health than if your cholesterol is higher. Second, this claim is often used without context. Although some studies have shown that people with low cholesterol have a higher risk of haemorrhagic stroke, these same people also have a significantly lower risk of having a heart attack or the much more common form of stroke, ischemic stroke (which accounts for 87% of all strokes, while 13% are haemorrhagic).[39,121-123] Because people with high cholesterol have more plaque in their arteries, they are likely to die from the types of cardiovascular disease associated with artery blockages before they have a chance to have a haemorrhagic stroke. If you ask me, that's hardly a reason to argue against having low cholesterol. Furthermore, having low cholesterol doesn't guarantee a higher risk of haemorrhagic stroke. A 2020 study in Taiwan showed that vegetarians with low cholesterol, low blood pressure and low alcohol consumption actually had lower risk of both forms of stroke when compared with meat-eaters.[124]

High blood pressure

When our blood pressure increases, our heart has to work harder to pump freshly oxygenated blood through our bodies. This increased pressure is one of the mechanisms that makes our artery walls more susceptible to atherosclerosis.

So to lower our risk of CVD, we need to lower our blood pressure. Which food choices do so? An overwhelming amount of evidence from observational research favours diets that get all or most calories from whole plant foods. For example, in both the EPIC-Oxford and AHS-2 populations, vegans had the lowest blood pressure.[125,126] It makes sense that the same foods that are naturally good at promoting a healthy body weight are also good for achieving healthy blood pressure, as being overweight or obese significantly increases a person's blood pressure.[127] What's interesting is that even when body weight is controlled for (which means comparing people with the same body weight so the only difference is their diet), people eating more calories from whole plant foods still have lower blood pressure.[125,128] Plants keep our blood pressure down – especially dark leafy greens, such as spinach.[129]

These findings are consistent with a large body of literature that clearly shows the consumption of animal flesh is associated with higher blood pressure.[130–132] The CARDIA hypertension study for example, which followed 4304 healthy subjects for over fifteen years, found those consuming greater amounts of processed and unprocessed meat had higher blood pressure, while the more nuts, fruits and whole grains subjects ate the lower their blood pressure was.[133] This is supported by three large observational studies from 2015 with a combined 188,518 subjects, which also identified consumption of processed or unprocessed red meat and poultry, and to a lesser extent seafood, as leading to higher blood pressure,[130] and a large study out of France observing 80,426 adults in 2017, which found consumption of animal protein, both processed and unprocessed, significantly increased the risk of developing hypertension.[134]

A 2014 meta-analysis looking at thirty-two observational studies involving 21,604 subjects identified that, on average, vegetarians' systolic blood pressure (SBP) was 6.9 mmHg lower and their diastolic blood pressure (DBP) 4.7 mmHg lower compared with omnivores.[135] This same meta-analysis included seven clinical trials which also showed that, compared with omnivores, vegetarian subjects had lower SBP (-4.8 mmHg) and DBP (-2.2 mmHg). While these numbers may sound small, it's thought that just a 2 mmHg reduction in the population's average DBP could result in a 17% reduction in hypertension, a 15% reduction in stroke and a 6% reduction in heart disease![136]

The evidence is so compelling, in fact, that the DASH diet (Dietary Approaches to Stop Hypertension), which was specifically designed to be a good dietary pattern for lowering blood pressure, was inspired by the observation 'that vegetarians have lower average blood pressure levels than do comparable non-vegetarian populations'.[137] Like the Mediterranean diet, the DASH diet is low in saturated fats and emphasises the consumption of whole foods – fruits, vegetables, whole grains, legumes, nuts, seeds, omega-3-rich fish, lean meats, low-fat dairy and eggs. DASH also emphasises a reduction in sodium, and the consumption of potassium- and magnesium-rich plant foods such as bananas, oranges, avocados, pumpkins, green leafy vegetables, nuts and whole grains. It is undoubtedly a predominantly plant-based diet – while it recommends two or fewer serves of lean meat products a day, it recommends five servings of fruit, five servings of vegetables and seven servings from a mix of dark leafy greens, whole grains and legumes.[138]

Overall, what seems to be most important about diet and hypertension is that, as we have seen elsewhere, there are several variations of the same theme that can work.[130,134,135,139] This theme is a way of eating that moves away from animal-products and ultra-processed foods towards getting all or most of our calories from whole or minimally processed plant foods. When we do this, our diet naturally becomes low in sodium and saturated fat, while being rich in plant protein, fibre, magnesium and potassium. All good things when it comes to our blood pressure!

Other dietary risk factors for cardiovascular disease

Heme iron

You've likely heard of the mineral 'iron' before. There are two types of iron: heme iron found only in animals (red meat, poultry, fish, etc.), and non-heme iron which is found in plants and animals.[140,141] While heme iron is more rapidly absorbed into our blood, our bodies are better able to regulate absorption of non-heme iron to prevent it rising to harmful levels.[142,143] An increased absorption rate is not always a good thing! In fact for a long time high levels of iron, particularly heme iron, were thought to promote the production of harmful molecules that would make LDL-C more likely to get lodged in the artery wall.[144] A hypothesis that today is supported by science. A 2015 meta-analysis of thirteen observational studies, involving over 250,000 subjects, found that for every 1 mg of heme iron consumed per day, subjects would increase their risk of cardiovascular disease by 7%, even after controlling for saturated fat intake.[145] That's not a lot of heme iron, given a 250 g beef sirloin alone contains about 5 mg.[146,147]

Animal protein

Several large observational studies and meta-analyses have identified that animal protein itself, independent of the saturated fats that it comes packaged with, appears to heighten the risk of dying from cardiovascular disease.[148–154] Specifically, each of these studies has identified a lowering of cardiovascular disease when one swaps animal protein for plant protein. For example, in a study published in 2019 that followed 70,696 Japanese subjects for over sixteen years, swapping just 3% of calories from red meat protein for equivalent calories from plant protein resulted in a 42% reduction in risk of dying from cardiovascular disease.[152] Practically speaking this swap could be as simple as making your favourite lasagne with lentils rather than beef mince.

While the precise mechanism explaining how animal protein affects our cardiovascular system has not yet been elucidated, a recent study, published in 2020, may shed some light. In this study, using a mice model, researchers were able to show that certain amino acids (the building blocks of protein), particularly leucine which is considerably higher in sources of animal protein compared with plant protein, directly impact the development of atherosclerotic plaque.[155] We'll come back to this in Chapter 8. Spoiler alert: animal protein is not the key to a long life.

Additional benefits of whole, plant-based foods

While a plant-based diet is naturally low in saturated fats, dietary cholesterol, trans fat, refined carbohydrates, sodium and heme iron – dietary components that we've seen increase CVD risk – plant foods have a few more tricks up their sleeve. They're also full of fibre, and rich in protective antioxidant compounds, both of which support a healthy heart.

Antioxidants

Plant-based foods contain a high number of the antioxidant molecules vitamin E, vitamin C, beta-carotene, lycopene and polyphenols, which are thought to prevent the damage that leads to atherosclerosis.[156–161] Think of these antioxidant molecules as bodyguards that protect the LDL particles in your blood from unstable molecules, called free radicals, which can hasten the hardening of LDL particles that become embedded in the arterial wall. It is not surprising that a plant-based diet is protective here, given that major sources of dietary antioxidants are fruits, vegetables, whole grains and legumes.[158] A meta-analysis involving seventy-one papers and 387,569 subjects identified that a specific antioxidant, 'lutein', known to be considerably higher in vegetarian diets, is particularly beneficial for protecting against atherosclerosis.[158,162] Kale, spinach and broccoli are great healthy sources of lutein. But rather than relying on them (antioxidants) to constantly protect you against the damage that excessive consumption of animal products and/or ultra-processed foods brings about, we would be far better off conserving them so they can protect us from threats to our cardiovascular health outside of our diet, and control, such as air pollution.[163,164]

Fibre

Consuming adequate dietary fibre is an important aspect of an optimal diet for human health. Unfortunately, while it's true that Australians consume slightly more fibre per day than people from the United Kingdom or United States, 72% of us fail to meet the adequate intake recommendations for dietary fibre (25–30 g per day) – an amount that was merely set with the aim of achieving regular bowel movements![165–167] The recommendation for dietary fibre intake based on avoiding chronic disease, referred to as the suggested dietary target (SDT), is 28–38 g per day, somewhat higher than the adequate intake level.[166] More than four out of five Australian adults fail to meet the SDT level.

How important is dietary fibre with regards to lowering our risk of cardiovascular disease? A 2014 meta-analysis that reviewed forty-two cohorts involving more than 1.7 million subjects looked at exactly this and concluded that for every additional 10 g per day of dietary fibre, people could lower their risk of cardiovascular disease by 17%.[168] This was based on fibre consumed from whole plant foods, not supplements. Two of the major mechanisms believed to be at play here are fibre's ability to lower LDL-C and blood pressure – as confirmed by many RCTs.[169] This is one reason I have porridge on the regular – just three-quarters of a cup of rolled oats with half a cup of blueberries and a tablespoon of chia seeds offers 15 g of fibre – and that's before you add anything else! It's also why lentils, beans and other legumes are the perfect swap for meat – they've been consistently shown to help lower LDL-C and blood pressure, and reduce the risk of developing cardiovascular disease.[89,170,171]

Eat plant-based for heart health

At the beginning of this chapter I mentioned that cardiovascular disease is practically non-existent in the Okinawans of Japan, the Tsimane people of Bolivia, rural Chinese and the Tarahumara Indians of Mexico – all populations that eat an abundance of whole plant foods, minimal animal foods and almost no ultra-processed foods. But you might be wondering: what about people from the same culture, with the same genetics and overall lifestyle but who eat differently? Can I really make that much difference if I move from the standard Western diet to a plant-predominant one? The answer is a resounding yes. Two meta-analyses of large observational studies, one from 1999 with 76,172 subjects and the other from 2012 with 124,706 subjects, found that among people from the same population, vegetarians, including vegans, had a significantly lower risk of dying from heart disease than non-vegetarians. Anywhere from 24–29% less risk![39,121] More recently a new meta-analysis has been performed with updated data from almost 250,000 subjects, again finding that vegetarians, including vegans, have better cardiovascular health – this time a 25% lower risk of developing and of dying from heart disease.[172]

Given we are talking about what is, statistically speaking, our most likely cause of death, this should be enough for plant-based dietary patterns to be the default way of eating in our communities. The fact that this is the same diet that's great for maintaining a healthy body weight and preventing several other chronic diseases is an added bonus.

CHAPTER 6

Eating to prevent cancer

Cancer is a scary and often misunderstood disease which can manifest in several different forms, some more aggressive and life-threatening than others, and some better understood than others. Globally, cancer is the second or third most common cause of death, responsible for approximately one in six deaths.[1]

Cancer is so ubiquitous that most of us view it as an inevitable part of ageing – it's almost impossible not to when nearly everyone you know is affected by some form of cancer once they reach a certain age. We often see cancer as 'bad luck', 'fate' or 'random'. Fascinatingly, however, only 5–10% of all types of cancer are driven by genetic defects.[2] That means that 90–95% of cancers are *not* predetermined by our genes. In other words, we have some power to prevent it.

So if not genes, what specifically in our lives is causing all of these incidences of cancer? For several of the leading forms of cancer affecting Western populations, such as colorectal, breast and prostate cancer, the science is pretty clear – the food we consume significantly increases our risk of developing them.[2,3] In fact, it's estimated that dietary choices may be linked to as many as 50–75% of all deaths by breast, prostate, colorectal, endometrial, pancreatic and gallbladder cancers.[2] Other factors known to contribute to developing cancer include smoking (the top risk factor for lung cancer), obesity, alcohol consumption, sun exposure (the top risk factor for skin cancer), contaminant and radiation exposure, infections, lack of physical exercise and chronic stress.[2]

Dietary risk factors for cancer

There is evidence to suggest that regular consumption of processed meat, red meat, ultra-processed foods and excessive salt is associated with a higher risk of developing various types of cancer.[4] Whether or not dairy should be included on this list is hotly debated, with evidence both in support of and against its consumption depending on the cancer you're looking at. On the other hand, whole plant foods, and specific compounds they contain, have been consistently shown to have anti-carcinogenic effects – that is, they protect against certain forms of cancer.[4] When you consider that 95% of Australians fail to meet national recommendations for daily fruit and vegetable intake while consuming three times the recommended amount of red meat, and too much ultra-processed food and salt, it is no wonder that one in two Australians is diagnosed with some form of cancer in their lifetime, with colorectal, prostate and breast cancer being the most common.[5]

With this in mind, it is *also* unsurprising that Cancer Australia's position statement, largely based on the recommendations of the World Cancer Research Fund (WCRF), advises the adoption of a dietary pattern that consists of mainly whole plant foods with adequate amounts of dietary fibre, while limiting consumption of ultra-processed foods, processed and red meat, and added salt.[6]

Why is consuming animal products a risk factor for developing cancer?

Years ago, it was theorised that the association between the consumption of animal products and increased risk of cancer was primarily due to a higher intake of dietary fat. However, based on results from large observational studies over the past two decades, this theory has all but been put to rest, with the science now indicating that there are non-fat components of animal products, particularly in red and processed meat, that better explain this risk.[3]

Red and processed meat

Meat is a part of many iconic aspects of Western culture – barbecued steaks, bacon-and-egg big breakfasts, Sunday roasts, Christmas ham and Easter lamb are all familiar parts of pretty much every gathering, holiday or celebration. Although there's been a slight shift away from red meat to white meat over the past few decades (Australians, for example, are consuming about 6 kg less red meat and 20 kg more white meat per year than twenty years ago),[7] our red meat consumption is still causing unnecessary disease and loss of life. The World Health Organization (WHO) classified processed meats (bacon, salami, sausages, beef jerky, ham, etc.) as Group 1 carcinogens in 2015, putting them alongside tobacco smoking and asbestos as agents known to cause cancer.[8] The International Agency for Research on Cancer (IARC), the cancer research agency of the WHO, came to this conclusion by reviewing over 800 scientific papers and determining that there was sufficient evidence of the carcinogenicity of processed meats in human diets.[8,9] From this it's been estimated that approximately 34,000 cancer deaths per year are attributable to diets high in processed meats.[8]

As part of the same review, the WHO classified unprocessed red meat – flesh from cows, pigs (yes, pork is considered red meat, despite what you may have heard), sheep, horses and goats – as a Group 2A carcinogen, which means that, based on strong mechanistic data, and the limited studies we have on humans, it is '*probably* carcinogenic to humans'.[8] The WHO use the word 'probably' because scientists cannot be as definitive in their conclusions about red meat as they can about processed meats based on the data available today. However, if the relationship is in fact causal, and red meat causes cancer, 50,000 cancer deaths a year could be attributed to overconsumption of eye fillets, pork belly, veal and so on.[8]

The WHO stressed that *the risk of developing cancer was shown to rise as the amount of red meat consumed rose* – in other words, there is a cumulative effect. However, the data available didn't allow them to conclude if there was any safe level of consumption.[8] The WCRF has a slightly different recommendation, stating that people should limit their red meat consumption to three small portions per week, equivalent to 350–500 g per week – around 60 g per day, or a steak approximately the size of a deck of playing cards.[10] Its rationale is that although red meat is not an essential part of a healthy diet, it is a good source of protein, iron, B_{12} and zinc. While this is indisputable, why take the risk when these nutrients can easily be obtained from a well-planned diet free of red meat and processed meats that features an abundance of whole plant foods – foods not associated with increased cancer risk?[11]

One meta-analysis, which looked at colorectal cancer, the type of cancer most associated with the consumption of red and processed meat, found a 17% increase in risk for every 100 g of red meat consumed per day, and an 18% increase in risk for every 50 g of processed meat per day.[12] Similar findings have been reproduced time and time again.[12–18] When diets make red meats the hero, and have them be the star of the plate, it's easy to understand why colorectal cancer is the second most common type of cancer that can affect both men and women in Australia and the United States.[19,20]

It is thought that the carcinogenic effects of these meats are in part due to several non-fat compounds that are either present in the meat (namely, heme iron, nitrates, nitrites, neu5Gc and N-nitroso-compounds) or are produced during cooking (such as heterocyclic aromatic amines and polycyclic aromatic hydrocarbons).[9,21,22] Mechanistic studies suggest these compounds are either themselves carcinogenic or promote the formation of carcinogenic compounds. Take heme iron, the form of iron only found in animal products and abundantly found in red meat. Studies show that heme stimulates the production of N-nitroso-compounds that damage the lining of the gut and subsequently may contribute to the development of colorectal cancer.[23]

Interestingly, the effect of some of these compounds seems to be determined by what comes along with them for the ride. For example, nitrates and nitrites are also naturally present in the human body and in health-promoting vegetables, such as dark leafy greens.[24] How can they be healthy when found in vegetables but carcinogenic when found in processed meat? Researchers have suggested that it's not so much the nitrate or nitrite compounds themselves but what they are packaged with that matters, and whether or not they are converted to a compound that is unhealthy (nitrosamines) or healthy (nitric oxide). Rather incredibly, the polyphenols and antioxidants in plants, particularly vitamin C, *inhibit* the production of the unhealthy, carcinogenic nitrosamine compounds, favouring the production of nitric oxide, which helps boost cardiovascular health.[25,26] Dark leafy greens, beetroot, cabbage and parsley are particularly good for boosting nitric oxide levels.[27]

Dairy

The biggest cause for concern when it comes to cancer and the consumption of dairy products is that they may increase the risk of developing prostate cancer, as consistently found in large meta-analyses.[28–31] However, it must be said that the WCRF considers this evidence to be 'limited – suggestive', which means that while there is a clear association the relationship isn't strong enough to warrant telling people to give up, or dramatically reduce, their dairy intake based on today's science.[32] While there is certainly more to be learned about the mechanism behind this relationship, there is some research that implicates a hormone called insulin-like growth factor 1 (IGF-1). The amount of this hormone in our circulation increases following the consumption of both low-fat and full-fat dairy products, and has been shown in animal studies to promote proliferation of prostate cancer cells and prevent their breakdown and elimination.[30,33–36] In the year 2000, researchers took 750 male subjects from the EPIC-Oxford study, some non-vegetarians, some vegetarians and some vegans, and compared their hormone levels. The findings? Vegans had the lowest levels of IGF-1, 9% lower than the meat-eaters and 8% lower than the vegetarians. Another interesting observation from that study was that despite the researchers' hypothesis, and perhaps contrary to what many outside of the science world presume, vegan men had the highest levels of testosterone, the major sex hormone in males, which plays an important role in building strong bones and muscle, as well as in sperm production and sex drive.[37]

Milk and acne

An emerging area of research is drawing the link between dairy consumption, particularly milk, and acne, the most prevalent inflammatory skin condition in the world. A study looking at 24,452 French adults, of which almost half had current acne or had experienced acne in their lifetime, identified that for each glass of milk consumed per day, subjects had a 12% higher risk of developing acne.[38] Given we know that low IGF-1 levels prevent the occurrence of acne, and that milk increases IGF-1 levels, this is not surprising.[39]

While this link between dairy and prostate cancer is something of a concern, and may well be a good enough reason for many to say goodbye to dairy, when it comes to looking at dairy and other forms of cancer, the evidence suggests it is neutral or, in some cases, beneficial. For example, there is strong evidence to suggest that dairy consumption *reduces* the risk of developing colorectal cancer and perhaps even premenopausal breast cancer.[40,41] Adequate calcium intake via food or supplementation is also associated with reduced risk of these two cancers, so it may well be that calcium is the protective factor here rather than dairy itself.[40–42] The inconclusiveness around dairy is most likely a result of two things. First, there are many different forms of dairy – full-fat versus low-fat, fermented versus unfermented, butter, cheese, milk, etc. – which have varying nutritional properties. The second factor is context. Where a population's diet is suboptimal – for example, people living below the poverty line eating an overwhelming amount of refined carbohydrates – dairy may be a healthy addition to the diet. In such populations, the addition of vitamin D, calcium and protein to their diet will likely be protective and lower their overall risk of certain types of cancer, other chronic diseases and premature death despite the presence of hormones, antibiotics and other substances commonly found in dairy.[43–45]

However, given that dairy is not an essential food group most people in the Western world need to survive, that it can be a significant source of saturated fats and cholesterol, that most of us have a degree of lactose intolerance (see below), and that there is cause for concern with regard to its potential promotion of prostate cancer, it certainly seems a reasonable option – for males in particular, and anyone prone to acne – to avoid it or to significantly reduce consumption and source adequate amounts of protein, calcium and vitamin D elsewhere (which we will address in Part Three). In other words, just because the science on dairy and cancer to date is somewhat inconclusive does not mean its removal from or addition to your diet will have no effect on your health. Rather, that effect is determined by what it is displacing or what you replace it with. Replace dairy with whole plant-based foods and you're likely to do better. On the other hand, replace dairy with red meat or sugary drinks, and you're likely to do worse. You are either trading up or trading down.[43,46]

Why are (most) humans lactose intolerant?

In most mammals except humans, the gene that produces the enzyme lactase, which allows the digestion of milk, is turned off after infancy and weaning. This symbolises that the animal no longer has a biological requirement for milk.

However, because our ancestors bred animals for dairy production, some of them developed genetic adaptations that allowed them to digest lactose beyond infancy. This is called lactase persistence. This likely occurred as a survival adaptation during a period of time when food was scarce and dairy offered a good source of calories and nutrients.

Today, about 30% of people across the world have a better ability to digest lactose, while 70% have reduced levels of the enzyme lactase, varying degrees of lactose intolerance and experience pain, discomfort and bloating when consuming dairy.[47]

One option for trading up, particularly for men, is swapping dairy milk for soy milk. A recent meta-analysis of thirty observational studies found that consumption of soy was associated with significantly lower risk of developing prostate cancer.[48] This finding may help explain why vegan men in the AHS-2 cohort have lower risk of developing prostate cancer compared with vegetarians and meat-eaters.[49] It's also one of the likely reasons for the increase in prostate cancer incidence in Japan and other Asian countries, where Westernisation is seeing people there swap traditional foods such as soy for dairy.[50] What's the mechanism at play here? Evidence suggests that the isoflavones genistein and daidzein, phytonutrients found in soy, preferentially bind to oestrogen receptors, which reduces cancer cell proliferation.[48] For women, despite widespread confusion and plenty of misinformation on social media, the highest-quality studies performed to date suggest that soy products are either protective against breast cancer or, at a minimum, seem to have no negative effect.[51–54] The general consensus today is that soy foods, in a whole or minimally processed form, such as tempeh, tofu, miso, edamame and soy milk, can be part of a healthy, well-diversified diet rich in whole plant foods for all men and women.[55,56] *

Eggs

An increased risk of prostate cancer features again in observational studies looking at regular consumption of eggs.[57,58] One study in particular, published in 2011, observed 27,607 American men for about two decades and identified that men who consumed more than two and a half eggs per week had an 81% higher chance of developing prostate cancer.[57]

* The exception here is soy isoflavone supplements, because these are much more concentrated sources of isoflavones, which haven't been proven to be safe. More research is needed before they can be recommended.[56,57]

Various studies have also identified associations between egg consumption and gastrointestinal cancer (cancers affecting the digestive system). A 2014 meta-analysis looking at 424,867 subjects and 18,852 cases of gastrointestinal cancer found that consuming five eggs per week increased the risk by 19%.[59]

It is worth taking these findings with a grain of salt. Is it the eggs or is it that these studies didn't fully account for the fact that the average Western person eating eggs also enjoys bacon and milk? According to the WCRF, it's the latter.[60] When it comes to deciding whether or not to include eggs in our diet, what's potentially more helpful is knowing that while some of the populations around the world who exhibit exemplary health and longevity do consume eggs in modest amounts (usually one every other day from cage-free hens that eat natural foods and are not given antibiotics), others don't.[61–63]

Bile acid and cancer

There is evidence that compounds formed in our digestive system called 'secondary bile acids' are carcinogenic, increasing our risk of developing colon cancer.[64] Numerous studies on humans show us that the best way to dial these down is through a combination of increasing our fibre intake and decreasing our consumption of animal products.[65,66] In fact, when you switch someone to a high-fibre, plant-rich diet, their microbiome alters so quickly that in just two weeks their body is already producing 70% fewer secondary bile acids![67] Too much saturated fats and insufficient fibre is a recipe for disaster for your gut,[68] one of the primary reasons I am not an advocate of the ketogenic diet for long-term health.

Why is consuming ultra-processed foods a risk factor for developing cancer?

Ultra-processed foods are high in calories, hyper-palatable and easily overconsumed but low in fibre and micronutrients that are known to protect our cells from damage.[69] They are typically rich in salt, sugar and fat, and may contain any number of additives such as preservatives, flavourings, emulsifiers, humectants, colourants, sequestrants, non-sugar sweeteners and firming, bulking, de-foaming, anticaking and glazing agents.[69]

Regularly consuming these foods significantly increases our risk of developing cancer. A 2018 study from France that looked at 104,980 subjects found that for every 10% increase in the consumption of ultra-processed foods, there was a 12% overall increase in cancer risk and an 11% increase in breast cancer risk.[70] What was neat about this study was that, among other things, it was able to control for body mass, giving strong reason to believe that these foods promote cancer not just via weight gain, but also through their inherent properties. In addition to these findings, the WCRF states that diets with high glycaemic load, which is to say diets featuring a lot of ultra-processed foods low in fibre, probably increase the risk of endometrial cancer.[71,72]

Understanding the inherent properties of ultra-processed foods that increase our risk of developing cancer is still a work in progress, and future studies will likely offer more clarity here. A few proposed mechanisms have focused on food additives (such as sodium nitrite), processing contaminants (e.g. heterocyclic amines) and endocrine-disrupting chemicals that can make their way into these foods via leaching from packaging.[70] However, the ongoing debate and research shouldn't distract us from the fact that we are better off without these foods in our diet, particularly given many of these ingredients are relatively new to our food system and we do not fully understand how they impact human biology over the long-term.

Diet quality is incredibly important if you are looking for optimal health. Eating ultra-processed foods once in a while isn't going to kill you, but when you are sacrificing calories that could be coming from extremely healthful foods in favour of ultra-processed foods on a daily basis, the science suggests you are increasing your risk of developing cancer.[70,73] While it may feel as if you would need to make major sacrifices to minimise these foods in your life, it doesn't have to be that way. We'll look at simple swaps and satisfying alternatives in Part Three.

Salt

There is convincing evidence that links excess salt consumption with stomach cancer.[74–77] A few possible mechanisms have been proposed to explain this. The first is that excessive salt consumption can directly damage the stomach lining, which, if left untreated, may eventually cause the development of cancerous cells.[78] The second is that *Helicobacter pylori*, a type of bacterial infection common in parts of Asia which also damages the stomach lining, may become more virulent in the presence of salt.[79] In fact, this is thought to be one of the reasons why certain Asian countries that consume more salt than the average Western diet, such as Japan, have a higher incidence of stomach cancer.[80]

In Australia, the best estimate for salt consumption is 9.6 g (3840 mg of sodium) per day, which is nearly double the National Health and Medical Research Council's recommendation of 5 g (2000 mg of sodium) per day.[81,82] Around 80% of this sodium is *not* coming from our salt shakers but from animal and processed foods – bread, unprocessed and processed meat, savoury sauces, dairy and cereal products derived from heavily refined grains, such as biscuits and pizza.[83] That's right – salt is hidden in foods that you are likely unaware contain it. The remaining 20% is from salt that naturally exists in other whole foods, as well as salt added during cooking or serving.

Alcohol

The honest lowdown on alcohol brings both good and bad news. I'll start with the good: evidence suggests up to two alcoholic drinks per day will decrease your risk of kidney cancer. The not-so-good news? While it takes a few alcoholic drinks to increase the risk of developing liver or colorectal cancer, alcohol at any level increases the risk of developing several cancers, such as breast cancer and oesophageal cancer. In a report in 2018, the WCRF declared there is 'strong' evidence of this.[84] A common question is, 'Does the type of alcohol matter?' Evidently not, with research suggesting that it is ethanol, the part of alcohol that makes it alcohol, which is responsible for the carcinogenic effects.[84]

When alcohol is metabolised, a toxic molecule called acetaldehyde is produced which impairs the body's ability to synthesise and repair DNA, which is thought to kickstart the cancer process.[24,85] Ethanol can also directly damage our cells and increase inflammation,[86] and alcohol increases oestrogen levels in the body, a known risk factor for breast cancer.[87] Further, alcohol directly affects our gut microbiome and promotes dysbiosis (more on this in Part Three), which means fewer good gut bugs and more bad gut bugs. The downstream effect of this is an impaired gut lining, allowing bacterial endotoxins – inflammatory molecules – to enter the bloodstream. We know from various studies that people who have elevated levels of these endotoxins in their blood are more likely to develop certain cancers.[88,89]

Why whole plant foods are *protective* against developing cancer

There are hundreds of identified phytonutrients and antioxidants in whole plant-based foods that, along with dietary fibre, are thought to protect against the development of cancerous cells.[2] These compounds are often referred to as *chemoprotective*.

Some of the most studied chemoprotective compounds include carotenoids, vitamins, resveratrol, sulphoraphane, quercetin, catechins (green tea), curcumin (turmeric), diallyl disulfide (garlic), piperine (pepper) and gingerol (ginger). For more about anti-cancer powerhouse sulfphoraphane, see Part Three.

There are mountains of evidence supporting the consumption of many different whole plant foods to reduce the risk of various forms of cancer. What seems to be more important than any one particular food is getting your daily dose of whole grains, fruits, vegetables and dietary fibre.[90] The strongest evidence of these protective properties is related to colorectal cancer, the third most common form of cancer in the world.[40,91,92] For every 90 g of whole grains consumed, the risk of colorectal cancer is lowered by 17%. For every 10 g of additional fibre per day, the risk of colorectal cancer is lowered by 9%.[90] This is a good reason to make friends with beans and brown rice!

In addition to this, there appears to be specific benefit in consuming plant foods rich in vitamin C (e.g. strawberries, broccoli, citrus fruits) and specific phytonutrients (carotenoids, beta-carotene and isoflavones), all of which are in abundance in a diet that emphasises a wide variety of whole plant foods.[93] This brings me to an important point – although we often want to find the silver bullet or one specific superfood, your diet quality ultimately boils down to its *diversity*. We'll come back to this from a practical angle later when we talk about gut health and the #plantproof40 challenge in Part Three.

Why whole grains, not refined grains?

You may wonder why this distinction is so important. During the refining process, much of the nutrition from the outer layers of the grain are lost. For example, approximately 92% of all vitamin E is lost during the refining of grains, leaving a much smaller amount of this known chemoprotective compound.[2,94] The refining process strips out many of the antioxidants (which whole grains actually have more of than many fruits and vegetables), vitamins, minerals, other chemoprotective compounds, fat and protein while concentrating the carbohydrate. With each mouthful of refined grains, you're missing out on a lot of nutrition that could have been enjoyed. This is certainly not an issue if it happens sporadically, but think about the cumulative effect of those lost nutrients over time. This is no doubt a major reason why people who consume whole grains and over 25 g of dietary fibre per day have lower risk of not just colorectal cancer but also breast cancer, cardiovascular disease, type 2 diabetes and premature death.[95]

Why is fibre so important when it comes to colorectal cancer? First, fibre helps to decrease the transit time of food through your digestive system, which inadvertently decreases the time that the gut is exposed to potential carcinogens in your meals.[96,97] Second, and perhaps most importantly, a specific type of fibre known as *prebiotic fibre* acts as a food source for the healthy, or 'good', bacteria that live in our colon. We need these bacteria, and the prebiotic fibre helps them proliferate and work optimally. This means that when you regularly consume enough fibre – at least 28–38 g per day – the good bacteria grow in numbers and outnumber the bad (pathogenic) bacteria that are inevitably always lingering around. As the good bacteria feed away on the prebiotic fibre, they create short-chain fatty acids, an example of which is *butyrate*, the primary energy source for the cells in your colon and an anti-inflammatory compound.[98,99] When you consider that inflammation is a hallmark feature of cancer, it's not surprising that butyrate protects against colorectal cancer.[99]

What's great is that we can make changes to our dietary pattern in order to fire up these butyrate-producing bacteria in a matter of days. In 2015, noting a thirteen times higher incidence of colon cancer among African Americans compared with native Africans, researchers analysed the microbiomes of African Americans who consumed a high-fat, low-fibre diet, and rural Africans who were consuming a low-fat, high-fibre diet.[66] The researchers had these subjects undertake a two-week diet switch and found that the African Americans who adopted the low-fat, high-fibre native African–style diet quickly developed higher numbers of bacteria that favoured butyrate production, had fewer markers of inflammation, and fewer bacteria producing carcinogenic compounds such as secondary bile acids.[100] Unsurprisingly, they found the opposite for the rural Africans who adopted a high-fat, low-fibre Western-style diet.

This study, along with others looking at native Africans who have tremendously low risk of developing colon cancer, suggests that rather than targeting 28–38 g of fibre per day, as suggested by the typical dietary guidelines, targeting at least 50 g per day is even more beneficial.[101,102] And we've had clues pointing to this ever since 1969 – the same year Neil Armstrong landed on the moon! It was that very year when scientist Denis Burkitt, famously known for Burkitt's hypothesis, wrote an article based on his observations in rural Uganda, where he identified that the local diet, which contained well over 50 g of fibre per day from an abundance of colourful whole plant foods, while being super low in animal products, was associated with absence of disease. At the same time, rates of colon cancer and other chronic diseases in Britain, where people were eating just 15 g of fibre per day, were increasing rapidly.[102]

T. Colin Campbell, author of *The China Study*, identified a similar pattern to Burkitt in the 1970s and 1980s when examining the relationship between dietary patterns and risk of chronic disease across sixty-five geographical regions of China. Various cancers, diabetes and cardiovascular disease were all associated with diets that had higher intakes of meat, eggs, dairy and total animal fat, while diets emphasising whole plants were associated with lower risk of developing these diseases.[103,104]

With this in mind, perhaps you're wondering if people who adopt vegetarian and vegan diets fare better when it comes to cancer. In short, yes they do. A 2017 meta-analysis that included 96 observational studies with subjects from all over the world found that, compared with a diet containing meat, a vegetarian diet reduced the risk of developing all forms of cancer by 8%, and a vegan diet reduced the risk by 15%.[46]

With regard to site-specific cancers, while we need longer studies with more plant-based subjects to draw more definitive conclusions, there is a growing body of research suggesting diets that de-emphasise animal products are protective against prostate cancer, breast and ovarian cancers, gastrointestinal cancers, stomach cancer, pancreatic and lymphatic cancer.[49,61,105–107] Perhaps the strongest evidence to date relates to hormone-dependent cancers. In 2012, a study looking at the AHS-2 cohort identified that vegetarian women were 34% less likely to develop breast, ovarian or uterine cancers compared with meat-eaters, while vegan males in the same cohort had a 35% lower risk of developing prostate cancer compared with meat-eaters.[49,105,108]

Importantly, it seems the benefits of these plant-based diets depend greatly on the quality of the foods they include. In studies where subjects are known to eat fruits and vegetables in abundance, and high amounts of fibre, the protection against these site-specific cancers is more obvious.[61] As we discussed earlier, consumption of ultra-processed foods, whether vegan or not, heightens the risk of developing cancer – if you're adopting a plant-based diet to lower your risk of developing cancer, the science emphatically supports the inclusion of whole plants, not junk food.

There is also a considerable amount of evidence, from both observational studies and clinical trials, demonstrating a protective effect for site-specific cancers, including breast, prostate, colorectal and even lung cancer, in another plant-based dietary pattern: the Mediterranean diet. For example, in the Lyon Diet Heart Study that we spoke about in Chapter 5, subjects randomised to the Mediterranean diet group had 61% lower risk of developing cancer compared with those eating the control diet, and therefore more meat and fewer whole plants.[109] A 2017 meta-analysis that included 83 studies looking at this relationship attributed the protective effect of the Mediterranean diet to its focus on fruits, vegetables and whole grains. [109–111]

Why coffee and tea are protective against cancer

I've got to let you in on a little secret: I love coffee. I love tea, too, but having grown up in Melbourne, the coffee capital of Australia, I have a special soft spot for coffee. Which is why I was pleased to discover that the WCRF found strong evidence that coffee decreases the risk of developing cancer, specifically liver and endometrial cancer. For each cup of coffee we have, we can lower our risk of liver cancer by 14% and endometrial cancer by 8-9%; on the other hand, there is also evidence showing that both green and black tea help to reduce the risk of bladder cancer.[112] Personally, I consume coffee in the morning and decaffeinated tea in the afternoons, with both being a tremendously rich source of specific antioxidant and anti-inflammatory polyphenols, which emerging evidence suggests protects our healthy cells from damage and stops the proliferation of cancer cells.[113,114]

You might be thinking, perhaps we could bottle up the nutrition from whole unrefined plants and take them in capsules or powder form – antioxidants from berries, for example? However, isolating certain compounds is no match for how they act in combination in their original, unadulterated form. Given the enormous amount of chemoprotective phytonutrients and antioxidants that are packaged into whole plant foods – more than 5000 phytonutrients have been identified to date[115] – and the high likelihood that they contain many more protective compounds we are yet to identify, dietary supplements are not recommended in place of consuming fruits, vegetables, whole grains and legumes when it comes to cancer prevention. Not only is the science not there to support it, but taking certain supplements like vitamins A and E may even increase the risk of certain cancers.[96,116]

The only exception to this is calcium supplementation, which evidence suggests can reduce the risk of colorectal cancer if it helps you reach the recommended intake level.[96] That's not to say a few supplements in other circumstances – for example, taking folate during pregnancy, or B_{12} for vegans or people aged over fifty – are not warranted. But what it does mean is that there are no shortcuts to a cancer-protective dietary pattern. Taking a multivitamin doesn't excuse us from eating the recommended servings of fruits and vegetables per day. (We'll talk more about these serving recommendations and specific information on supplements in Part Three.)

Overall, based on the lower risk of developing cancer among vegetarian and vegan populations and those eating a high-quality Mediterranean diet, it seems the protective effect of these dietary patterns is likely a combination of the chemoprotective compounds they contain, combined with the fact they eliminate or greatly reduce intake of red meat, dairy and ultra-processed foods, and promote a healthy body weight.[3] Of course, eating this way will not guarantee that we will avoid this devastating group of diseases, especially not the forms of cancer that are driven by genetics. But while there is no such thing as a miracle food or miracle diet that guarantees cancer immunity, it's nice to know that through our food choices we have the power to greatly reduce our risk of developing several of the most common forms of cancer that exist today.

Organic versus conventional produce and cancer

Whether or not we should be buying organic produce to lower our risk of cancer and improve our health in general is widely disputed and, to be honest, somewhat unclear. Despite what many would presume, there is very little research assessing the difference between organic and conventionally-grown produce consumption and cancer risk. Running a long-term RCT is cost-prohibitive and will more than likely never occur. However, we do know that eating more conventional produce increases synthetic pesticide exposure, and two large prospective studies, one out of France and one out of the United Kingdom, suggest that it may be better to err on the side of caution where possible, with both finding that those who regularly consumed organic produce had less chance of developing non-Hodgkin's lymphoma (a form of blood cancer).[117-119]* Specifically, it is thought that three common pesticides used in conventional farming (glyphosate, malathion and diazinon) are responsible

* Interestingly, while the French study found women eating more organic food had a lower risk of developing postmenopausal breast cancer, the UK study found the opposite – an increased risk of breast cancer with organic food consumption. The researchers of the UK study noted that this may be explained by the fact that the women in their study consuming organic foods also consumed more alcohol and had fewer children – both are known risk factors for breast cancer. They were also of a higher socio-economic class, and thus may have had better access to health care and increased cancer screening.

for this increased risk, with the IARC classifying each of them as *probable human carcinogens*.[96,120] Additionally, while organic and conventional produce contain similar amounts of vitamins and minerals, organic fruits and vegetables contain higher amounts of antioxidant compounds such as polyphenols, which have anti-cancer properties, though whether these differences are sufficient enough to make a tangible difference to an individual's cancer risk remains unknown.[121] Before we get too carried away, I want to make it super clear that this evidence is relatively weak and the benefits of eating fruits and vegetables, even if conventional, clearly outweigh the possible risks – something that is often missing from this conversation in communication to the public.[96,122] However, until we have more data, I personally believe it's a good idea to buy organic where it makes sense. Although this is based on limited data, I see it as playing things on the safe side until we have a better understanding of how chronic exposure to these synthetic compounds, which are relatively new to our food system, affect our long-term health. This precautionary approach was the conclusion of a 2020 systematic review on this very topic.[119]

CHAPTER 7

Eating to keep your brain young

Most of us will agree that we want to improve or at least maintain our brain capacity for as many years as possible. This is especially true for those of us who have witnessed someone affected by dementia. My grandmother suffered from vascular dementia when I was a teenager, and it was devastating to see her struggle to recognise the people who loved her.

Dementia is the second leading cause of death in Australia but is not in fact a disease itself. Instead, dementia describes a collection of symptoms that are caused by diseases and disorders affecting the brain. People with dementia may experience difficulty with memory, comprehension, calculation, learning capacity, judgement, language and performing everyday tasks, and may become confused or experience personality change.[1,2] Alzheimer's disease and vascular dementia are the most common forms of dementia, which account for about 70% and 15% of all cases respectively.[3]

The statistics are pretty startling. Globally, although reported figures are slightly variable, it seems approximately one-third to half of all people aged eighty-five or older have dementia.[4,5]

As frightening as these numbers are, it's highly likely these statistics are actually underreported, with many cases of dementia going undetected because people think their fading memory or slowing brain activity is simply a part of normal ageing.[6]

The economic burden of dementia is also staggering, with annual healthcare costs for patients with dementia currently estimated to be AU$15 billion in Australia, US$100 billion in the United States, and over US$1 trillion globally.[1,7,8]

So, is dementia and a decline in our cognition part of our genetic fate that is simply becoming more prevalent due to the fact we are living longer? Or is there anything we can do to prevent the effects of dementia?

The good news is only about 3% of all Alzheimer's disease cases, the most common form of dementia, are categorically determined by the person's genes.[9,10] These are rare conditions, like early onset Alzheimer's, which affects people between thirty and sixty years of age.[11] In saying that, there are certain genes which may *predispose* one to developing dementia. For example, APOE4, which approximately 25% of the population carry, can predispose a person to Alzheimer's disease.[9,12] However, even then, studies of identical twins have shown that it is not uncommon for only one twin to develop Alzheimer's, shedding light on the importance of lifestyle.[13] In fact, even with genetic predispositions, neurologists now estimate that approximately 90% of Alzheimer's disease is preventable within a normal life span by adopting a healthy lifestyle.[14] What about other forms of dementia? Same story. While some of us may be predisposed to dementia, it is our lifestyle that dictates whether or not those genes are expressed (or turned on).[9] The genes themselves represent a risk, but for almost all of us, whether that risk turns into disease is within our control.

While billions of dollars have been spent by pharmaceutical companies, and plenty of people selling magic pills, there is no solid evidence to date that advanced dementia, including Alzheimer's disease, can be reversed.[15,16] On the bright side, there is evidence suggesting dementia can be prevented or delayed, and the progression of early stage Alzheimer's disease slowed, through the adoption of a healthy lifestyle. By early stage, I mean routinely forgetting small things like names or phone numbers, or where you put your keys. On the other hand, forgetting who someone is or how to drive your car is typically what we see with more advanced disease, and by that stage, it seems the cell damage has progressed to a point where it can no longer be reversed. However, just a few simple dietary changes, like adding dark leafy greens and berries to your day and eating less red meat and dairy, may help to keep our brains youthful.[17–19]

Rather than hope for a 'cure', the most important thing we can do is adopt a lifestyle that reduces our exposure to known risk factors for dementia. Adopting lifestyle changes aimed at minimising these risk factors will not only reduce your chance of developing dementia, but also help grow the capacity of your brain. That's right – building what is called your *cognitive reserve* creates a brain that is more resilient against dementia.[20] Think of it this way: dementia is a progressive neurological disorder that starts with mild cognitive impairment – pre-dementia. It's a spectrum. So, if you do the right thing by your brain today, not only will you increase your chances of preventing dementia, but you will also maximise your brain's potential. A win-win. This is one positive to come from the heartbreaking dementia epidemic we are confronted with today – it has resulted in a great amount of scientific investigation, producing data that we can use to enhance everyday functioning of arguably our most important organ and keep it stronger for longer. Retaining good brain function, including our memories, thoughts and personality traits, seems to me to be an integral part of extending our health span, not just our life span.

Risk factors for dementia

The major modifiable risk factors for developing dementia include high blood pressure, high cholesterol, insulin resistance and diabetes, vascular disease (atherosclerosis), inflammation, obesity and smoking.[21–27] As we've seen, aside from smoking, these are all risk factors that respond positively to dietary patterns that favour the consumption of whole plant foods.

Other risk factors which should be considered as part of a holistic approach to reducing the chance of developing dementia are: depression, sleep deprivation, chronic stress, excessive alcohol consumption and physical inactivity, as well as traumatic brain injury, such as could be developed by playing contact sports.[28–33]

Saturated fats, cholesterol and dementia

We've already seen the dramatic impact that diet has on cholesterol and blood pressure, and scientists have shown a further link between both of these and dementia. A fascinating study measured the cholesterol levels of nearly 10,000 people between 1964 and 1973 and then followed them for more than forty years to see the effect that those levels had on their brain health as they aged.[34] They found that high cholesterol midlife increased the subjects' chance of developing Alzheimer's and vascular dementia three decades later by 57% and 26% respectively. Another study found that subjects with both raised systolic blood pressure of 160 mmHg or greater and total cholesterol over 251 mg/dL (6.50 mmol/L) had 3.5 times the risk of developing Alzheimer's later in life, even after controlling for age, weight, smoking and other lifestyle factors.[27] It makes sense – these modifiable risk factors affect vascular health, and in the same way that they affect blood vessels supplying oxygen and nutrients to your heart, they affect blood vessels and vital tissues in your brain. And, like cardiovascular disease, just because it's uncommon to experience the symptoms of dementia in our midlife, it doesn't mean we aren't laying down the foundations for it to emerge in the future.

You will recall that two dietary factors that negatively influence our cholesterol levels are saturated fats and, to a lesser extent, dietary cholesterol. Based on this, I am sure you would agree it makes sense to de-emphasise these in our diet in order to protect our brain from cognitive decline. However, my low-carb friends will often suggest we should be doubling down on them by pointing to the fact that 20% of the body's cholesterol is found in the brain, and that 60% of our brain is fat.[35,36] By their logic, our brains are made of fat and cholesterol, therefore our diets should contain foods rich in saturated fats and dietary cholesterol.

Understanding the difference between *essential* and *non-essential nutrients* will help us see why this logic is flawed. An essential nutrient is something our bodies cannot make on their own, so we must get it through our diet. Non-essential nutrients can be made by our body without any help. Polyunsaturated fats, such as omega-3s and omega-6s, are considered essential nutrients. Both saturated fats and dietary cholesterol, on the other hand, are non-essential nutrients. Our bodies can produce the required levels of these without dietary input. When it comes to cholesterol, the cholesterol in the brain does not come from any cholesterol in our diet – it is exclusively made by cells in our brains.[36] In fact, research clearly shows that not only do the cells in our bodies make the cholesterol and saturated fats they require, but that diets rich in these damage the millions of arteries supplying oxygen to the brain and increase the risk of developing cognitive impairment and dementia.[35-44] One study looking at 6183 elderly women found that those who consumed higher amounts of saturated fats had 70% faster decline in memory while women consuming low amounts of saturated fats had brains that behaved as if they were six years younger.[41] We also know from both lipid-lowering trials and studies of people who have genetic mutations that even when people have super-low cholesterol levels – far lower than what could be achieved through diet alone – they still produce healthy amounts of hormones.[45-47] This again reiterates that the idea we need to eat dietary cholesterol or focus on foods rich in saturated fats for good health, be it brain health or hormone health, is simply not true, and in fact extremely dangerous advice.

And, despite the hype on social media, there is no evidence to suggest that coconut oil is any different to animal foods rich in saturated fats when it comes to risk of cognitive impairment.[48,49] Coconut oil is not a superfood – we'll talk more about why in Part Three.

How plants protect your brain

Based on what we have already seen about diet and modifiable risk factors for cardiovascular disease and type 2 diabetes, you may suspect that people who eat a predominantly or entirely whole-food plant-based diet and have lower risk of developing these risk factors would also have less incidence of dementia. If so, you would be correct – observational studies have consistently shown a positive association between such dietary patterns and the prevention of dementia-related conditions. In the AHS-1 cohort, subjects eating meat (including fish and poultry) were two to three times more likely to develop dementia compared with vegetarian counterparts matched for age and gender.[50]

A multi-decade study published in 2019 that followed 16,948 Chinese subjects living in Singapore identified that subjects who best adhered to plant-based dietary patterns (including the Mediterranean and DASH diets) had 18–33% less risk of developing cognitive impairment later in life compared with subjects eating more meat, more processed foods and fewer whole plants.[51] Several meta-analyses and large observational studies looking at cognitive function and diet have come to similar conclusions – the Mediterranean and DASH diets are both good options when it comes to preserving brain function.[52–56]

In recent years, new observational research has come out in support of a third diet that is associated with significantly better results, called the MIND diet, a hybrid of the Mediterranean and DASH diets, created by leading Alzheimer's researcher Dr Martha Clare Morris for preserving brain function.[17,57,58] Specifically, Dr Morris and her team found that while the Mediterranean and DASH diets were only associated with decreased risk when strictly adhered to, just moderate adherence to the MIND diet decreased the risk of developing Alzheimer's by 35%, while high adherence decreased the risk by 53%![17] The main differences to the Mediterranean and DASH diets are that the MIND diet further de-emphasises red meat and cheese, minimises fish intake to just once or more per week, and places greater emphasis on dark leafy green vegetables and berries, both of which have been associated in various studies with slower cognitive decline.[16,18,59,60]

Specifically, it is the polyphenols and carotenoids in berries and dark leafy greens (which is what gives them their vibrant colours) that are believed to be neuroprotective compounds, both having antioxidant and anti-inflammatory properties.[18,60–64] It's now understood that in order to reap the benefits of these polyphenols, we need to have a healthy gut (which we'll discuss in Part Three). About 90% of all polyphenols we eat pass from our small intestine to our large intestine, where they act as a source of food for good bacteria, promoting the production of molecules such as caffeic acid and ferulic acid, which emerging science suggests may have an anti-depressant effect, reduce inflammation and protect the brain from degeneration.[65–68] It's interesting to note that these polyphenol compounds are also found in olive oil, which may be another reason why the Mediterranean and MIND diets are thought to be protective against dementia.[69]

In spite of an overwhelming amount of observational evidence in support of these plant-based dietary patterns for protecting our brain function, there is a paucity of clinical trials looking at dietary interventions and cognitive function. Where trials have taken place, almost all of them have used the Mediterranean diet, and results have been underwhelming, with most studies finding no benefit.[70] The most promising findings are from a small sub-study of 334 subjects from the PREDIMED trial (which we spoke about in Chapter 5). In the PREDIMED trial the major differences between the Mediterranean diet groups and the control group's diet were that the latter were consuming less unsaturated fats, less fruit and vegetables and more refined carbohydrates. The researchers found that over a four-year period subjects following the Mediterranean diet, with either added extra-virgin olive oil or nuts, had significantly better cognitive function including better memory.[71]

There are a few possible explanations for why there is, to date, such limited support from clinical trials for the Mediterranean diet being preventative of dementia. First, it may be that we simply need longer trials, with more people – people may need to eat this way for decades to see a benefit. Second, it could be that diet alone is not powerful enough to prevent cognitive decline and dementia, and that we need a more holistic intervention that includes healthy amounts of sleep, exercise, cognitive activity and so on. Third, it may be that the Mediterranean diet itself is inferior to dietary patterns such as the MIND diet or a WFPBD, which place greater emphasis on foods known to be protective against dementia (dark leafy greens, berries, legumes, whole grains, nuts and seeds, etc.).

While there are currently no published clinical trials assessing the effectiveness of the MIND diet or a WFPBD for preventing or reversing dementia, there are a few underway that are likely to be published in coming years.[72–74] Until these appear, though, we can take comfort in the fact that a plant-based diet, be it plant-predominant or plant-exclusive, has time and time again been shown to lead to favourable outcomes with regard to body weight, blood pressure, cholesterol levels, insulin resistance, atherosclerosis, depressive symptoms and inflammation – all risk factors for cognitive impairment and dementia.[75–84]

Overall lifestyle and Alzheimer's

While this book is focused on diet, it's of course important to remember that our lifestyle extends beyond the food we put into our mouth. In 2020 an interesting study was published in the *Journal of Neurology* that speaks to this. Researchers in the United States took a total of 2765 subjects from two cohorts in their seventies and eighties and observed them over time to see how various lifestyle factors affected their risk of developing Alzheimer's.[85] Subjects were given a lifestyle score from 0–5, with higher scores representing a healthier lifestyle, based on five lifestyle factors:

1. diet quality (scored based on proximity to the MIND diet)
2. physical activity (150 minutes or more of moderate or vigorous activity per week being optimal)
3. smoking (never or former being optimal)

4. cognitive activity (daily engagement in reading, writing, playing games like chess etc., being optimal)
5. alcohol consumption (research shows very small amounts of alcohol per day may be protective against dementia,[86] so the MIND diet gives a high score for one standard drink per day for women and two per day for men, and a low score for consumption above or below this).

Here's what they found. Compared with people who had one or fewer healthy lifestyle factors:

- those with two to three had 37% lower risk of developing Alzheimer's
- those with four to five had 60% lower risk of developing Alzheimer's.

This represents a huge opportunity for each of us.

Berries are brain food

A study published in 2020 that followed 921 elderly subjects without dementia identified that those with the highest intakes of flavonols, a specific group of polyphenols with antioxidant and anti-inflammatory properties, had 48% lower risk of developing Alzheimer's than those with low flavonol consumption.[87] Some of the best dietary sources of flavonols include berries, broccoli, beans, tomatoes, kale, spinach, onions, apples, pears, oranges, olive oil, green tea and black tea.

Of these, berries are my favourite. Not only are they packed with flavonols, they also contain anthocyanins, another group of polyphenols which animal studies suggest promote the growth of neurons in the hippocampus, the part of the brain responsible for learning and memory.[88] The idea that berries are good for our brain has also been validated in studies on humans. In 2012, researchers published data from the Nurses' Health Study, which included over 16,000 female subjects who had been followed for decades, showing that compared with women who rarely consumed berries, women who consumed one or more servings of blueberries per week, or two or more servings of strawberries per week, experienced a delay in cognitive ageing of up to 2.5 years.[60] More recently, in 2019, Dr Martha Clare Morris and her team from the Rush Memory and Aging Project (MAP) published similar results after following 925 subjects over two decades. Specifically, they identified that compared with people who rarely ate strawberries, those consuming strawberries once per week had 24% lower risk of developing Alzheimer's.[19] Imagine what a daily serve or two could do!

The benefits of berries for brain health don't stop there. Not only does it seem that berries are protective against cognitive decline over the long-term, but a 2019 RCT showed that compared with a placebo smoothie, a mixed berry smoothie prevented cognitive fatigue over a six-hour period.[89] You might be wondering how berries can have such an immediate effect. One of the current hypotheses is that they promote increased blood flow to the brain and neuroplasticity (growth and reorganisation of our brain cells).[90] Whatever the reason, there's a strong case for a handful of berries on your morning oats, or a berry smoothie to fire up your brain for the day ahead.

Fish, omega-3s and DHA

You've likely heard that fish is good for brain health, but is there a benefit to consuming fish over plant sources of omega-3s, such as nuts and seeds? Some studies show protection and others do not.[53,91,92] It really depends what the fish is replacing in your diet. If you put down a piece of red meat for a piece of salmon, that's going to shift your diet towards a dietary pattern associated with lower risk of dementia. That's certainly a good move, and one I strongly encourage! In fact, Dr Morris and her team have shown that including just one piece of fish per week in your diet can lower your risk of dementia by 60%, a finding that her team puts down to DHA (the main type of omega-3 found in fatty fish).[93] More than one piece of fish per week was not shown to offer any extra benefit. This benefit was only observed when comparing fish-eaters with people consuming almost zero plant-based sources of omega-3s per day. The good news for those who would prefer to avoid fish for environmental or ethical reasons is that omega-3s are not unique to the animal kingdom, and there is zero evidence to suggest the addition of fish to a WFPBD that provides adequate amounts of omega-3s would offer any additional protection against dementia. In other words, a diet that's good for brain health may or may not contain fish. Personally, I choose to get mine from walnuts, flaxseeds, chia seeds and algae oil, which we will discuss in more detail in Part Three.

Daily dose of leafy greens

As mentioned earlier, the MIND diet places great emphasis on dark leafy greens (e.g. spinach, kale and rocket). In 2018, data from the MAP study provided compelling evidence to consume a daily salad including these. Specifically, compared with those who rarely consumed dark leafy greens, those who had about a serving a day had brains that performed as if they were eleven years younger. The researchers believe these benefits can be explained by the neuroprotective nutrients that these leafy greens contain, such as folate, vitamin E, beta-carotene and lutein.[18]

Our diet affects our mood

Something the world needs less of that we haven't yet discussed is anxiety, depression and stress. In 2018–2019, 4.3 million Australians were prescribed with mental health-related medications.[94] That's almost 20% of our population, and it fails to include those with undiagnosed conditions.

While there are a variety of reasons for this high prevalence of mental health conditions, it cannot be denied that the food we eat affects our psychological state. Data from observational studies involving more than 200,000 people from all across the world shows that people who eat more fruits and vegetables tend to be more optimistic, have higher self-efficacy and are less likely to experience depression.[95,96]

But is this cause or effect? Does eating these plant-based foods create a better mood, or does a better mood lead to people eating healthier foods? The only way to truly understand this relationship would be via a clinical trial, which we now have – two, in fact. The first was a small study out of Arizona State University, which randomised 39 omnivores to an omnivorous diet, a pescetarian diet or a vegetarian diet. In just two weeks, subjects randomised to the vegetarian diet experienced significantly improved mood compared with subjects eating meat and fish.[83] The second study was bigger – it included 292 subjects from across the United States who were randomised to either a WFPBD group (with a multivitamin to ensure sufficient vitamin B_{12} intake) or a group that maintained their existing diet. At eighteen weeks, those randomised to the WFPBD group experienced fewer symptoms of depression and anxiety, and improved productivity.[82]

The most likely explanation for why plant foods correlated with improved mood in these trials is that the plant foods restored healthy gut function, leading to greater production of feel-good hormones such as serotonin.[97] Our gut and brain are very much connected! We'll talk more about restoring healthy gut function in Part Three when we look at the importance of having a diversity of plants in our diet.

Spotlight on specific nutrients

The science shows some nutrients are particularly important for preventing cognitive decline, with foods rich in unsaturated fats, B vitamins and antioxidants (particularly vitamin C, vitamin E, polyphenols and carotenoids) related to decreased risk of developing dementia.[53] There is also evidence to suggest we should ensure we are getting adequate levels of vitamin D, 90% of which comes from exposure to sunlight.[98,99]

However, as we saw with cancer, preventing cognitive decline and dementia won't come from a supplement. Several meta-analyses of controlled trials and a World Health Organization review have concluded this.[100–103]

And just as there is no magic pill, there is also no magic food. Walnuts and berries are both super healthful foods but a handful of each in an otherwise unhealthy dietary pattern isn't going to be your saving grace. Keeping your brain youthful and firing on all cylinders will depend on your overall dietary pattern, and consistency over time – a dietary pattern that emphasises calories from a diverse range of whole plant foods, bringing together a number of protective components like different instruments forming a symphony, to keep the brain sharp and healthy.

Podcast highlight: Episodes 65, 78, 97, 112 and 117 with neurologists Dean and Ayesha Sherzai

In these five episodes I sit down with the authors of *The Alzheimer's Solution* and talk at length about how diet and other lifestyle factors such as sleep affect brain health.

Healthy brain now and later

Despite the absence of specific and comprehensive RCTs, the totality of available science today strongly suggests that when it comes to food and cognitive function, our best bet is to adopt a diet that maximises calories from a diverse range of whole plant foods – fruits, vegetables, whole grains, legumes, nuts and seeds, with particular attention to regularly consuming berries, dark leafy greens and sources of omega-3s. These foods are rich in vitamins, minerals and compounds unique to the plant kingdom, such as polyphenols, that appear particularly important for keeping our brain young. By making whole plants the star of your plate you will be inadvertently reducing calories from meat, dairy and eggs – foods rich in saturated fats and cholesterol, which raise cholesterol levels and increase the risk of developing cognitive impairment and dementia.

Importantly, a plant-based diet doesn't just reduce your risk of losing the power of your most important organ in your later years – eating this way also improves the output of your brain in your day to day.[104] More brain power now and more brain power for longer, which will matter to you even more when you add years to your life.

FIGURE 7.1:

FOODS AND NUTRIENTS ASSOCIATED WITH DECREASED RISK OF DEMENTIA AND GOOD BRAIN HEALTH

NUTRIENT	GOOD SOURCE
Omega-3s	Chia seeds, ground flaxseeds, hemp seeds, small to medium-sized fatty fish, walnuts
B vitamins	Spinach, collard greens, turnip greens, romaine lettuce, small to medium-sized fatty fish, oysters, mussels, beans, lentils, chickpeas, sunflower seeds, whole grains
Vitamin C	Yellow capsicum (bell pepper), blackcurrants, parsley, mustard greens, kale, kiwifruit, broccoli, brussels sprouts, lemon, lychee, papaya, tomato, berries, orange, thyme, guava, chilli pepper, grapefruit, potato, cauliflower
Vitamin D	Sunshine with or without supplementation (see Part Three)
Vitamin E	Almonds, sunflower seeds, hazelnuts, pinenuts, avocado, mango, spinach, turnip greens, butternut squash, kiwifruit, broccoli
Carotenoids	Carrots, pumpkin, sweet potato, spinach, kale, collard greens, turnip greens, dandelion greens, mustard greens, squash, red capscicum (bell pepper), herbs and spices, asparagus, pistachios
Polyphenols	Berries, cherries, pecans, walnuts, cocoa, kale, spinach, olive oil, artichoke, red onion, pecans, ground flaxseeds, green tea, black tea, coffee, herbs and spices

CHAPTER 8

A diet for living longer

Reducing your risk of developing common diseases and maintaining a healthy body weight both increase your chances of enjoying a longer health span. The question is, can changing the foods you eat lead to a longer life span? And if so, how can we slow down our biological clock?

The short answer is yes, the food we eat multiple times a day directly affects how we age. The not-so-short answer involves looking at what's happening on a cellular level. Although research in the area of ageing, known as gerontology, is exciting and very promising, it is still in its infancy, and there are many theories about the primary biological basis of ageing. I say theories because, while new studies are rapidly being added to this area of science, there is still much research to be done, particularly in humans, before we are able to conclusively piece together all of the biological processes involved in ageing.

Scientists believe a central tenet of ageing is the process of something called *autophagy*, which is a cell's natural mechanism to remove unnecessary or dysfunctional components, like toxins or damaged molecules. It appears that a significant part of the ageing process is a result of cells being unable to read important epigenetic information (see Genetics and epigenetics 101 below) required for youthful gene expression.[1] When there is too much 'clutter', such as the damaged molecules mentioned above, the cell forgets how to remain youthful.

It's best to think of autophagy as a dial, where various stimuli, including what we eat, how much we eat and the timing of our meals, have the ability to turn the dial up or down. When the dial goes up, the cell shifts its focus from dividing and growing – the mechanisms of ageing – to autophagy, thus directly affecting the cell's life span. In contrast, when the dial is turned down, less house cleaning occurs and it becomes more difficult for the cell to stay young.

FIGURE 8.1:
THE AUTOPHAGY DIAL

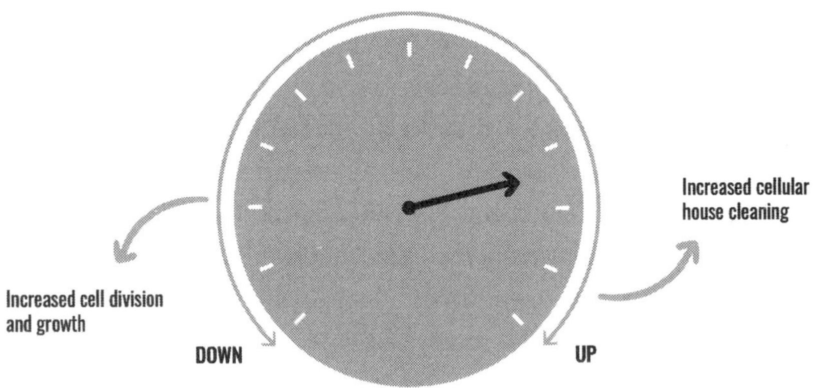

To increase our longevity, we want to explore which foods and dietary habits turn down the dial and which turn it up. We should also examine the lifestyle traits of populations who have been nurturing the biological processes responsible for optimal cellular ageing for centuries. Although understanding things at a cellular level can give you a deeper understanding about any lifestyle changes you may make, what's most important is immediately focusing on what these people, who are living proof of the impact of lifestyle on achieving a long healthy life, are doing *differently* to you, so you can appreciate just what changes to make. After all, I can almost guarantee that very few of these people understand the cellular mechanisms responsible for their own longevity.

This idea of eating like people who are living proof of longevity is not a new concept, and is in line with advice from world-leading longevity scientists such as Elizabeth Blackburn PhD, Valter Longo PhD and David Sinclair PhD. Eating more fruits, vegetables, whole grains, legumes, nuts and seeds, and good amounts of omega-3s from fish, nuts, seeds or algae, while minimising meat, dairy, eggs and refined carbohydrates, will not only improve your odds of living more years in good health, but will likely add more years to your life too.

Genetics and epigenetics 101

Epigenetics is the study of changes in organisms caused by modification of gene expression, rather than alteration of the genetic code itself. Think of your genes as instructions which tell your cells how to perform important tasks such as making proteins. Epigenetics is how your cells read those instructions. Picture epigenetics as two highlighters - a green highlighter telling your cells what to pay close attention to, and a red highlighter telling your cells what to ignore. These instructions determine which genes are turned on or off, which then determines a cell's function. It is why a liver cell is a liver cell and a brain cell is a brain cell.

When epigenetic information is lost, the cell has trouble reading its instructions. In relation to longevity, it specifically has trouble reading instructions that help the cell stay youthful.[2] Epigenetics can be influenced by a multitude of lifestyle factors including our diet, medications, UV exposure and environmental toxins, which is part of the reason why genetically identical twins can experience very different health outcomes.

Foods (and nutrients) associated with decreased life span

Animal protein

As we've seen, there are clear associations between animal protein intake and increased risk of chronic disease. Predictably, many large observational studies that have been going for decades, with subjects from all over the world, have shown that animal protein isn't our best choice if we're looking to extend our life span.[3–6] For example, a 2020 study involving more than 400,000 subjects found that swapping just 3% of calories from animal protein for plant protein lowered subjects' risk of death by 10% during the sixteen-year study period.[4] And it's not just the fact that animal protein often brings saturated fats along for the ride. Even when studies compare people consuming the same amount of saturated fats, subjects consuming more animal protein and less plant protein are still more likely to live a shorter life.[3] No wonder legumes are a hallmark of diets consumed by the longest-living populations.[7–9] In fact, the data suggests *avoiding* legumes is likely to shorten your life.[10] Given that around 70–85% of the protein in a typical Western diet is from meat, fish, dairy and eggs, this represents a big opportunity – that's an enormous amount of animal protein that can be traded for plant protein.[11]

The major reason why plant protein is thought to be favourable for our pursuit of longevity comes down to amino acids, the building blocks that make up protein. While all plants contain the nine essential amino acids that our bodies require, they have a much more optimal amino acid profile when it comes to nurturing the biological processes responsible for cellular ageing, whereas animal protein has an abundance of particular amino acids, such as methionine, that turn the autophagy dial down.[12–14] They do this by signalling to the body when consumed in plentiful quantities, 'times are good, let's focus on growing'. In contrast, when these amino acids are consumed in smaller quantities the body thinks food availability is not so good, so rather than focusing on growth it switches to 'house cleaning' mode in order to operate as efficiently as possible.

FIGURE 8.2:
FOODS ASSOCIATED WITH INCREASED AND DECREASED LIFE SPAN

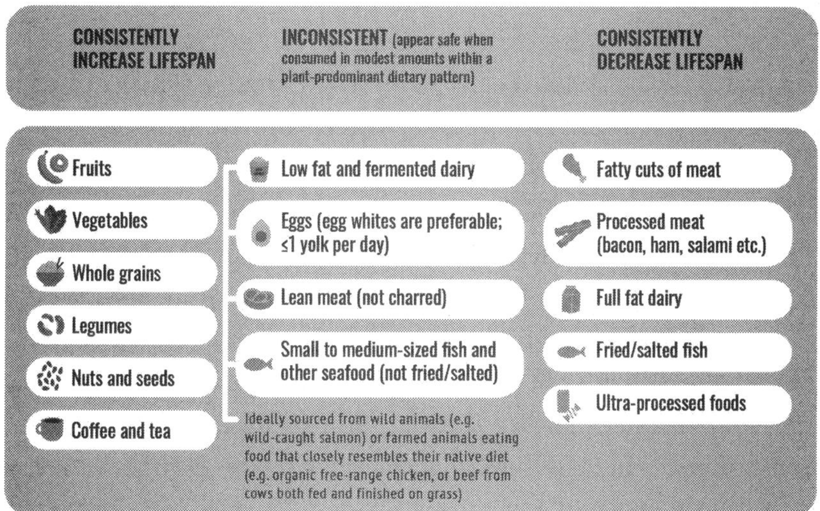

Based on findings from large observational studies and RCTs looking at individual nutrients, foods and dietary patterns.[3,4,6,15–38]

Many people claim how much you eat matters more than what you eat, but when it comes to how quickly your cells age, both are important.[39,40] While all calories are equal when it comes to energy, the same cannot be said for how you feel, your disease risk or your longevity. Where you get your protein from matters.

Science clearly shows that people choosing foods such as lentils and tofu instead of beef and eggs live longer.[3–6]

The Paleo myth

I understand the appeal of the low-carbohydrate Paleo diet at first glance – who doesn't like the idea of eating like a big, strong caveman? But when you dig into the science involved, it doesn't take long for Paleo to come unstuck.

Unlike some animals in the wild, *Homo sapiens* are not herbivorous or carnivorous. We are constitutionally omnivores, which means we are evolutionarily adapted to eat both animal- and plant-based foods. Our digestive system can process and absorb nutrients from both animal and plant matter, so we have a choice about how we fuel ourselves. Few people will argue with this idea of *Homo sapiens* being constitutionally an omnivore. Where debate begins to arise is how much animal and plant matter our ancestors ate, and how we can tell whether they were primarily hunters or gatherers.

It's generally accepted that the discovery of fire in the Stone Age, approximately 250,000 to 1.9 million years ago, by *Homo erectus*, our direct ancestor, enabled humans to consume a wider variety of foods, including root vegetables such as potatoes, carrots and beetroot and meat, and that these new, energy-dense food sources were responsible for the rapid development of the *Homo sapiens* brain that was to follow.[41] Where people disagree is whether these ancestors were eating more tubers or more meat.[42,43] Those who argue for meat lean on archaeological evidence of the remains of animal bones. This doesn't take into account that plant matter doesn't leave remains in the same way that bones do, so it's highly likely the amount of meat in the *Homo sapiens* diet has been overstated.[44-46] Realistically, the precise diet of a prehistoric human would have fluctuated according to their geographical location, the season and their level of hunting success, which would all dictate what foods were available. Whatever food they were eating, though, it was the discovery of fire and cooking that provided our ancestors with the ability to unlock more nutrition from their food, not the food itself.

Even if we accept that perhaps in certain locations meat provided more calories for *Homo erectus*, which it may well have, the modern Paleo diet seems to be a long way away from the foods traditional hunter-gatherer populations would have eaten. I'm talking about food quality. Many adopting the Paleo diet today seem to be attracted by its promises of health and vitality while still being able to consume plentiful amounts of the foods they enjoy – salami, sausage, bacon, eggs, factory-farmed grain-fed beef, etc. While the consumption of such foods may allow one to fall under the Paleo label, are they truly representative of what our ancestors ate? In short, no. These modern meats are nutritionally very different to the Stone Age meats like mammoth and antelope. These meats would have been far lower in saturated fats while being richer in unsaturated fats.[47] Typically, the meat from wild animals, often referred to as 'game', contains less than 10% of calories from fat and tiny amounts of saturated fats.[48,49] For example, 100 g of antelope contains just 0.9 g of total fat in 144 calories of meat. In comparison, for the same amount of calories, grass-fed beef today contains over ten times the amount of total fat (9.1 g), of which over 40% is saturated, while containing significantly less polyunsaturated omega-3 fats. Conventionally farmed beef fares even worse.

The other thing Paleo enthusiasts fail to consider is longevity. In the Palaeolithic era, most humans did not live long enough to experience chronic disease, thanks to high infant mortality, infectious diseases and predators. Focusing on calorie-dense foods, whether they were tubers or meat, or a combination, made sense for *Homo erectus* because they were simply eating for survival. Today, however, most people in the Western world are living longer and are more prone to chronic conditions, so a less calorie-dense, anti-inflammatory diet makes more sense so we can maintain our health for a longer period of time. Put simply, even if we did know what our Palaeolithic ancestors ate, it doesn't hold that this would automatically be the best diet for us today, because we have different goals.

Instead of looking back to the diet of our ancestors, it is more instructive to look at the science around the long-term health outcomes of modern-day humans eating different foods. How do people typically fare if they eat a diet rich in whole plants compared with those eating fewer whole plants? A diet rich in animal products compared with those eating fewer animal products? A diet rich in ultra-processed foods compared with those eating fewer ultra-processed foods? When we do this, it becomes very clear that a plant-predominant or plant-exclusive diet is the best diet for improving our chances of living a long healthy life.

Saturated fats

There are large observational studies showing us that consumption of saturated fats and trans fats are clearly associated with an increased risk of premature death.[17,50] Remember, the two major sources of saturated fats in the Western diet are dairy and red meat.[51] On the flip side, polyunsaturated and monounsaturated fats found in whole foods such as nuts, seeds and avocados are consistently associated with improved life span.[50]

Ultra-processed foods

In 2019, a study tracked nearly 20,000 Spanish subjects for fifteen years, looking at the relationship between the consumption of ultra-processed foods and premature death. Compared with those eating whole foods, subjects regularly consuming ultra-processed foods such as cookies, processed meats, muffins, doughnuts and sugar-sweetened drinks were 62% more likely to die during the fifteen year period – the most likely cause of death being cancer.[18] They found that for every additional serve of ultra-processed foods per day, there was an 18% increased risk of premature death. In 2020, a second study, this time out of Italy, with over 22,000 men and women recruited between 2005 and 2010, came to a similar conclusion.[19] The researchers from this study were able to attribute most of the increased risk of premature death seen in those eating more ultra-processed foods to higher consumption of refined sugars. So, if you are aiming for longevity, consider swapping a snack of biscuits for a handful of blueberries or nuts.

Foods (and nutrients) associated with increased life span

Dietary fibre

By now, given what we have learned about the ability of fibre to promote a healthy body weight and protect us against developing various chronic diseases, it's probably not surprising to learn that those who add more fibre to their diet also add more years to their lives.[15,24,52,53] In fact, a 2014 meta-analysis including over 1.7 million subjects showed that for every 10 g increase in fibre per day, the risk of premature death was lowered by 11%.[53] Given that fewer than 20% of Australians reach the suggested daily target for dietary fibre (28–38 g per day), this represents a great opportunity to make changes in our diet that will help us to live longer.[54] And the best place to get fibre is a wide variety of whole plant foods.

Legumes

If you take only one recommendation from this book (of course, I hope you take more than that!) it should be swapping as much as possible, preferably all, of your meat for legumes. This will instantly ramp up the amount of plant protein and fibre in your diet and improve your chances of living a longer, healthier life.[7,8]

For every 20 g per day increase in legumes, such as lentils, chickpeas and black beans, you could decrease your risk of premature death by 7–8%.[8] Just 20 g!

Fruits and vegetables

Do you want the good news first or the better news? Let's start with the good. Regular consumption of fruits and vegetables is associated with greater longevity, with a recent meta-analysis of ninety-five cohorts from around the world finding that for every 200 g increase in fruits and vegetables per day, subjects enjoyed 10% lower risk of premature death.[55] The better news? Maximum benefit was seen at 800 g per day – a 31% lower risk of premature death – with the overachievers being apples, berries, citrus fruits, cruciferous vegetables, leafy green vegetables, pears and potatoes.[55]

Nuts and seeds

There is overwhelming evidence showing nut and seed consumption is associated with a longer life.[25,26,56–59] Although nuts and seeds have often been demonised based on their calorie density, they are jam-packed with nutrition (heart-healthy unsaturated fats, fibre, vitamins, minerals and phytonutrients) and, despite what many may presume, their consumption is associated with a healthy body weight, decreased risk of chronic disease and a longer life.[25,60–61] How many serves per day or week is associated with benefit? One study that combined two cohorts with over 120,000 subjects followed for over two decades identified that, compared with subjects not eating nuts, those consuming seven or more 28 g serves per week had a 20% lower risk of premature death.[56] That is a small handful a day.

Two of my favourite nuts are walnuts and pistachios. Walnuts are rich in antioxidants – the richest of all the common types of nuts – and pistachios are a potent natural source of melatonin, a hormone that helps synchronise our sleep–wake cycle with the night and day, which is particularly beneficial for people experiencing insomnia and jet lag.[62,63]

Whole grains

Every three servings (of around 30 g each) of whole grains, such as oats, brown rice, rye, buckwheat and wild rice, was shown by a large meta-analysis of eleven observational studies to reduce the risk of premature death by 17%. This effect was observed up to a total of around seven servings per day.[36] Given that the average Australian consumes less than two serves of whole grains per day, and the average American less than one serve per day, I'm sure you will agree that this is another quick win on offer for our longevity.

Coffee and tea

One of the more frequent questions I get is, 'Is coffee healthy?' The good news for my caffeine-loving friends is that it certainly seems to be. Numerous meta-analyses of observational studies show regular consumption of coffee, up to four cups per day, is associated with reduced risk of various chronic diseases and improved life span.[28,64,65] As decaffeinated coffee is associated with similar improvements, the benefits of coffee have widely been attributed to its rich polyphenol content – molecules with antioxidant properties. In fact, in a study looking at 238 beverages, a double espresso had the highest antioxidant content – six times more than green tea and four times more than red wine.[66]

Trials conducted on mice have shown that polyphenols in coffee stimulate autophagy, providing a possible explanation for these observed findings.[67]

If you're not a fan of coffee, the good news is that the polyphenols in tea have also been shown to induce autophagy.[68] Freshly brewed green, black or matcha tea seems to be your best bet. If you want to take your tea longevity game to the next level, add some turmeric powder, which contains a potent polyphenol called curcumin, that will dial up autophagy even further.[69] *

Inconsistent foods

While there are foods that would be a valuable addition to, or deletion from, pretty much any diet, there are also some foods such as low-fat dairy and certain fish that may or may not feature within an optimal diet for human health. It's difficult to just say, 'All dairy is bad' or 'Fish is good' without understanding the context of a person's overall diet. What would these foods be replacing or displacing? For example, there's an overwhelming amount of science showing that by replacing ultra-processed foods or red meats with low-fat dairy and/or fish, you would be trading up and no doubt improving your chances of a longer, healthier life. Equally speaking, there's no solid evidence to suggest the addition of these foods (middle column of Figure 8.2) to a well-planned nutritionally adequate WFPBD would improve health outcomes

* Try adding at least one teaspoon of turmeric powder (typically contains about 200 mg of curcumin). Alternatively, make a turmeric latte using the same amount along with a few pinches of black pepper. Piperine, a compound found in black pepper, has been shown to increase the bioavailability of curcumin by 2000%![70] As curcumin is fat-soluble, I personally like to use cashew or macadamia milk (both good sources of unsaturated fats) when making a turmeric latte. Results from various clinical trials show us that two to five teaspoons of turmeric powder per day is needed to provide sufficient curcumin to experience the benefits it offers.[71–74] Hipster though they may be, turmeric lattes aren't so silly after all.

or longevity. Because of this inconsistency, you'll see some diet tribes saying they're toxic at any level and others claiming they should feature prominently within our diets, with each selecting only the data that supports their narrative. In reality, when it comes to these foods, like most things in life, the dose is likely to be the poison. As long as their inclusion in your diet is limited, and not taking you out of a whole-food plant-predominant diet (be it Paleo, keto, vegetarian or other), then we are probably splitting hairs. Based on the science we do have, if I were asked what animal products one could safely include in modest amounts within the context of a plant-predominant diet, these are the ones. Of course, to more closely approximate the types of animal products eaten by our ancestors, I would recommend sourcing these from wild animals (e.g. wild-caught salmon) or farmed animals eating food that closely resembles their native diet (e.g. organic, free-range chicken).

A good example of this is fish. A few pieces of small to medium-sized wild-caught fish a week is not going to derail the benefits of a plant-exclusive diet. The Blue Zones populations we will meet shortly and various pescetarian cohorts from large observational studies are evidence of this. At the same time, when a study with 12,654 subjects looked at which components of the Mediterranean diet improved life span, fish was not rated as 'important'. The most important dietary factors were low meat consumption and high consumption of vegetables, fruits and nuts, olive oil and legumes.[27] There are also no studies that show that the addition of fish to a nutritionally adequate WFPBD offers any extra benefit when it comes to our life span. So, while a modest amount of fish can certainly feature within a healthy dietary pattern, it seems that what matters most when it comes to increasing life span is the abundance of whole plant foods consumed with it.

Living proof of longevity

This brings me to the living proof – examples of people who eat a WFPBD and enjoy a long, healthy life span. After all, if all of this information about certain foods is true, then surely it plays out in real life. And if it's not, then surely we will see that people who live long, healthy lives eat diets rich in animal protein and/or ultra-processed foods.

Blue Zones

The Blue Zones are the locations of five populations, identified by American author Dan Buettner, that show extraordinary health and longevity.[75] They are in Okinawa (Japan), Ikaria (Greece), Nicoya (Costa Rica), Sardinia (Italy) and Loma Linda (California). People of these five populations enjoy more time in good health to do the things they love – essentially, what I am hoping this book offers you! These populations have the highest number of centenarians – people aged 100 or over – in the world, a feat a person from a Blue Zone is ten times more likely to achieve than the average American.[76]

One of the commonalities across these populations is that they all consume a plant-predominant or plant-exclusive diet.[76] While they also exhibit other healthy lifestyle choices, the remarkable similarities in the characteristics of their diets are undeniable; diets low in saturated fats and ultra-processed foods, with a focus on calories from whole plant foods and the optional inclusion of a small amount of protein from animals that themselves consumed natural diets. On average, the people in these populations who do eat meat would do so approximately five times per month, and the portion would only be about the size of a deck of cards.[76] So where do they get most of their protein from? Legumes! Soybeans, fava beans, black beans and lentils feature prominently in most centenarian diets.

Blue Zone population characteristics

- Approximately 85% or more of their calories come from plant-based foods
- They have culturally prevalent ways of reducing stress
- They perform regular, low-level exercise
- They develop close friendships with people who share a similar lifestyle
- They keep their families close
- They have life partners and invest time and love in relationships with their children.

In addition to the Blue Zones, you may have heard that Hong Kong has one of the longest-living populations in the world, with life expectancy of 81.3 years for men and 87.3 years for women. Besides comfortable weather all year round, an excellent public health system and a thirst for exercise, the Hongkongers who experience this longevity eat an Asian version of the Mediterranean diet – a diet rich in whole plant foods, and fish as their preference of animal protein due to location.[77,78] If they eat other meat, it is used to accompany dishes rather than as a meal itself – and those who consume a diet with less emphasis on meat tend to live longer.[79,80] However, based on recent data, the younger generations are beginning to be influenced by Western culture, and are eating more and more meat – since 2003, beef consumption has doubled – and as a population, they now have one of the highest rates of colorectal cancer in the world.[81–83]

As we covered in Chapter 6, with the study comparing the gut health of native Africans with African Americans, we know that a diet that emphasises meat is bad for gut health and heightens our risk of colon cancer. Given that this change in the Hong Kong diet is as recent as the last few decades, chances are their mortality rates and life expectancy will begin to change as the generation who have made these changes becomes elderly. This is similar to the 'French paradox' identified by researchers in the early 1980s.[84] Researchers were amazed to find that despite consistent findings from forty other countries to the contrary, the French consumed high amounts of saturated fats and had a relatively low incidence of heart disease. What the researchers didn't pick up on at the time was that the French had only recently increased the amount of saturated fats in their diet, in the 1970s, so the effects of this change were therefore yet to play out.[85] Quite simply, French people hadn't been eating a diet rich in saturated fats for long enough to clog their arteries. Marion Nestle PhD famously termed this the *time-lag effect*.[86]

Meat versus plants for longevity

What about observational studies that compare the life spans of people within the same population who eat varying amounts of animal and plant foods?

On the whole, people eating high-quality plant-based diets tend to outlive people whose diets are centred on animal foods. There are three major meta-analyses that combine data from the well-known observational cohorts looking at populations with subjects that adopt different dietary patterns.[87–89] Each of these analyses demonstrate the benefits to adopting a diet that limits animal products, specifically beef and poultry. Unsurprisingly, the reduction in risk associated with a plant-based diet is highly dependent on how well it is adopted. For example, while there appears to be no difference in premature death risk between British vegetarians and non-vegetarians, the vegans, vegetarians and pescetarians in the AHS-2 cohort had significantly less risk (12%) of premature death than those eating just small amounts of meat.[32,90] This is a reminder that the removal of animal products from your diet is not automatically healthful – it must make room for the consumption of whole plant foods.[91] Swapping bacon or pizza for doughnuts isn't really what we're after! If you make the swap to whole plant foods, the results will speak for themselves. Compared with the general US population, vegetarian Adventists (vegetarians, vegans and pescetarians) from Loma Linda, California, who also regularly exercise and do not smoke, enjoy around ten to fourteen extra years of life.[92,93]

Even though British vegetarians seem to have a less healthy diet compared with the American Adventist vegetarians, when researchers looking at the EPIC-Oxford cohort removed subjects who had jumped back and forth between diets during the observation period, they found vegans and vegetarians had a 14% lower risk of dying before the age of seventy-five and an 8% lower risk of dying before the age of ninety.[90] This lines up with the results from a large review of six vegetarian cohorts from around the world, which found those following a vegetarian diet for more than seventeen years lived almost four years longer than short-term vegetarians.[94] These results speak to the fact that the longevity benefits of adopting a plant-based diet are compounding, and lie in how well one can adhere to a diet centred around the consumption of plant foods in the long-term.[94] Rather than looking at it as a diet for a few years, if you're looking to add years to your life, it needs to become a lifestyle you can sustain.

While we'll never get a long-term RCT that allows us to clearly see the difference between optimally planned dietary patterns over complete life spans, one of the longer RCTs we have is the PREDIMED trial, as discussed in Chapter 5. You may recall that when researchers doubled back and looked a little closer at the way the subjects were eating, those who were consuming more whole plant foods and fewer animal foods (including less fish), a 'pro-vegetarian' diet as they labelled it, had 41% lower risk of dying during the course of the five-year trial.[35]

'But my grandmother lived to ninety-seven, and she ate whatever she wanted, smoked regularly and drank often'

We've all heard a story like this one! And I won't deny that it is possible for someone like this to live a long life and not experience chronic disease. Of course it's possible; it's just not *probable*. These anecdotal cases are not proof that drinking, smoking and poor diet are not risk factors for disease. All it proves is that occasionally, for the extreme minority, the human body can be incredibly resilient. This person got lucky and lived a long life in spite of their lifestyle, not because of it.

These outliers are also explained in the scientific literature. The simple fact is that for every outlier, there are significantly more people who could adopt the same lifestyle behaviours and experience terrible disease and shorter life spans.

FIGURE 8.3:

LIVING TO 97 IS POSSIBLE, BUT NOT PROBABLE

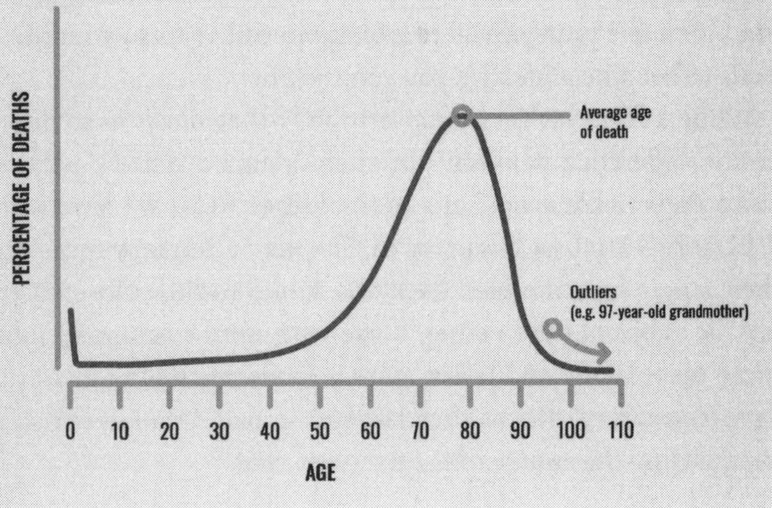

At the end of the day, your chances of being an outlier are slim, and adopting healthy lifestyle habits is clearly the safer bet. Even if it does turn out that you are genetically protected, a healthy lifestyle is only going to provide additional benefit. Imagine how long this hypothetical grandmother might have lived if her lifestyle hadn't included these known risk factors!

Low-carb or high-carb for longevity?

When it comes to life span, what we have previously seen on the question of carbohydrates holds true: the source of the nutrients we consume is of far greater importance than the macronutrient ratio of our diet.[95,96] A preference for unsaturated over saturated fats, plant protein over animal protein, and unrefined carbohydrates over refined carbohydrates matters more than the amount of carbohydrates in your diet. When you get all or most of your calories from fruits, vegetables, whole grains, legumes, nuts and seeds, the ratio looks after itself.

How much and when we eat

One of the most well studied mechanisms known to both improve health span and prolong the life of an organism is calorie restriction (CR) without malnutrition, which means consuming fewer calories than you habitually would without being deprived of essential nutrients.[97,98] It's believed the stress of CR activates autophagy. The first evidence of this was actually observed in yeast, where researchers saw that CR could increase the life span of yeast by two to three times.[99] Scientists found similar effects in mice that were fed a CR diet of 20–50% fewer calories than their daily requirement without malnutrition, and then lived 1.5 times their expected life span.[97]

But that's mice. Although their biological, genetic and

behavioural characteristics resemble those of humans, these studies provided a scientific model for further enquiry. Researchers from University of Wisconsin randomised seventy-six adult rhesus monkeys into two groups: a control group that maintained their current diet and a CR group that consumed 30% fewer calories than their maintenance level within a diet that ensured nutritional adequacy was achieved. The monkeys allocated to the CR group ate almost all of their daily calories in a single meal, which means they were essentially fasting for the rest of the day. Over twenty years, researchers were able to clearly see that CR delayed the development of age-related diseases such as diabetes, cardiovascular disease and cancer, and produced significantly better brain preservation and survival. In fact, over the course of the twenty years, 37% of the monkeys in the control group died while only 13% in the CR group died.[100,101]

We've seen this play out in Blue Zone populations that naturally consume a high-quality, nutrient-dense, calorie-restricted diet. In the Ikarian Blue Zone population in Greece, for example, most elderly people are free of chronic disease and typically enjoy eight more years of life than the average American.[76] For around 200 days of the year, Ikarians perform CR as part of their traditional religious practices. During these periods, they adopt an essentially vegetarian diet by removing energy-dense animal products from their diet.[102]

The Blue Zone population in Okinawa, Japan, home to the longest-living women in the world, is another example of life span promotion through CR.[103] Okinawans are four to five times more likely to reach the age of 100 than people in other industrialised nations, and compared with Americans have a 40% lower chance of dying from cancer and 80% lower chance of dying from heart disease.[97,104] In addition to eating a largely whole-food vegetarian diet (in which fewer than 1% of calories come from meat and over 95% of calories come from whole plant foods, mainly purple sweet potato, whole grains and legumes), these Okinawans also inadvertently practised CR.[29]

In Okinawan culture, the phrase 'hara hachi bu' is an instruction that means to finish eating your meal when you are 80% full. Physiologically, this allows for the fact that it takes about twenty minutes for your body to digest the food that you have eaten in order for you to feel 100% full. As a result, the Japanese from Okinawa following the traditional diet would consume approximately 300 fewer calories per day than Japanese from other regions, and on average fall into a 10–15% calorie deficit.[97,105]

If you practice hara hachi bu and push your plate away before you are full, or eat smaller serving sizes than you are used to, you are allowing for this delayed sense of fullness – something we do poorly in Western populations. And of course, like the Okinawans, the fewer animal products on that plate, the better, to promote longevity from two angles.

You may be thinking, *How am I going to adopt a CR diet long-term?* And, look, I agree. While for some this may be achievable without affecting their enjoyment of life, it will be unrealistic or a significant burden for others, particularly those who do not want to lose weight or muscle mass, or have a history of disordered eating.[106] Fortunately, the science also shows that going without food for a period of time turns on our autophagy even in the absence of weight loss.[106–109] In fact, adopting such practices may be just as beneficial or potentially even better when it comes to preventing disease and slowing down ageing, largely owing to greater adherence.[110,111] Scientists believe these periods of prolonged 'wanting', often referred to today as fasting, create a similar micro-stress to sustained CR. This healthy micro-stress is a form of *hormesis*, a scientific name for the idea that anything that doesn't kill you makes you stronger.[112]

Remember, autophagy is a dial, and one way of turning that dial up is by being hungry. Autophagy certainly increases during a caloric deficit and weight loss, but it's also possible to have periods of hunger and therefore times when autophagy is turned up within the context of a diet that is providing enough calories to maintain or even gain weight.[108] You just need to eat enough calories outside of the fasting window to ensure that your energy balance stays at an equilibrium or surplus. Preferably, with as much of these calories coming from whole plant foods as possible.

If you think about the history of *Homo sapiens*, this makes complete sense. It is only recently that we have had constant access to food and have made a habit of eating from the moment we wake to the moment we go to sleep. What we call fasting would have been a normal part of life for our ancestors. While it would be nearly impossible to reliably replicate *what* our ancestors ate, it's a different story when it comes to replicating *when* they ate.[101]

Eating stressed-out plants

There's a whole body of research surrounding what are called *CR or fasting mimetics*. Essentially, some plant compounds mimic the action of CR and fasting by creating healthy doses of micro-stress that activate disease resistance and longevity pathways.[113] This type of hormesis is called *xenohormesis*, and these molecules are part of the plant's natural defence mechanism. The emerging school of thought is that where possible, we want to eat fruits and vegetables that are grown under imperfect, organic conditions – exposed to insects, sun, wind, etc.[114] Ones that had to naturally defend themselves are more likely to be richer in these compounds. So what are these molecules, and what foods are they found in?[115,116]

- Curcumin (found in turmeric)
- Resveratrol (found in grapes, cocoa, blueberries, and red wine)

- Catechins (found in green tea, matcha, apples, dark chocolate and red wine)
- Sulphoraphane (found in cruciferous vegetables)
- lignan (found in flaxseeds, whole grains and sesame seeds)
- Quercetin (found in berries, cherries, apples, red wine, tomatoes and citrus fruits).

This might just be one of the keys to the Okinawans' longevity. When 138 foods from Okinawa were compared with the same foods from elsewhere in Japan, those in Okinawa were grown under more stressful conditions and were much higher in these phytonutrients.[117] So, if you can, try to find local suppliers who grow their produce under more natural conditions, or grow your own, and don't be put off by the fact organic produce doesn't always look as perfect as conventional fruit and veg.

Earlier I mentioned the study with the rhesus monkeys that showed calorie restriction improved the health of the monkeys and prolonged their life.[100] However, when a similar study was conducted in almost identical conditions, no benefit in life span was observed in the monkeys eating a CR diet.[118] While these conflicting findings may seem confusing, the different outcomes are thought to be explained by the studies' unique feeding protocols. In the study that found the increased life span, the monkeys ate almost all of their calories in their morning meal, whereas in the study that found no benefit, the monkeys ate twice a day. In other words, it was only the monkeys that were fasting, and therefore experienced periods of hunger, that lived longer.[101]

Today, there are many highly publicised fasting protocols or 'diets'. The most common forms are time-restricted eating (in which you typically eat within an eight- to twelve-hour window every day), the 5:2 diet (meaning five days of normal eating per week and two days restricted to around 500–600 calories) and alternate-day fasting (with a 500–600 calorie day every other day).[119] We'll talk more about what the best available science says about meal timing in Part Three, so you can add it as a tool in your toolbox if it is right for you. For now, though, it's worth noting that the degree of benefit derived from fasting will largely come down to the foods in a person's diet. Fasting with a diet that emphasises calories from whole plant foods is likely to be much more effective for slowing ageing and age-related diseases than a diet that is rich in meat, dairy and eggs.[107]

On the whole, what's important to take away here is that having periods of wanting within the context of a nutritionally adequate plant-predominant or plant-exclusive diet is beneficial for activating your longevity genes. It's okay to feel a little bit hungry from time to time, which in a world of food abundance is not something we are used to but is something we should become more comfortable with. The best part? It is absolutely free and you can start today!

Telomeres and ageing

One of the more studied hallmarks of ageing is attrition, or shortening, of our telomeres. In recent years, the science of telomeres has been documented by Nobel Prize winner Elizabeth Blackburn PhD and her team.[120] To learn the basics of telomeres, we need to understand a few fundamental parts of living cells. Our genes are contained within chromosomes, which are in long strands like a shoelace. Now, just like your shoelace, at the ends there are two caps that stop everything from unravelling. These are your telomeres.

Telomeres are important because they are representative of our biological age.[121] As our cells age, our telomeres become shorter in a process called telomere attrition.[122]

As our telomeres shorten, we become more susceptible to developing diseases such as cardiovascular disease, various cancers, dementia and depression.[123-126] What's fascinating is that just as there are ways to switch on autophagy, there are ways to stop telomere attrition and, in some cases, reverse it. If a person can slow down the rate at which their telomeres are shortening, they can literally slow down the ageing process.

Diet is one of the ways telomere attrition can be slowed down. Several studies show greater adherence to Mediterranean-type diets is associated with longer telomeres.[127-129] Specifically, Dr Blackburn and her team recommend a diet rich in whole plant foods and omega-3 supplements, with less meat and ultra-processed foods.[120]

Of course, there are other healthy lifestyle practices that can increase the length of your telomeres, one of the most powerful being exercise. Exercise can protect telomeres from the negative ageing effects of chronic stress – yet another reason to move every day.[130] Just fifteen minutes of vigorous exercise per day is associated with longer telomeres. When we zoom back out, this stacks up – a 2014 meta-analysis of studies looking at cardiovascular fitness, body weight and life span found exercise to be a better predictor of a long, healthy life than body weight.[131] While maintaining a BMI in the normal range is incredibly important to healthy ageing, so is our level of fitness.

The elixir of youth

While we wait for a scientific breakthrough and a magic anti-ageing pill to help us wind back the clock, the closest thing we have today to an elixir of youth is a healthy lifestyle that naturally slows down the biological ageing process. There's no reason you can't be fifty-five but feel forty, or be eighty-five but feel sixty-five – you just have to create a lifestyle conducive to prolonging cell life. Such a lifestyle should include eating a diet in which all or most calories come from whole plant foods and rich sources of polyphenols (such as berries, coffee and tea), calorie restriction and/or regular periods of wanting (fasting) without malnutrition, maintaining a healthy body weight, regular daily exercise, about seven hours of good sleep every night, good social support and friendships, and strategies to avoid chronic stress.[63]

Now that we have seen it's entirely possible to increase the years of your life and the life in your years, think about what makes this important to you. What do you want to do with that extra time? Ultimately, whatever you decide will be part of the driving force behind your decision to live a healthier lifestyle.

CHAPTER 9

The optimal diet for all life on the planet

When I first became passionate about diet and food, discovering that a plant-based diet in which all or most calories are derived from whole plant foods is the optimal diet for human health was enough for me to change to a plant-exclusive diet. I chose to go 'all in' because with my personality, trying to limit myself to small amounts of animal products would have likely seen me fall back into my old habits of a diet that focused on meat as the star of the plate. When it's off the menu, it's much simpler to stay on track – for me anyway. Looking back, however, I now know that I had a somewhat narrow view of health, and there was an arguably more important reason to adopt a plant-exclusive diet. Once I understood the concept of planetary health – a concept that explains the inextricable link between our health and that of the planet – I saw that my definitions of *health* and the *optimal diet* needed expanding. This concept was born out of the realisation that 'human health and human civilisation depend on flourishing natural systems and the wise stewardship of those natural systems'.[1] The problem is, we humans haven't been the greatest stewards.

By almost all measures, human progress in the past century or so has been formidable. At a global level, we are living longer than ever before, rates of poverty have steadily declined, and more of the world has access to education than at any point in history. In the process, however, we have collectively abused our planet and its resources. We have emitted reckless amounts of greenhouse gases (GHGs) into our atmosphere, poisoned waterways, degraded soils, and cleared old-growth forests and their fauna to make space for our cities, industries and agriculture.[2–4] This has led to the current climate crisis and the unquestionable abnormalities we are witnessing in catastrophic weather events, rising air and ocean temperatures, and widespread melting of snow and ice, leading to rising sea levels.[5] And while this crisis is by no means just about the food we eat, our agricultural system is a significant contributor.

Before I became aware of this, my ethos had been shaped by nutrition science alone. But now I asked, what good is a healthy diet if we cannot survive on a planet threatened by climate change? We simply cannot be healthy without the planet on which we are dependent also being healthy. With this in mind, I once again began to research, this time focusing on a single question: what is the optimal diet that we can adopt to preserve our ecosystem and help mitigate the existential threat posed by climate change and environmental degradation? What I found proves our interconnectedness with Mother Earth: according to the best available environmental science, the diet that is great for human health is also great for all life on the planet. We can curb chronic disease and heal our planet all at once. The science is so clear that independent of their own diets, scientists from around the world conducting and reviewing environmental science have acknowledged that the cheapest, easiest, fastest and most effective action that can be taken on a personal level to help mitigate climate change, restore biodiversity and save freshwater is to shift to a plant-predominant or plant-exclusive diet.[1,6–9] But time is running out, so we have to move quickly.

The importance of a plant-based diet for planetary health was beautifully summarised by the EAT-*Lancet* Commission in 2019 – a collaboration between thirty-seven world-leading doctors, scientists and food systems experts backed by both the United Nations Intergovernmental Panel on Climate Change (IPCC) and *The Lancet*, one of the most highly regarded academic journals in the world. This commission worked to determine how we will feed a population of 10 billion people by 2050 within nine 'planetary boundaries' – meaning the sustainable limits of systems and processes like climate change, freshwater use and biodiversity loss, to preserve the Earth for future generations.[10]

The consensus of the commission was that we *can* achieve a future where people's health and the environment are not irreversibly damaged, but to do so, we will need to significantly change our food systems and the way we eat, including halving all food waste. They describe this as a 'Great Food Transformation'. The report states, 'Transformation to healthy diets by 2050 will require substantial dietary shifts. Global consumption of fruits, vegetables, nuts and legumes will have to double, and consumption of foods such as red meat and sugar will have to be reduced by more than 50%. A diet rich in plant-based foods and with fewer animal source foods confers both improved health and environmental benefits.'[11]

FIGURE 9.1:
EAT-*LANCET* COMMISSION PLANETARY HEALTH PLATE

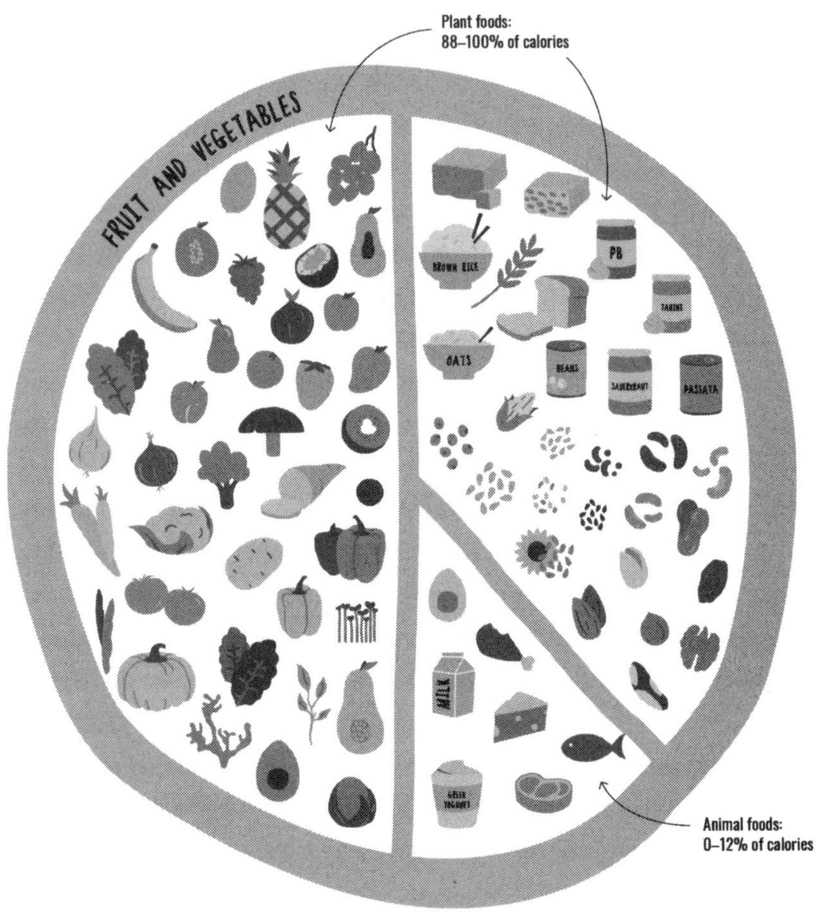

Adapted from the EAT-*Lancet* Commission on Healthy Diets From Sustainable Food Systems[10]

If the entire world were to shift to this diet, we would cut at least a quarter of the world's GHG emissions while simultaneously improving all other measures of planetary health at the same time.[12,13] Adopting this diet and halving our food waste would be equivalent to the GHG reduction that would be achieved by removing 2.7 billion cars from the road,[14] approximately double the cars on planet Earth today. That's no small feat.

You may be wondering, why didn't the EAT-*Lancet* Commission simply recommend a plant-exclusive diet for everyone? The aim of their report wasn't to necessarily state what is optimal for planetary health, but to provide a solution that, if widely adopted by people all over the world from different cultures and with different levels of food access, would ensure both climate goals and improvements in human health. As such, they recommended a diet that consists of 88% or more calories from whole plant foods, allowing room for a modest amount of animal products. However, it's worth noting that a 2019 meta-analysis comparing the environmental impact of various dietary patterns, the most comprehensive analysis of its kind to date, identified that a plant-exclusive diet consisting of fruits, vegetables, whole grains, legumes, nuts and seeds in their whole or minimally processed form is the single best dietary pattern for the planet.[15]

Global warming is a threat to life on Earth

Before we look at the science that led the EAT-*Lancet* Commission and other experts to these conclusions, we should address the scientific consensus behind global warming in order to appreciate what we are trying to avoid through making changes to what we eat. This is one of the biggest issues facing the world today and its importance cannot be overstated.[16]

A note on the science

While there are a number of ideological viewpoints on climate change, there is really only one *scientific* position. The figures below are backed up by the highest level of research and academia. They were sourced from the

International Energy Agency, the IPCC, the Food and Agriculture Organization of the United Nations (FAO) and other United Nations organisations, and large peer-reviewed studies published in world-leading academic journals such as *Science*.

Our planet is surrounded by atmosphere, which largely acts as a greenhouse, just like one you'd have in your backyard if you lived in a cold climate and needed a temperature-controlled environment to grow veggies. In this atmosphere are gases – greenhouse gases (GHGs), to be precise – which effectively trap the heat coming from the sun and make our planet inhabitable. The *greenhouse effect* is vital to life on Earth, maintaining temperatures that allow the species that live here to survive. Without it, our planet would be freezing. However, if the amount of these gases in our atmosphere rises above normal levels, then too much heat is trapped and the planet warms beyond optimal levels – a phenomenon known as *global warming*. This is precisely what's happening today.

While global warming is very much a modern human problem, the scene was set a long time ago. During the Neolithic era, approximately 8000 years ago, humans started clearing forests and domesticating animals for the first time, unknowingly releasing carbon dioxide (CO_2), nitrous oxide and methane, the three major GHGs in the atmosphere today.[17–20] This change in human activity paved the way for a future in which humans were responsible for atmospheric greenhouse gas concentrations well above levels that would have otherwise naturally occurred.

In the 1700s came the Industrial Revolution – a time when we started burning an extraordinary amount of fossil fuels like coal, oil and gas to power our modern industries, homes and cars, and we intensified animal agriculture. While atmospheric CO_2 has naturally gone up and down over the course of history, as you can see in Figure 9.2, it had never exceeded 300 particles of CO_2 per million particles of air (ppm) until after this period of industrialisation. Today, it sits above 400 ppm.[21–24]

FIGURE 9.2:

ATMOSPHERIC CO_2 LEVELS OVER THE PAST 800,000 YEARS

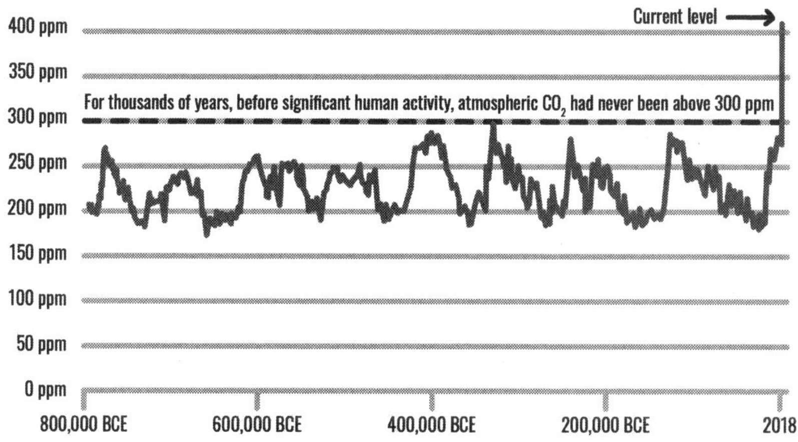

Adapted from Our World in Data[21]

In the same time period, levels of methane and nitrous oxide, GHGs that are significantly more potent than CO_2, have also increased substantially (Figures 9.3 and 9.4).[25–27]

FIGURE 9.3:
METHANE LEVELS SINCE THE PRE-INDUSTRIAL ERA

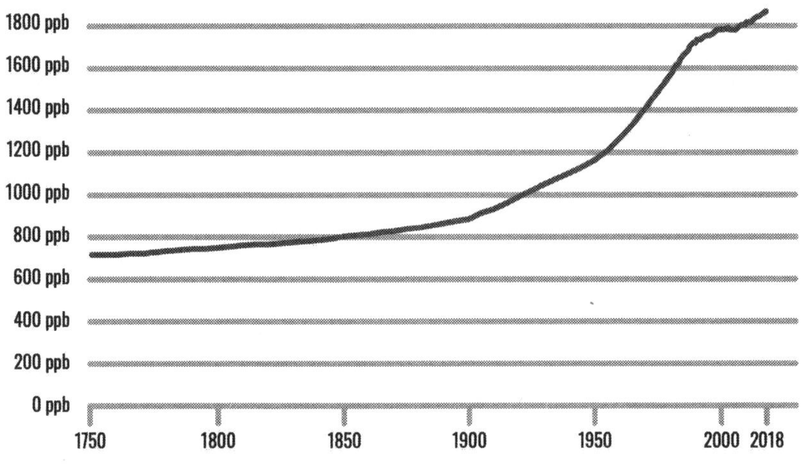

Adapted from Our World in Data[26]

FIGURE 9.4:
NITROUS OXIDE LEVELS SINCE THE PRE-INDUSTRIAL ERA

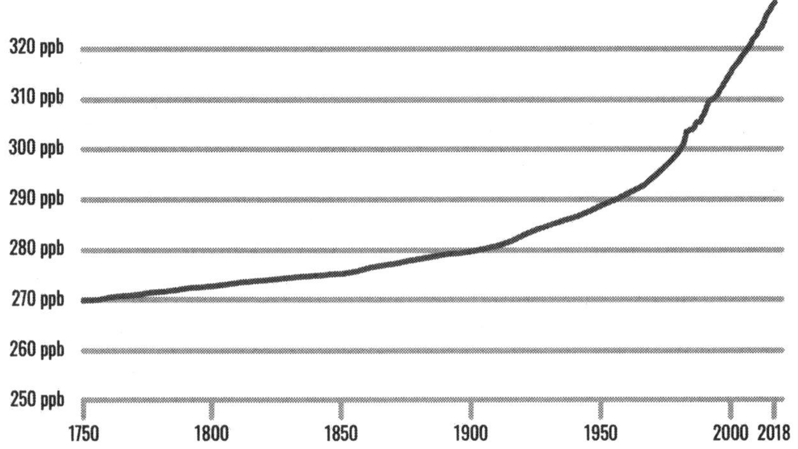

Adapted from Our World in Data[26]

While these statistics are interesting, what's most important is how they have affected the average temperature of our planet, and what that means for us. Since pre-industrial times, our planet has warmed roughly 1–1.2°C.[21,28] As you can see in Figure 9.5, most of this increase has occurred in the past few decades, as our population has exploded and our energy and food requirements have greatly increased.

FIGURE 9.5:

AVERAGE GLOBAL TEMPERATURE INCREASE ABOVE PRE-INDUSTRIAL LEVELS

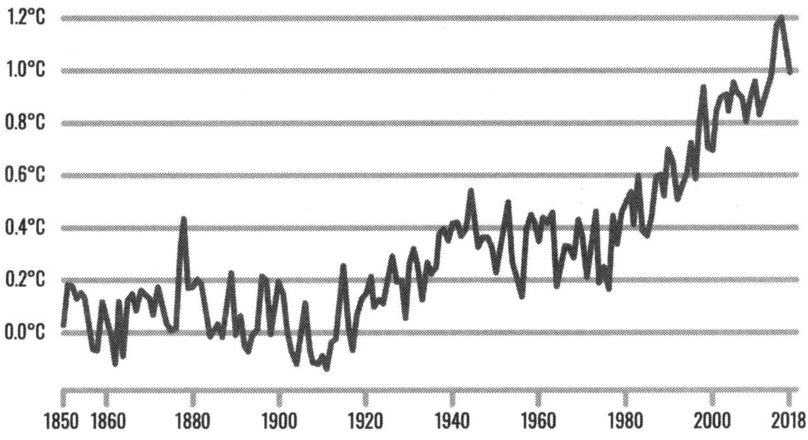

Adapted from Our World in Data[21]

These numbers might sound small, but their effects are truly frightening. The Paris Agreement, which was signed by world leaders in 2015 to pledge their united fight against climate change, aims to limit warming to 1.5–2°C above pre-industrial levels.[29] Climate change is literally a matter of degrees! Even at these temperatures, climate experts expect we will experience:

- deadly heatwaves
- extreme precipitation in some parts of the world and severe drought in others

- food and water shortages in developed countries
- increased deforestation and wildfires
- more ocean 'dead zones' – areas of the ocean that no longer support aquatic life
- all coral reefs 70–90% deteriorated at 1.5°C, and non-existent at 2°C
- climate refugees
- huge global economic implications.[30]

According to the best available climate modelling, published by the IPCC, which looked at more than 6000 independent resources, we can avoid this if we choose to, but we only have until 2030 to change our ways and limit the Earth's warming to 1.5°C.[31,32] However, warming doesn't occur evenly around the planet. Many parts of the world are already experiencing average temperatures above 1.5°C.[30] In other words, climate change is already here.

Should we fail to act, continued warming at the current rate will see a rise in average global temperatures of at least 3–5°C by 2100.[33,34] A 3°C increase could bring 'outright chaos' to our societies, sparking a global water crisis, causing flooding of entire regions and provoking a widespread failure in our global food production. A warming of 4°C could result in a reduction of the human population by 80–90%, largely due to regular heatwaves with temperatures exceeding 55°C. Above that, the temperature would simply become incompatible with human life.[34]

Focusing on energy alone is not enough to reach net zero

Given the attention that is paid to the energy sector in conversations about climate change, you may be surprised to learn that agriculture ties with the production of electricity as major contributors to global warming. Together, these two are responsible for around 50% of the world's GHG emissions.[35] It's true that if we are to limit global warming, we must find ways to power our lives and industries through greener sources of energy, like the sun and wind, rather than with fossil fuels such as coal or gas.[36] Having said that, focusing on energy alone won't be enough to help us stay under a 3-4°C warming scenario. Just as we need to move to green energy, we need to move to green food. If countries address CO_2 emissions from fossil fuels but meat and dairy consumption continues to grow, animal agriculture could take up almost half of the allowable GHG budget for the 1.5°C threshold of warming by the year 2030.[37] To meet the goals set out in the Paris Agreement and reach *net zero*, a point where GHG emissions from human activity are balanced by an equal amount of natural carbon removal, will require changes to the way we eat.[21,38,39]

What we eat matters

What is it about plant-based foods that make them such an integral part of our fight against global warming? To answer this question, we need to zoom in on two fundamental aspects of agriculture – the amount of land required to grow certain foods and the amount of GHGs that the production of different foods is responsible for.

Our food and greenhouse gas emissions

It is estimated that the cumulative emissions generated by agriculture, forestry and other land use account for 21–37% of the world's yearly global emissions.[40] This large share of emissions is primarily driven by an increase in both agricultural emissions from livestock and from deforestation, which is itself driven by the livestock sector's growing need for land.[41] When you add up the carbon-generating inputs required by animal farming (e.g. feed production), the methane produced by these animals as they digest their food, and the nitrous oxide produced by decomposing manure, the 1.4 billion livestock that are on the planet at any one time are alone said to be directly responsible for at least 14.5% of global emissions each year.[23,36,42,43]

While it's true that GHG emissions from animal agriculture in developed nations like Australia and the United States are moderately lower than the global average of 14.5%, this should not be confused with the idea that people in these countries are eating a more environmentally friendly diet. A lower percentage does not mean lower total emissions. All this really tells us is that developed nations are burning far more fossil fuels for things like electricity, transportation and industry, than developing nations, where agriculture makes up a greater share of their total emissions because of the lower demand for fossil fuels.

The methane myth

You may have heard, perhaps from those involved in animal agriculture, that methane is less of a worry for climate change than CO_2, because while each CO_2 molecule released into the atmosphere has a life span of 100 years, a methane molecule only lasts twelve years. This might sound convincing, but it fails to take into account that over a 100-year period, each molecule of methane is twenty-eight times more powerful at warming our atmosphere than CO_2, and twelve years doesn't matter as much as the fact that we continue to replace whatever methane falls out of the atmosphere with more and more, year after year.[27] The total amount grows regardless of what amount might be falling out.[44,45]

On the flip side, the short life span of methane molecules means we could clear a large amount of this highly potent GHG from our atmosphere in just twelve years if we completely stopped, or at least dramatically reduced, the human activities responsible for methane emissions. This represents an enormous opportunity for tackling the climate emergency.[46]

No matter where you pull your data from, or whether you look at per unit of food or per unit of protein, the simple fact is plant agriculture results in significantly fewer GHG emissions than animals raised for food.[15,47–53] Figure 9.6 is based on perhaps the most comprehensive summary of the data we have available today, a 2018 study from a group of researchers at Oxford University who compiled data on the environmental impact of different foods from around 38,700 farms in 119 countries, including Australia and New Zealand, the largest study of its kind to date.[49,54] Red meat and dairy are clearly responsible for the most emissions: producing 100 g of protein from beef is responsible for more than 113 times more GHG emissions than producing 100 g of protein from peas.[54] With findings like this, it's no surprise that a 2020 study published in the journal *Global Environmental Change*, analysing the environmental footprint of specific dietary patterns in 140 countries, identified that a plant-exclusive diet reduces GHG emissions by 70% compared with the typical omnivorous diet.[52]

When it comes to GHG emissions, even the least sustainable plant-based foods are still significantly more sustainable than the best environmentally performing animal-based food products – even almonds and avocados.[7,55,56]

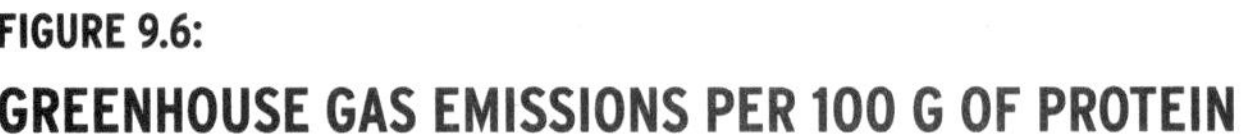

FIGURE 9.6:
GREENHOUSE GAS EMISSIONS PER 100 G OF PROTEIN

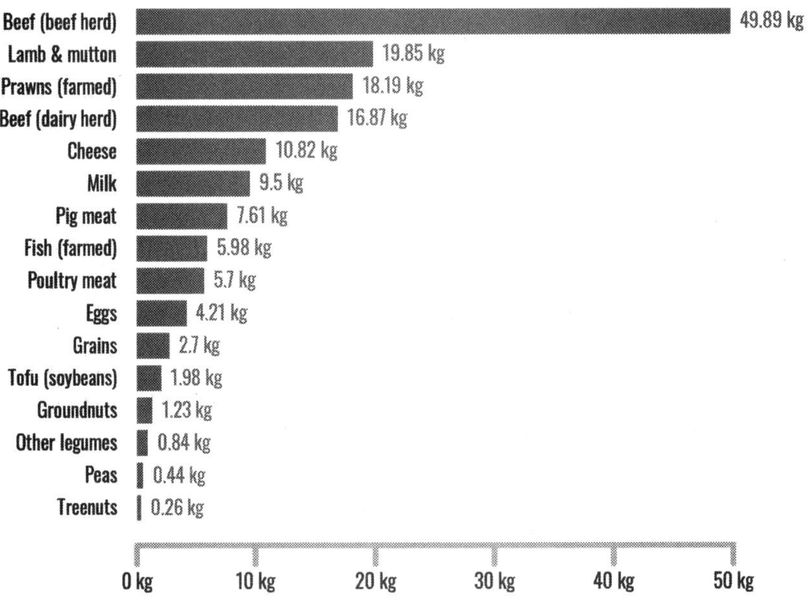

* Carbon dioxide, methane and nitrous oxide combined to form a single measure (kg CO_2 equivalents) of GHGs associated with the supply of that food.
Adapted from Our World in Data[54]

No, cows can't save the planet

We will see the world's population swell to about 10 billion people by 2050. Our challenge lies in feeding more people than ever before in a way that substantially reduces the emissions generated by global food systems.

To achieve this, many proposals and ideas have been put forward across the world. One of these is the concept of regenerative agriculture, which is a principle of farming that seeks to nurture ecosystem services and produce food in a way that is not just sustainable, but regenerative. At its heart, regenerative agriculture seeks to restore health to dying soils, enhance biodiversity and make crops more resilient to droughts. These principles apply to both plant agriculture and pastoralism. The latter form, which is most commonly referred to as *regenerative* or *holistic grazing* (a particular method of rotating livestock over pasture), has garnered increasing international attention, with its proponents stating that it should be seen as a key solution to climate change, and essentially a reason for people to double down on their consumption of red meat.[57]

While this form of animal husbandry is arguably better for soil quality and a step in the right direction when compared with more intensive forms of animal agriculture, the largest meta-analysis looking at animal grazing and climate change to date, *Grazed and Confused* by the Food Climate Research Network, found that, despite anecdotal claims, it is still very much a net CO_2 emitting practice.[44,45] Even though specific forms of grazing can help sequester CO_2 in the soil, the practice as a whole emits significantly more GHGs than it stores.

Furthermore, what's often conveniently left out of this conversation is that any shift towards holistic grazing, away from the significantly more efficient intensive practice of factory farming, would mean a dramatic reduction in overall meat supply of around 75% or more.[58] Based on basic supply and demand, this would see the prices of animal products like beef and eggs rise dramatically. If we maintained the same budget we had been using to buy such foods and made a decision to only support regenerative farms that were not decimating our planet, we would naturally consume just a fraction of the animal products we do today. In other words, by taking a stand against intensive animal agriculture and supporting holistic grazing, you are inadvertently advocating for a transition to plant-predominant diets.[59]

The bottom line is that, yes, holistic grazing may be better than factory farming, but presenting it as the answer to global warming is greenwashing and clearly a last-ditch attempt to keep meat relevant. It's not a silver bullet climate solution and is a distraction from what matters most: people eating more plants.[59]

Our food affects the natural world's ability to draw down carbon

It's not just the direct emissions from animal agriculture that deserve our attention. This industry is causing our planet to warm in a more indirect manner too, through taking away Earth's natural carbon sinks and reducing its biodiversity.

Producing animal-based food products at a mass scale for human consumption is a highly inefficient process, one that requires considerably more land compared with growing plant-based foods (Figure 9.7).[49] As an example, to produce an equal amount of protein, seventy-four times more land is required for beef compared with tofu.[60] Seventy-four times! That's a tremendous amount of land across the globe that, if restored to its natural state, could be sequestering CO_2 out of our atmosphere (see 'Forests cool our planet' below).[61,62] This is one of the major reasons that the emissions from animal agriculture are still widely debated, with many climate scientists suggesting that they are 39–90% underestimated, largely because calculations fail to comprehensively account for this carbon opportunity cost.[63,64] While we often just assume that grasslands are meant for livestock grazing, much of this land was originally forests that were cleared for agriculture.[65–67] When looking at the carbon footprint of foods that come from such land, we have to factor in not only direct emissions related to each food type, but also the fact that forests are far more powerful than pasture at pulling carbon out of the atmosphere and securely storing it.[68]

FIGURE 9.7:

LAND USE PER 100 G OF PROTEIN

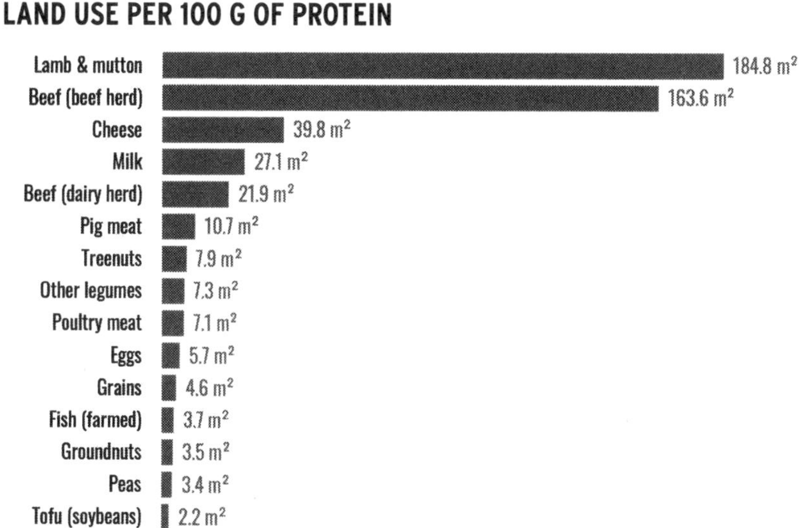

Adapted from Our World in Data[69]

To give you an idea of just how inefficient producing animal foods is the FAO states the animal agriculture industry takes up over 75% of all land dedicated to food production across the world, yet only provides 18% of the world's calories and 37% of the world's total protein.[49,69,70] If that's not staggering enough, every year approximately 72 billion farmed land animals are sent to slaughter – about 200 million per day – in order to provide milk, eggs and meat for human consumption.[71] To make room for these animals, 83% of wild animals have been killed off, to the point where today just 4% of all land mammals on Earth are wild, with 36% being human and the remaining 60% being livestock that we exploit.[72]

The problem is that humans are reliant on Earth's biodiversity. Wild animals are crucial to nourishing our soil, drawing down carbon from the atmosphere, preventing wildfires and generally creating a more resilient environment that can adapt to changes in our climate.[73–76] So reliant are we on this biodiversity that many environmental researchers are calling for *trophic rewilding*, a strategy where livestock are replaced with wild herbivores such as rhinos, horses, donkeys, zebras and kangaroos, that emit significantly less methane while helping to restore the surrounding ecosystem.[75]

FIGURE 9.8:

POPULATION BREAKDOWN OF ALL MAMMALS ON EARTH, 10,000 YEARS AGO AND TODAY[72]

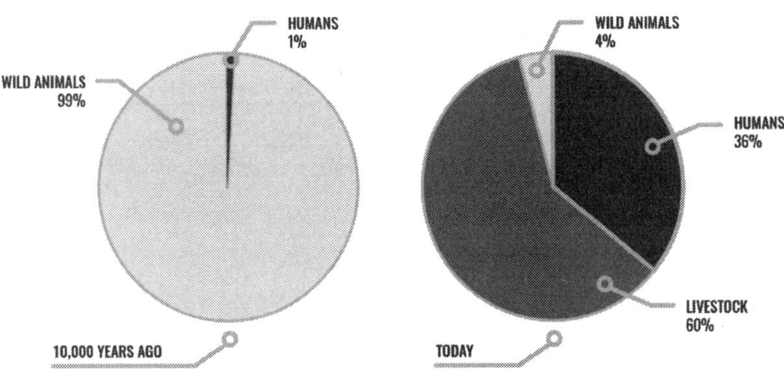

We have a food system that fails to see the value of a healthy planet rich in biodiversity and inflicts incredible amounts of pain, suffering and death, all for just 18% of the world's total calories. The point of sharing these numbers is not to induce shame but to illustrate how problematic our current agricultural system is, and also why there is reason for all of us to have hope. If we flip these FAO numbers on their head, this means that from just one quarter of all land dedicated to food production, plant-based agriculture is supplying 82% of the world's calories and 63% of the world's protein![49] All while only being responsible for about one-third of food-related GHG emissions.[60] Scaling this up and scaling back animal agriculture would mean less land dedicated to food production, which in turn would mean we could restore natural carbon sinks and biodiversity, and significantly decrease the number of animals that we're exploiting.[77] All while upgrading our health at the same time. It's a win-win-win situation.

The typical Western diet today requires 3 billion hectares of grasslands to produce red meat and dairy; a plant-exclusive diet would require zero. Restoration of just 1 billion hectares of this land would draw down two-thirds of all carbon emissions released since the pre-industrial era.[78] This is why major climate change reports such as the Drawdown Review by environmentalist Paul Hawken place a strong emphasis on global shifts towards plant-rich diets.[9] Of course, part of this reforestation working on a global scale will rely on incentives and subsidies for farmers to value conservation and carbon sequestration over livestock production.[79] An example of this is the Carbon Farming Initiative in Australia.[80]

FIGURE 9.9:

TOTAL GLOBAL AREA OF GRAZING LAND REQUIRED TO SUPPORT DIFFERENT DIETS[78]

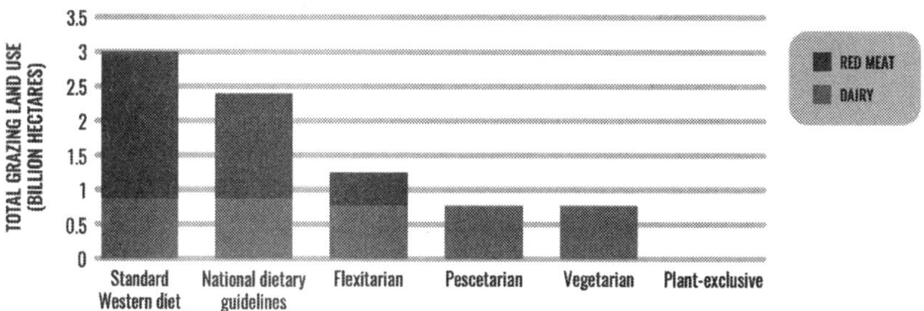

Forests cool our planet

Plants are able to convert sunlight, water and the CO_2 that we and other animals exhale into oxygen and sugars through a process called *photosynthesis*. The plant uses the sugars for growth and repair, releases the oxygen into the air and stores varying amounts of CO_2 in its leaves, branches, trunk, roots and the soil beneath it - nature's way of balancing CO_2 and oxygen in our atmosphere.

The problem is, this masterful balancing act is being greatly jeopardised by humans. Every time we knock down a forest, we are not only immediately releasing the trees' stored CO_2 into the atmosphere but we are also decreasing our planet's ability to suck existing CO_2 out of the atmosphere and into the soil, both of which contribute to the warming of the Earth. Currently, it's estimated over 15 billion trees are cut down per year across the world, and compared with 12,000 years ago, the total number of trees on Earth has decreased by around 50%.[81] This twofold effect of deforestation is why protecting our existing forests and regenerating damaged land is such an important part of the IPCC's recommendations to stop our planet warming to dangerous levels.[29]

The major driver of deforestation is undeniably our growing demand for meat.[82,83] We are clearing millions and millions of hectares from forests rich in biodiversity, such as the tropical rainforests of the Amazon, to create pasture for more cows, and increased space for crops such as soy to feed these animals. Just 6% of soy is grown to make minimally processed foods for human consumption, like edamame, tofu, soy milk and tempeh, while more than three-quarters of global soy crops is used as animal feed.[84,85] And this isn't just happening in the Amazon, it's truly a global problem. Despite the widely held view that Australia's grazing land has always been arid, that's not entirely true. Beef production in Australia is actually the number one driver of deforestation and land clearing. One report analysed more than 1.6 million hectares of land that had been cleared in Queensland between 2013 and 2018 and found that 73% of this occurred to make space for a growing beef industry.[66]

The next greatest driver of deforestation is the production of vegetable oils, such as soybean and palm oils, which are widely used in ultra-processed foods.[83]

Our insatiable appetite for both animal products and ultra-processed foods is impairing the planet's natural ability to cool itself. Making matters worse, this deforestation, and subsequent rise in temperatures due to global warming, increases the frequency and intensity of devastating bushfires, as we saw in Australia in 2019–2020 and in California in 2020, which causes greater overall forest loss and CO_2 emissions.[86,87]

The good news? If we get out of the way, we still have time to regenerate the vast amounts of forest we have cleared. A beautiful example of this is the rainforests in Costa Rica. After decades of logging that decimated two-thirds of trees, in 1996 the Costa Rican government stepped in and restricted logging while incentivising landowners to conserve land and actively participate in reforestation of pasture. The outcome? In just two decades, they have doubled the size of their tropical rainforests while creating thousands of jobs, reducing their livestock industry by one-third and improving their economy at the same time.[65,88]

There's really no way around this. If we are to get anywhere close to meeting climate goals, we must hit the brakes on deforestation. That is why every cent I receive from sales of this book is being donated to Half Cut, a not-for-profit organisation that is actively protecting the world's oldest intact tropical rainforest – the Daintree in Northern Queensland (which is around 180 million years old) – from clearing, along with the ambitious goal of helping to reforest Earth by working with international reforesting projects to plant 1 trillion trees by 2050.

Animal agriculture's impact on our planet's natural ability to cool itself extends beyond what occurs on land. Our ocean, which covers 70% of the Earth's surface, is also crucial to keeping our planet at an optimal temperature for human health. In the same way that forests can absorb and store CO_2, sea grass, kelp, microscopic algae and ocean forests are able to draw down enormous amounts of CO_2 from the atmosphere and store it in the sea floor for centuries. However, for this to be effective, a thriving marine ecosystem rich in biodiversity is essential, specifically a fully functioning food chain all the way from the surface algae that absorb billions of tonnes of CO_2 to the small fish feeding on the algae through to whales and other large marine animals. Disturbing this food chain through overfishing and plastic pollution affects the ocean's natural ability to transport CO_2 from the surface waters to the deep ocean floor.[89–94] While the strong movement against single-use plastics is great to see, it's actually fishing nets and other gear left behind by commercial fishing fleets that are the biggest source of plastic pollution in our ocean.[95] So, if we are truly concerned about plastic in our ocean, we should be focusing on reducing the consumption of fish just as much as we try to reduce plastic straws and cups.

FIGURE 9.10:
VARIETY OF LIFE IN OUR OCEANS IS CRUCIAL TO COOLING OUR PLANET[89-94]

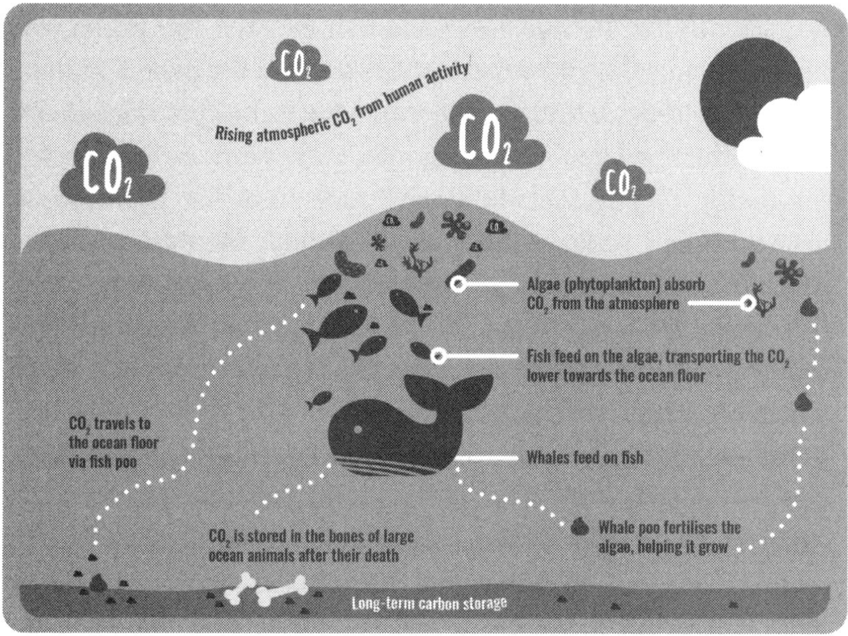

Less than 3% of the world's ocean is protected from fishing. Thanks to a doubling of fishing fleets since 1950, humans have been taking out many more fish than those that remain can replace,[96] so commercial fishing operations are now turning to the deep sea, where they use a destructive technique called *bottom trawling* which involves a heavy net being scraped along the ocean floor, indiscriminately trapping whatever is in its way while simultaneously releasing CO_2 that nature had so cleverly locked away.[97–100] When our ocean's natural carbon sequestration system is broken and we fail to get transfer of CO_2 from shallow to deep waters, the surface water temperature rises and the ocean becomes less capable of drawing down CO_2 from the atmosphere. We lose it as an ally in our fight against global warming. At the same time, more CO_2 in the shallow parts of the ocean creates more acidic water, which has serious implications for marine life, such as coral bleaching.[101–104]

We've been so good at emitting CO_2 and disturbing marine ecosystems, that it's now predicted that by 2100, our ocean will be more acidic than it has been at any point in the past 20 million years.[101] And while farmed fisheries, which now provide almost half of the 2 trillion fish consumed each year, are known for promoting their sustainability and may seem like the obvious answer to this problem, they aren't without their faults either. More than two-thirds of all fishmeal and fish oil derived from fish caught by ocean trawling is used as feed for the farmed fish industry, depleting the ocean of smaller fish low in the food chain which are vital to marine ecosystems.[105]

So while our oceans can be a solution to climate change, they are currently a victim. Much like our forests, we need to realise that the biodiversity in our ocean is essential to cooling our planet. If we stop disrupting the finely tuned natural world and allow our ocean to rewild, it will be able to extract enormous amounts of CO_2 from our atmosphere and safely deposit them in the deep sea floor.

Zoonotic diseases

As our demand for animal products has increased and we've progressively torn down more and more forests, both humans and farm animals have become closer to the habitats of wild animals, increasing the risk of zoonotic diseases - diseases that transmit from animals to humans. Approximately 60% of all known infectious diseases, and 75% of emerging infectious diseases, including viruses such as Covid-19, MERS and SARS, are considered to be zoonotic.[106] While there are different ways zoonotic diseases can spread from animals to humans, farmed animals are perfect intermediary or reservoir hosts, helping a virus to spill over to humans.

One Australian example of this is Hendra virus, a virus discovered in the suburb of Hendra in Brisbane, Queensland, in 1994. As a result of deforestation and the expansion of animal agriculture, horses involved in the racing industry were stabled near the habitat of bats, which act as a reservoir host for many viruses. Horses are thought to have picked up the virus via food that was contaminated with bat urine, and in turn transmitted the virus to humans who worked with them.[107] The Hendra virus has a 50% fatality rate in humans and 70% in horses, but is fortunately not very contagious.[108] In contrast, a more contagious virus that we are all well aware of is influenza A, or seasonal flu, which is commonly transferred from wild birds to poultry to humans, sometimes via intermediate animals such as pigs.[109] Given what we know about social distancing from our recent experience with Covid-19, it's not surprising that factory farms (where animals such as cows, chickens and pigs live on top of one another under enormous amounts of stress that impairs their immune system) are breeding grounds for these infectious diseases and quite possibly for the next global pandemic.[110,111]

Should we buy local?

We've all heard this catch-cry, but if you're like me, you may have wondered about the actual environmental impact of these choices.

When it comes to eating locally produced food, it's important to understand that for most foods, transportation emissions only make up a small amount of the food's total GHG emissions – typically less than 10%.[50] The main drivers of emissions in our food system, accounting for 80% of most foods' environmental footprint, is land use change (e.g. deforestation) and farming (including emissions from animals, farming equipment, fertilisers, etc.). If we want to lower the emission impact of our meals, what we eat is far more important than where our food has travelled from.[50,112,113] For example, 99% of the GHG emissions from beef are not transport related, so buying beef from a local farm rather than somewhere far away has a tiny overall effect on our environmental footprint.

FIGURE 9.11:

SOURCE OF GREENHOUSE GAS EMISSIONS PER KG OF FOOD PRODUCT[49,50,114]

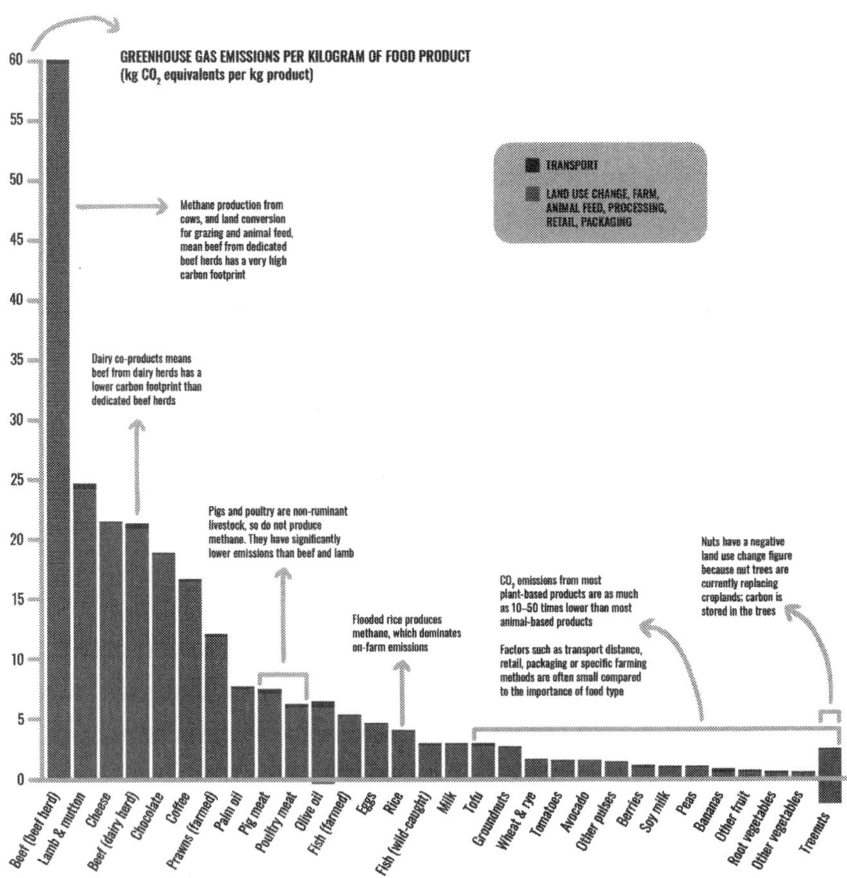

* Carbon dioxide, methane and nitrous oxide combined to form a single measure (kg CO_2 equivalents) of GHGs associated with the supply of that food.

Supporting local business often gives you the opportunity to find out what practices farms are using so you can buy from those who are dedicated to looking after their land and nourishing the soil. However, it's important that we don't let the feel-good aspect of this distract us from the fact that the percentage of animal products in our diet, particularly red meat and dairy, is single-handedly the most important contributor to the total GHG emissions related to our food consumption, regardless of whether they were farmed locally, conventionally, free-range or organically.[51] However, in the words of environmental geoscientist Dr Hannah Ritchie, 'Whether you buy it from the farmer next door or from far away, it is not the location that makes the carbon footprint of your dinner large, but the fact that it is beef.'[50] If you are already consuming a plant-based diet, then buying local produce will help further lower your emissions slightly.

Should we buy organic?

Similarly, the 'organic versus conventional farming' debate detracts from what is most important – the percentage of animal-based foods in our diet. There is actually no clear winner when it comes to the environmental impact of organic versus conventional food. For example, based on data from 742 agriculture systems and over ninety foods, while certain food groups such as fruits produce fewer GHG emissions when organically grown, others such as vegetables produce fewer GHG emissions when conventionally grown.[51,115] Furthermore, while organic farming typically uses less energy because it does not require the same energy-intensive chemical inputs, it requires substantially more land to produce the same amount of food because the yield is lower, and it is responsible for greater pollution of our waterways due to nitrogen and phosphorus that leaches from manure, its primary fertiliser.

This extends to animal foods as well. Unfortunately, many of the claims about the environmentally friendly nature of organic animal products are not supported by science. Like we saw with holistic grazing, this is another case of greenwashing. Animals raised on organic farms take longer to grow to slaughter weight, produce less meat, and require more land. As a result, the GHG emissions from grass-fed organic beef, lamb, chicken, pork and eggs are typically greater than their conventional counterparts.[53]

The point here is not to write off organic food altogether but to remind us not to lose sight of the forest for the trees. When it comes to lowering the environmental footprint of our diet, the biggest difference we can make is through eating more whole plant foods and fewer animal foods. Not through buying organic or local.

This doesn't mean that once you are getting most or all of your calories from whole plant foods it's not a good idea to get to know where your food comes from – it is. If you are interested in this, I recommend seeking out biodynamic or, better yet, regeneratively grown plant foods, which are forms of farming that are becoming more widely used and focus on improving soil health and biodiversity. Food that gives back to the Earth! Whether you choose conventional, organic, biodynamic or regenerative, nothing beats talking to the farmers at your local market or friends in your community who have already explored this area. If you can, get to know where your produce is grown and the practices the farmers use on their land. Ideally, support farmers who use reduced tillage practices, employ crop rotation and use inputs such as green manure and vegetable compost to nourish their land.[116,117] Depending on where you live, you may also have room to grow some of your own food too.

The ethics of higher-quality animal products

As more and more people have become aware of the cruelty of the livestock industry, there has been an exponential rise in animal products marketed as organic, grass-fed, free-range, humane or ethical. These products often attract a premium price, and their rise in popularity is indicative of changing consumer desires: people are willing to pay significantly more for products they deem to be more ethical and that involve less cruelty towards animals. But do these products really afford a better life to the animals?

There are two main considerations. The first is that definitions of grass-fed, free-range, humane and organic are loose and subject to interpretation. There are very few standards and certifications around using these descriptors, and even when use of a term is regulated, it does not necessarily mean that the animals have had a better quality of life as the certification process is based on a slew of arbitrary requirements. For example, the official definition of free-range eggs in Australia allows for hens to be kept at a stocking rate of 10,000 birds per hectare and requires that they must have 'regular and meaningful' access to the outdoors, but there are no rules about what 'regular and meaningful' actually translates as, and it is left up to the interpretation of individual farmers.[118]

So even if we were to spend extra on 'free-range' eggs, this is no guarantee that the hens laying those eggs have anything close to what you and I would deem a decent life. Perhaps, more importantly, these eggs only come from egg-laying hens – females. Male chicks from this industry are different to the chickens bred for meat, and because they cannot lay eggs, they are considered useless and are shredded alive shortly after birth.[119] This is considered the most humane way to kill them.

The second and perhaps most important point to be made is that regardless of how well these animals may have lived, how much land they roamed and how much fresh air they inhaled, they suffer the same fate as factory-farmed animals. Their lives are still taken against their will, well before what their natural life span would have been under normal conditions. If anything, animals raised in these less intensive conditions have even more reason to want to stay alive.

FIGURE 9.12:

NO MATTER HOW THEY ARE FARMED, ALL ANIMALS GROWN FOR FOOD EVENTUALLY MEET THE SAME FATE

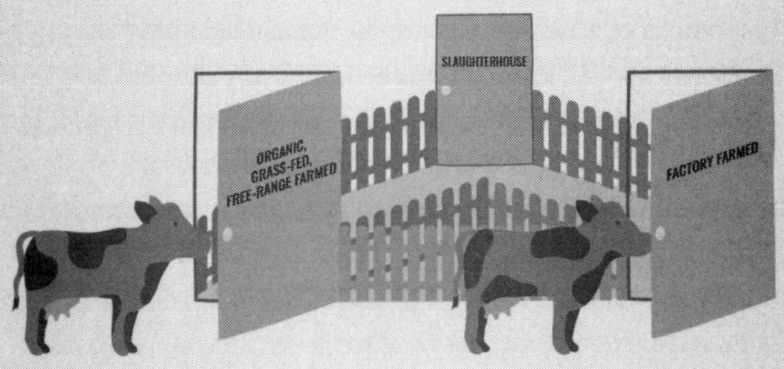

This is not to say that there is zero benefit in paying for higher-quality animal products. Anyone who acknowledges the atrocities happening in factory farms and decides to no longer support such practices should be congratulated. It is, however, important to be realistic about what we are buying, and to at no time be under the impression that these higher-quality animal products are truly cruelty-free options. Hidden behind these labels – ethical, humane, free-range, organic – is an industry that few of us could voluntarily bear witness to. Are these labels there to protect the animals, or our conscience?

Food and water security

The warming of our planet is just one facet of environmental health that deserves our attention. Our food choices have consequences far beyond this, also contributing to food insecurity and freshwater scarcity.[46,50] For many of us, it can be difficult to imagine what it's like to be unsure about when our next meal or sip of clean water will be. Speaking personally, I know this is something that I gave little thought to for over two decades of my life. I still have to consciously remind myself to be grateful for having access to nutritious food and being able to stay hydrated with uncontaminated water. Unfortunately, some humans do not have this privilege. Food and water insecurity is a daily reality for over 2 billion of our fellow humans.[49,120] While that should be enough for us to roll up our sleeves and do what we can to improve food and water supply across the globe, it's unfortunately difficult to get people to act when we feel so disconnected from what's taking place somewhere distant to where our reality lies. If it's not our supermarket shelves that are empty or our taps running dry, changing our behaviour seems less meaningful, or at least less urgent.

However, developed nations are by no means immune to food and water insecurity. In the next thirty years, our global population is expected to reach 10 billion people. To feed this many people, we will need to make available around 50% more calories than we do today while tackling extreme weather (floods, droughts, storms, etc.) and reduced crop yields.[121,122] This isn't hypothetical, but a reality that we face.[123] Climate change is already affecting our ability to produce food for human consumption, and if we don't change the way we're living and stop our planet warming, a global food crisis looms.[123,124] At the same time, the World Health Organization (WHO) predicts that by as early as 2025, more than half the world's population will live in water-stressed areas.[125] We need to realise that our access to food and water is only as safe and guaranteed as our planet is healthy.

So how do our food choices affect food and water security? Let's take a look.

When we hear 'food waste', most of us probably think about the excess food that enters our homes and restaurants and ultimately makes its way to landfill. But what if I told you there was another, far more significant source of wasted calories within our food system?

As Dr Jonathan Foley, an environmental scientist and author of a *National Geographic* article titled 'A five-step plan to feed the world' put it, we could easily feed the entire population of humans on Earth, and stop deforestation in its tracks, 'if more of the crops we grew ended up in human stomachs'.[126] Currently, approximately 36% of the world's edible crops are fed to farm animals. In this process, for every 100 calories of crops that could have been fed to humans but are instead fed to livestock, we get only 40 calories of milk, 22 calories of eggs, 12 calories of chicken, 10 calories of pork or 3 calories of beef.[49] Put simply, many more calories go into making the animal products than the calories made available to the end consumer.

FIGURE 9.13:

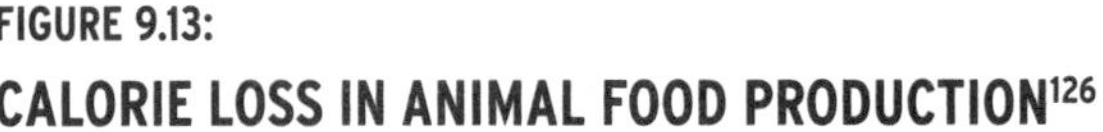

CALORIE LOSS IN ANIMAL FOOD PRODUCTION[126]

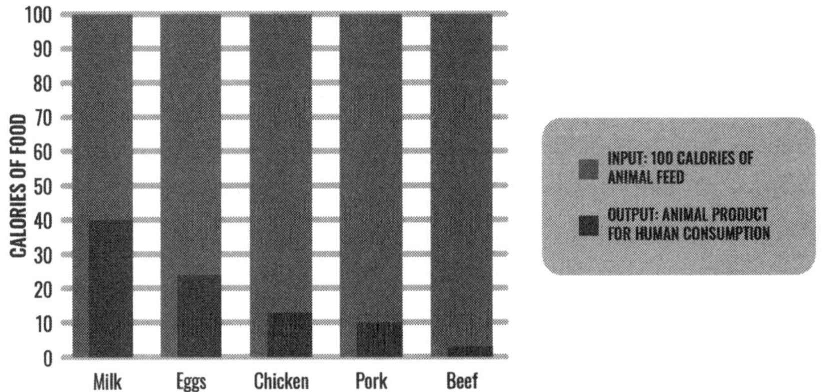

That's right – 97% of the calories fed to a cow are lost in the production of beef. Think about the extreme inefficiency of this practice. Even if we take chicken, one of the most efficient meats, to produce a 200 g chicken breast containing about 340 calories, you have to feed that chicken nearly 3000 calories of plant food! If we shifted to growing food exclusively for humans, not only would we require significantly less land for agriculture – freeing up vast amounts of land that could be regenerated into powerful carbon sinks – but it's been estimated that there would be an approximately 70% increase in available calories in our food system, which could feed an extra 4 billion people.[49,127] In other words, there is no good reason why over 800 million people today are undernourished and more than 150 million children are stunted.[128,129] Improving our food system is not just about respecting the environment and improving the lives of those of us in developed countries, but about creating a more equitable system so all humans can have access to adequate nutrition. This should be a basic human right.

Although the calories we are losing inside the current agricultural system are significant, food waste at the consumer end – which you and I are responsible for – also matters. About a third of all calories produced for human consumption end up wasted.[130] Food that is produced but never makes its way into a human's mouth. To put this in perspective, if food waste were a country it would be the world's third largest emitter of GHGs behind China and the United States.[130] This is three times the emissions of air travel! This represents an opportunity not only to free up calories for people going hungry, but also to reduce global GHG emissions at the same time.[131] To make matters worse, when food is not disposed of correctly, it ends up in a landfill, where it rots and produces methane.[132]

If we want to contribute to less food waste, we need to be conscious of two areas. First and foremost, we should be focusing on the foods we buy as this is the primary source of wasted calories. More plants and fewer animal products. And then, we should be looking at how much food we buy and create a plan to minimise the amount of food that we send to landfill. Other than only buying what we need and finding shops that sell 'imperfect' fruits and vegetables, another great strategy is using your food scraps to make compost, which can then be used to nourish soil.[133] If you do not have your own garden, a number of cities around the world, including Sydney, San Francisco, Los Angeles, Seattle and Copenhagen have compost services to help you get your food scraps from kitchen to farm.[134] By doing this, you will reduce the amount of methane released into the atmosphere while helping the carbon in your food make its way to our soil – not into our atmosphere.

There are similar losses and inefficiencies in the freshwater used by animal agriculture, as we can see in Figure 9.14. Over 70% of the typical person's freshwater footprint comes from the food they eat, with household use being responsible for only a few per cent.[135,136] Despite the fact that nuts require a relatively large amount of water to produce, it's been calculated that shifting from a standard omnivorous diet to a balanced whole-food plant-exclusive diet that includes a significant amount of calories from nuts would still save a great deal of freshwater.[49] We have to realise that water, something that's so easy to take for granted, is a finite resource and our reservoirs of freshwater are fast disappearing,[135] so much so that water scientists have estimated that, to avoid catastrophic shortages and global conflict (known as 'water wars'), the entire world needs to adopt a diet that is at least 95% plant-based by 2050.[137] Eating more plants means we can conserve and restore more forests, which are absolutely crucial to preserving healthy freshwater supplies. Unlike bare or hard ground, where rainfall tends to run off and evaporate, forests are very good at ensuring that precipitation ends up being absorbed into soil to replenish our water tables.[138,139]

FIGURE 9.14:

WATER REQUIREMENTS PER CALORIE OF FOOD PRODUCT

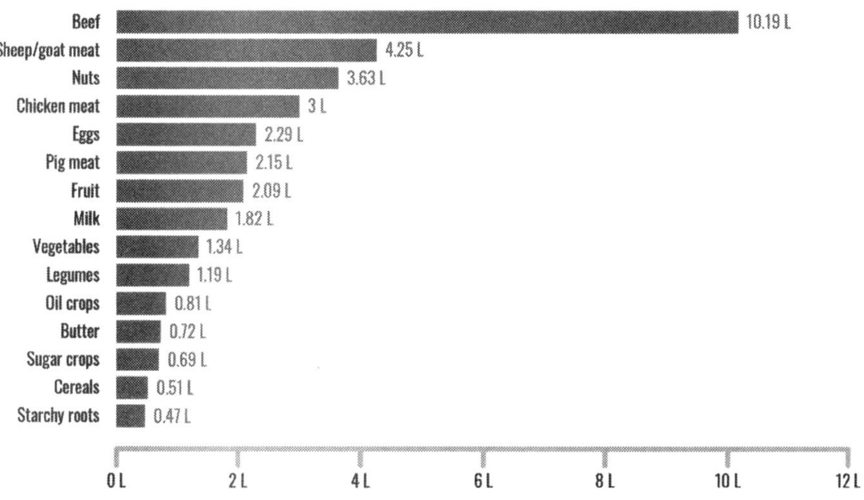

Adapted from Our World in Data[140]

More frequent catastrophic water and food shortages, causing widespread poverty, hunger, displacement, conflict, death and disease, spell disaster for global health, standards of living and economies. As a 2019 report written by United Nations expert Philip Alston stated, we are headed for a 'climate apartheid', where wealthy people pay to escape rising temperatures, hunger and water scarcity at the expense of everyone else. The decisions we make on a daily basis affect not just our own health, but the health of all life around us, including our fellow humans from less privileged populations.[141]

Australia's share of GHG emissions

If you're from Australia you may be thinking, *This is interesting, but our emissions are low compared with other countries. Why should we make change?*

First, it's true that in absolute terms, Australia's GHG emissions seem low, comprising only 1.3% of all global emissions.[142] However, this is because our country has an extremely small population rather than because it is environmentally friendly. Australia actually has one of the highest GHG emissions per person of any country in the world, and that's without even factoring in emissions related to the fossil fuels and meat we export.[143,144] Why so high? Because we are losing our forests, eating more meat than just about any other country, prefer to drive rather than use public transport, and we don't use enough green energy.[145–148]

If you factor in our export emissions, Australia accounts for 5% of global GHG emissions while being home to only 0.3% of the world's population.[149] We could be leaders in tackling climate change, particularly given the vast amount of land we have that has the potential to draw down CO_2 from the atmosphere. Instead, we are currently showing the world what *not* to do.

If wealthy countries like Australia cannot improve our emissions, how can we expect developing countries to do so?

Antibiotic resistant 'superbugs'

Planetary health and animal welfare aside, there is another important reason why we should be doing our best not to support intensive farming of animals. I'm talking about antibiotic resistance. You may be surprised to know that the majority of the world's antibiotics are actually fed to farmed animals.[150] This is a lucrative market for the pharmaceutical industry. These animals, mostly in factory farms, are routinely fed antibiotics to prevent them from getting sick in the overcrowded and dirty environments they are confined to.[151] By doing this, farms can be more productive, keeping more animals in a given amount of space, and animals free from disease will reach slaughter weight more quickly. But while it makes sense from a business point of view, the widespread use of antibiotics comes at an enormous biological cost, one that I do not think many of us are aware of. In short, when we overuse antibiotics, they become less effective and certain bacteria known as superbugs become resistant to their effects. Between the years 2000 and 2018, the amount of antibiotic resistance in farm animals has nearly tripled.[152] This is incredibly dangerous for humanity. As of today some 700,000 people die per year as a result of infections that no longer respond to antibiotics.[153] Like climate change, antibiotic resistance is not speculative – it's already arrived, and based on predicted rates of antibiotic use in coming years, things are set to get a lot worse.[150] Relatively routine surgical procedures that we now take for granted, such as caesarean sections, could quickly become too risky to perform if antibiotics are no longer effective at safeguarding patients against infection. And life-saving interventions such as heart or kidney transplants could be off the table too. As terrible as it has been, if you think Covid-19 has been a challenge for humanity, think about this: by 2050, it's predicted that more than 10 million people per year will die from superbugs globally.[154]

The writing is on the wall here but experts believe there is time to avoid this threat, which has been described by the WHO as one of the greatest threats to global health today.[155] Not only do we need to reduce our own antibiotic use, but we need to cut down the use of antibiotics fed to chickens, cows, sheep, fish, etc.[150,155,156] By eating more plants and less meat, fish, eggs and dairy (particularly products sourced from factory farms), we can be part of the solution to combating this threat.

Taking action

If the science is so clear about the planet-saving potential of a plant-based diet, why are there not more people talking about this? Why instead does the conversation on climate change mitigation and concern for the environment in general mostly revolve around energy, reducing air travel and single-use plastics?

From a policy perspective, talking about diet and food has always been somewhat taboo. Most political parties prefer to ignore or avoid the topic, for fear of public backlash. Telling people what to eat is seen as too personal or not the role of a democratic government, so few politicians are willing to tackle it. Imagine the public – and industry – upheaval if the government outlawed or rationed meat consumption! It's a topic that even prominent environmentalists steer clear of.

On an individual level, it's also a big ask to get someone to consider what the health of the planet will be like in thirty to eighty years' time when many of them will not be around to deal with the repercussions of the irreversible damage that is being done. Earlier, we spoke about our genetic wiring and how our gravitation towards energy-dense foods, once a helpful trait for the survival of our ancestors, fails us in the modern developed world, where food is abundant and chronic disease is rife. Like chronic disease, climate change is typically viewed as a slow-to-develop condition, one that doesn't require our immediate attention.

Just as it's hard to look at a beef burger and see the system it is a part of, and its effect on our personal health, it's difficult to see its effect on the planet's health. And even if we do understand its effect, we are simply not wired to prioritise the long-term health of our planet over the immediate pleasure we derive from the foods we eat three or more times a day.

Nevertheless, the truth is that climate change is real and rather than it being something that our species will have to deal with in hundreds or thousands of years, it's knocking on our door and needs our immediate attention. As a result of our ancestors' lifestyles, particularly since the industrial era, and our lifestyles today, we find ourselves living on a planet that's on the precipice of experiencing its own irreversible chronic disease. Although greenhouse gases are invisible to the eye, we cannot deny that present levels are at an all-time high, well above natural levels observed in the past 800,000 years. We also cannot deny that the warming induced by their presence has been affecting our weather, with increasing frequency and intensity of hurricanes, wildfires, floods and other extreme events being experienced across the world in recent years.[157,158] Events that historically were thought to be natural disasters are now believed to be greatly influenced by human-inflicted climate change.

Because we have these scientific truths, many of which have been strengthened by large studies in just the past five years, unlike our ancestors, who weren't to know that their innovations were damaging the planet, it's us who will be judged by how we respond. And when it comes to the lives we live today, it's clear that for too long we've been feeding humans at the expense of our environment. In the process, we have been destabilising the climate, so much so that our policymakers and politicians, and we as individuals, can no longer ignore it, particularly in developed countries like Australia and the United States, where we consume more red meat and emit more GHGs per person than just about any other population in the world.[143,144]

Should we reduce our driving and air travel, live in smaller homes, purchase fewer things and consider having fewer children to combat the effects of global warming and climate change? While these are somewhat sensitive topics, each of these does make up a considerable portion of our personal emissions.[159] But the fact we are responsible for emissions through various sources doesn't mean we should only focus on one. In order to meet the climate goals laid out in the Paris Agreement, we need to fiercely defend the natural world wherever we can – and as we have seen, science shows us that animal agriculture has impacts upon our planet's health far beyond emissions. The same goes for advocating for political change. While fighting for top-down change is a worthy cause, and one I am strongly in favour of, making changes to our plate is cheap, easy, fast and effective. Plus, if we want to ask for change from our political leaders, we really should walk the walk, right?

This is where you and I come into the picture. Although the science about human health says the best diet is one that consists of 85–100% of calories from whole plant foods, if you factor into the equation the enormous environmental advantages of feeding the world with plants, it makes an extremely compelling case for adopting a diet that is as plant-exclusive as possible – one that is based on whole foods and minimises food waste. Each time we choose plants over animals, we are voting with our dollar for a system that favours the production of more calories from less land so we can rewild the Earth and cool the planet while providing a growing population with ample amounts of healthy nutritious food and clean water. Each time we choose plants over animals, we are voting to let our greatest ally, nature, do what we know it's so capable of – creating an environment that allows humans, and all life on the planet, to thrive. If that doesn't give added meaning to the food we put on our plate, I'm not sure what will.

I'm not saying that each of us needs to execute this perfectly, but time is of the essence, with less than ten years to prevent irreversible damage. And given what we've been doing hasn't been working out so great, why not aim high?[160] Not only will this in part offset the emissions caused by those who will continue to regularly consume animal foods but it will come with a side of undeniable personal health benefits.

Podcast highlights: How our food choices affect planetary health

In Episode 104, I sat down with environmental researcher Nicholas Carter to discuss how our food choices affect planetary health. This conversation is then continued, and expanded on, in Episodes 119 and 120, with climate and environmental scientist Dr Jonathan Foley and environmental geoscientist Dr Hannah Ritchie.

In Episode 109, I sat down with Bruce Friedrich, co-founder of The Good Food Institute, to discuss the role of plant-based meat and cellular or 'cultivated' meat in transforming our food system to meet climate goals and improve planetary health. A fascinating area of innovation that stands to shape the future of food.

All four of these episodes consolidate many of the learnings from this chapter.

PART THREE

MAKING THE SHIFT

NOW WE'VE CUT THROUGH THE CONFUSION AND UNDERstood the science, it's time to learn how to make the shift to a diet that is as plant-exclusive as possible. As an individual, this means living in alignment with your values and beliefs while tapping in to the health-promoting benefits of plants, whether you're hoping to add more years of good health to your life, tread more lightly on the planet or be kinder to the other species we share it with.

Once you understand the eight Plant Proof principles I've established to help you make the shift, have stocked up your pantry and fridge and make a few new habits, you will be well on your way to this new way of living. While it may seem like there are a lot of things to keep track of, over about three to six months, as you start to make changes to your plate and make adjustments based on how your body is responding, all the information will become more meaningful and easier to recall. So take your time and enjoy the changes you are making without feeling pressure to do everything perfectly from day one. You can (and should!) go at your own pace, follow your tastebuds and customise the recommendations to suit your lifestyle.

Despite how motivated we may be, shifting to a plant-exclusive diet can feel daunting – after all, it's an entirely new way of fuelling our bodies. So, whether you're new to this approach or a long-time vegan wanting to place greater emphasis on your health, I understand that you likely have a bunch of questions: *Am I going to feel full? Will I get enough protein? How will I get enough calcium without drinking cow's milk? Is the sugar in fruit healthy? What about my iron levels? How do I handle an increase in fibre? Should I take any supplements?* This part is about addressing all of these questions and many more, so you understand the foundations of a well-planned, nutritionally adequate dietary pattern that excludes, or greatly minimises, animal products, and have all the best tips and tricks to make a sustainable lifestyle change.

As you consider making the shift, it should be comforting to know that the majority of dietetic associations across the world, including the US Academy of Nutrition and Dietetics (AND) and the British Dietetic Association, support a plant-based diet, including a vegan diet, for all stages of life.[1–6] As the AND – the world's largest nutrition association, representing over 100,000 nutrition professionals – stated in their 2016 position paper: '*appropriately planned vegetarian, including vegan, diets are healthful, nutritionally adequate, and may provide health benefits in the prevention and treatment of certain diseases. These diets are appropriate for all stages of the life cycle, including pregnancy, lactation, infancy, childhood, adolescence, older adulthood, and for athletes. Plant-based diets are more environmentally sustainable than diets rich in animal products because they use fewer natural resources and are associated with much less environmental damage.*'[2] This was actually quite a big moment for the AND – an association that has a well-documented history of accepting sponsorship money from organisations such as the National Cattleman's Beef Association, the National Dairy Council, Coca-Cola, Mars, McDonald's and Nestlé.[7] For them to honour the science and endorse a vegan diet, and specifically emphasise the importance of whole foods – fruits, vegetables, whole grains, legumes, nuts and seeds – was pleasing to see.

'Appropriately planned' is a key phrase in the AND's statement. *Any* diet that is not appropriately planned can go wrong. We need to be informed and to focus on key food groups and micronutrients to fully unlock the health benefits of this powerful lifestyle. Thankfully, as I am going to show you, this is easily achieved.

How I define 'processed' foods

The idea of 'processed' food should be approached with a degree of common sense. Not every processed food is harmful. Take wholemeal bread, beans or nut butter for example. While these foods undergo a degree of processing, often in order to make them edible, they are extremely health-promoting and from food groups that we need to be eating more of. Or vinegar, processed by definition yet great for improving blood sugar and lowering cholesterol.[8] Essentially, by 'unprocessed' or 'minimally processed' whole plant foods, I'm talking about foods that are free from or contain minimal added sugar, salt, fat and artificial ingredients. This includes foods like tofu, plant-based milks and even olive oil for those who use cooking oils. It's the ultra-processed foods, such as biscuits, cookies, cakes and sugary breakfast cereals, that have had a lot of their nutritional value stripped away, and usually contain a bunch of not-so-healthy additives, which we want to minimise.

A reminder here before we get into the chapter: you should regularly consult with a doctor in matters relating to your health, and particularly with respect to an existing condition or to any symptoms that may require diagnosis or medical attention. ●

CHAPTER 10

The eight Plant Proof principles of a healthy WFPBD

There are eight main principles that create the foundation for a successful whole-food plant-based diet (WFPBD). Together, they make up the Plant Proof Food Pyramid. Decades of research has shown that a WFPBD is one of a few diets that fits the theme of optimal eating for *Homo sapiens*, and these principles are a distillation of that evidence. I am confident that no matter what nutrient or diet is in the headlines at a given moment, these principles will stand the test of time. They are:

1. **FOCUS ON FOOD GROUPS, NOT MACRONUTRIENTS.** When we focus on food groups, given there is enough diversity in our diet, the macronutrients (carbohydrates, protein and fat) take care of themselves. These food groups include fruits, vegetables, whole grains, legumes, nuts and seeds in their whole or minimally processed forms.

2. **BE FIBRE-OBSESSED (AND PROTEIN-AWARE).** Aim for at least 28 g per day of fibre if you're a woman or 38 g per day if you're a man.

3. **DIVERSITY IS KEY FOR GUT HEALTH.** Aim for over forty unique plants per week with plenty of different colours. In doing so, you will feed your healthy gut microbes and help them grow stronger.

4. **CONSIDER NUTRIENTS OF FOCUS.** Paying attention to specific micronutrients will allow you to experience the full benefit of a WFPBD. The nutrients of focus are omega-3s, vitamin B_{12}, vitamin D, calcium, iodine, iron, selenium and zinc.

5. **WHEN WE EAT MATTERS (NOT JUST WHAT WE EAT).** Optimising meal timing based on our bodies' natural clock, or circadian rhythm, may help renew our energy levels, promote a healthy body weight and improve our mood while also decreasing our risk of chronic disease and possibly even adding years to our lives.

6. **DRINK WATER FOR THIRST.** And minimise alcohol consumption.

7. **CUSTOMISATION IS KEY.** Adapt to a way of plant-based eating that works for you.

8. **DON'T LET PERFECTION BE THE ENEMY OF GOOD.** Keep in mind that this is a lifestyle, and therefore it needs to come with a degree of flexibility. What's most important is incorporating as much of this information as possible into your lifestyle in a sustainable and enjoyable manner. Consistency over time matters far more than what you eat in one particular day.

FIGURE 10.1:

THE PLANT PROOF FOOD PYRAMID

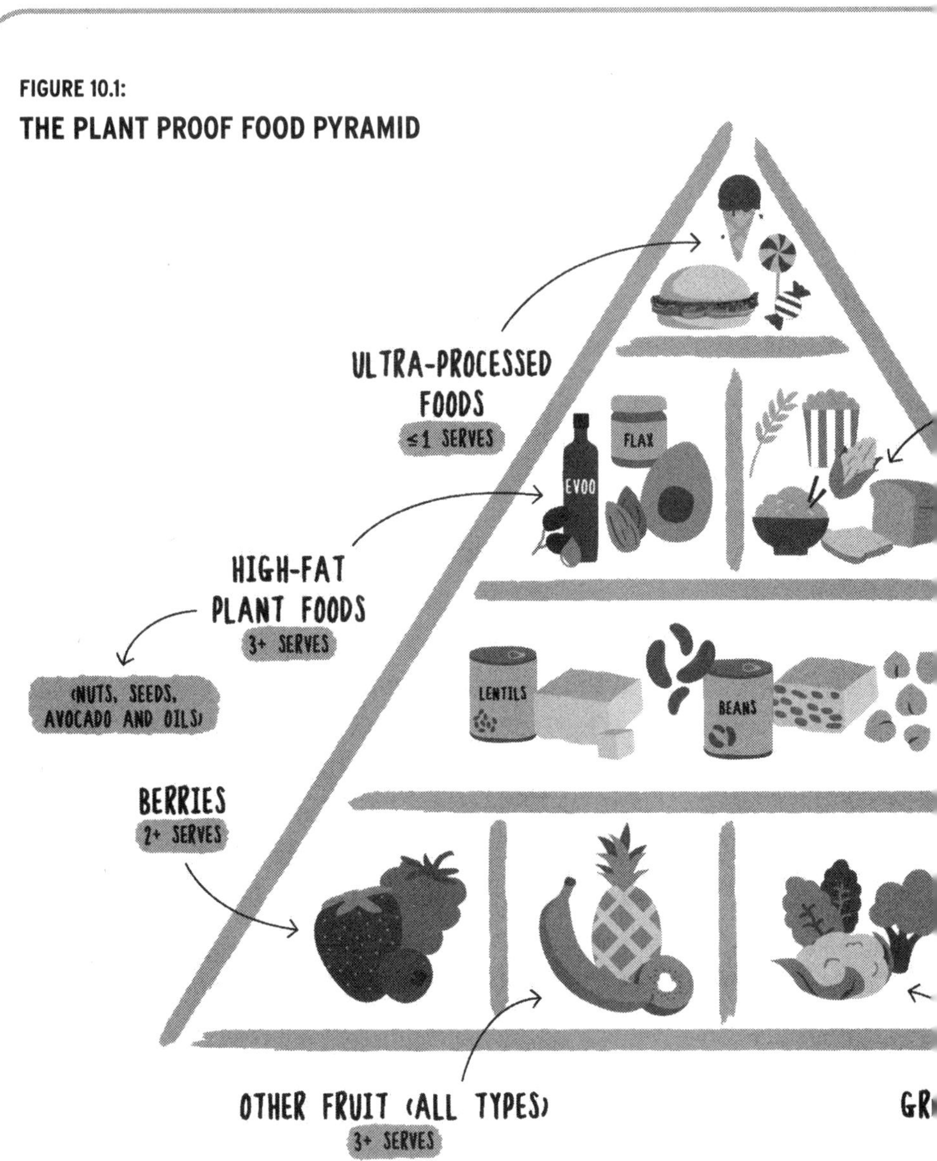

SERVING SIZES

Cooking oils: 1 tbsp (≈100–120 calories)

High-fat plant foods: ⅓ medium avocado, 30 g nuts/seeds or 1 tbsp oil

Legumes: ½ cup cooked or 150 g tofu/tempeh

Whole grains: ½ cup cooked or 2 slices of whole grain bread

Berries: ½ cup

Other fruits: 1 medium fruit or ½ cup chopped

Greens and cruciferous vegetables: ½ cup chopped

Other vegetables: 1 medium vegetable or ½ cup chopped

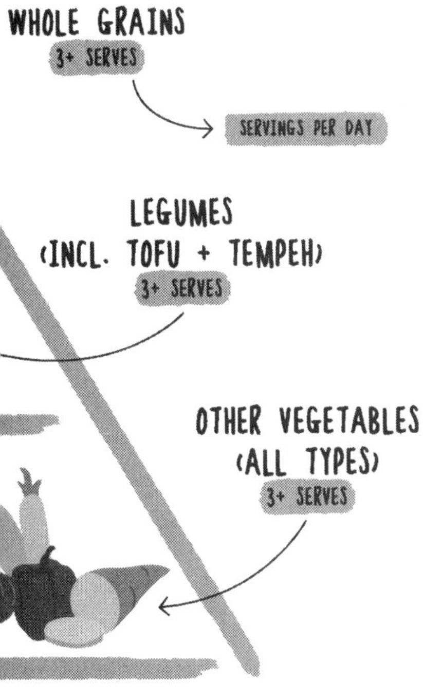

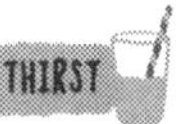

THIRST

Plain water for thirst: Best indicator of hydration is clear to light straw coloured urine

Alcohol: Avoid alcohol or minimise to 1 drink per day for women or 2 drinks per day for men

Calcium-fortified plant milk: Fortified plant milk with at least 100–150 mg of calcium per 100 mL Aim for 1.5 cups per day

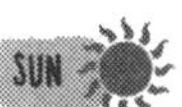

SUN

20 mins of sun daily

TRY NOT TO MISS

Ground flaxseed or chia seeds: 1 tbsp/day for women, 2 tbsp/day for men

Brazil nuts: 1 per day

Seaweed: 2 tsp of dulse or wakame flakes

Enhance iron absorption: Lemon juice, onion and/or garlic

Enhance zinc absorption: Onion and/or garlic

Soaking and sprouting grains, legumes, nuts and seeds significantly increases nutrient levels and makes them easier to absorb

MEAL TIMING 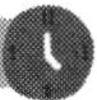

Eat within a 10–12 hour window (e.g. 7am–7pm). Enjoy a hearty breakfast and lighter dinner. Try to avoid food a few hours before bed

SPICES, FRESH HERBS OR OTHER

Sprouts, nutritional yeast, turmeric, oregano, garlic, parsley, coriander, chives, black pepper, etc.

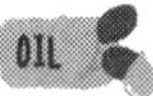

OIL

If choosing to cook with oils, be mindful of the high caloric density, especially if your goal is weight loss. For oil recommendations see the Plant Proof Oil Pyramid

SUPPLEMENTS

1. Vitamin B_{12} (everyone following a WFPBD)
2. Vitamin D (if not getting 20 mins of sun daily)
3. Omega-3 DHA/EPA algae oil supplement (not essential but recommended)

For dosage amounts along with more details, see **Principle 4: Consider nutrients of focus**

Principle 1: Focus on food groups, not macronutrients

Unless you have a very specific body composition goal or you have a disease such as diabetes, it makes more sense to pay attention to food groups than macronutrients. Yes, you need a balance of macronutrients – carbohydrates, fats and protein – but when you focus on food groups, the macros will take care of themselves.

Around the Plant Proof Food Pyramid, you will see the names of the eight food groups: fruit, greens and cruciferous vegetables, other vegetables, legumes (including tofu and tempeh), berries, high-fat plant foods, whole grains and ultra-processed foods, as well as spices, fresh herbs or other. As with any food pyramid, those that you should consume the most of form the base. When you're planning a meal, work up from the bottom of the pyramid to plan your servings for each group.

FIGURE 10.2:

EXAMPLE PLATE WHEN EATING ACCORDING TO THE PLANT PROOF FOOD PYRAMID

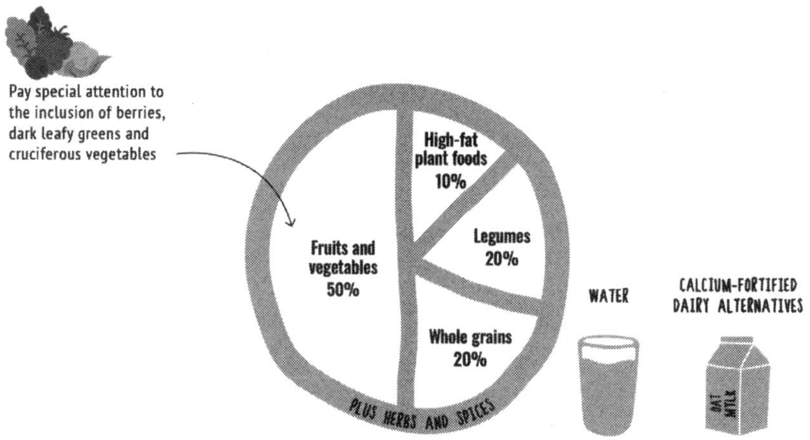

For example, if I am thinking about what I need to make tacos for dinner, I first think about the delicious fruits and vegetables I'll be working with – this could be purple cabbage, fresh jalapenos, zucchini or mango. After fruits and vegetables, it's time to think about whole grains – perhaps whole wheat or corn tortillas, or corn as a side dish. Next is legumes – black beans, kidney beans or tofu/tempeh all go well in tacos, and while all plants contain protein, legumes are where a significant amount of your daily protein will come from. Finally, I would add a source of plant-based fat – perhaps a spicy cashew cheese or some avocado salsa, and a few fresh coriander leaves.

To work with the food pyramid, in Figure 10.3 I've listed some common, delicious foods that fall within each of the food groups. As we saw in the principles above, while we will all have our favourites, diversity is key.

Nut allergy and a WFPBD

Can a WFPBD be done if someone is allergic to nuts? Absolutely. Neither the avoidance of tree nuts or peanuts inhibits someone from consuming a nutritionally adequate WFPBD. However, because nuts are rich in certain key nutrients such as omega-3 fats, selenium and zinc, anyone who's excluding them should pay particular attention to what they eat instead. Eating more legumes, mushrooms and seeds (e.g. ground flaxseeds and sunflower seeds) will help to ensure these nutrients are consumed in the required amounts for optimal health.

FIGURE 10.3:

PLANT PROOF FOOD PYRAMID FOOD GROUPS

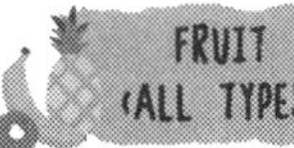

Apple, apricot, banana, cantaloupe (rockmelon), cherries, chestnut, dates, grapefruit, grapes, guava, honeydew melon, jackfruit, kiwifruit, mandarin, mango, nectarine, orange, papaya, passionfruit, peach, pear, persimmon, pineapple, plum, watermelon

GREENS + CRUCIFEROUS VEGETABLES

Bok choy, broccoli, brussels sprouts, cauliflower, chinese cabbage, collard greens, kale, kohlrabi, lettuce, mustard greens, pak choi, red cabbage, rocket (arugula), spinach, swiss chard (silverbeet), watercress, white cabbage

OTHER VEGETABLES (ALL TYPES)

Artichoke, asparagus, beetroot, capsicum (bell pepper), carrot, celeriac, celery, corn, cucumber, eggplant, green beans, kimchi, leek, mushrooms*, onion, parsnip, potato, pumpkin, radish, rhubarb, sauerkraut, snow peas, squash, swede, sweet potato, tomato, turnip, zucchini

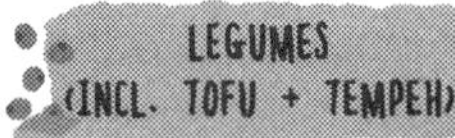

Adzuki beans, black beans, black-eyed peas, borlotti beans, broad beans, brown lentils, butter (lima) beans, cannellini beans, chickpeas**, edamame, green peas, kidney beans, lupini beans**, mung beans, navy beans, pinto beans, red lentils, soy beans, split peas, tempeh, tofu

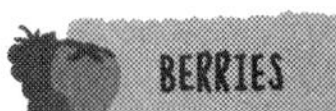

Acai berries, blackberries, blueberries, cranberries, goji berries, raspberries, strawberries, mulberries

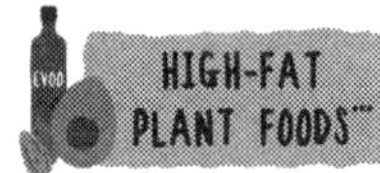

Almonds, avocado, brazil nuts, cashews, chia seeds, flaxseeds, hazelnuts, hemp seeds, macadamia nuts, olives, peanuts, pecans, sesame seeds, tahini, walnuts

WHOLE GRAINS

Amaranth** (GF), barley**, black rice (GF), brown rice** (GF), buckwheat** (GF), millet** (GF), oats**, quinoa** (GF), rye**, spelt**, teff** (GF), wheat**, wild rice (GF)

SPICES, FRESH HERBS OR OTHER

Basil, black pepper, cardamom, chilli, cinnamon, chives, cloves, coriander, cumin, dulse, garlic, ginger, lemon, lime, marjoram, mint, mustard, nori, nutmeg, nutritional yeast, oregano, paprika, parsley, rosemary, sage, sprouts, thyme, turmeric, wakame

*Like plants and animals, mushrooms belong to a kingdom of their own – fungi! However, based on their nutritional properties, and for the purposes of our diet, we can think of them as a vegetable

**Also available in flour form

***Including cooking oils (see the Plant Proof Oil Pyramid)

(GF) = Gluten Free

The food pyramid also includes a daily serving recommendation for each of the food groups. As caloric intake can differ greatly between individuals based on their age, gender and lifestyle, the number of servings you have per day will likely differ to those of your partner, friends or parents. With that in mind, take the serving recommendations in the pyramid as a minimum. It might seem like a lot of servings, but the serving sizes listed (e.g. half a cup of cooked rice, or a small handful of nuts) are achievable and will help you to ensure diversity.

FIGURE 10.4:

MINIMUM DAILY SERVINGS TARGETS ACCORDING TO THE PLANT PROOF FOOD PYRAMID

FOOD	MINIMUM DAILY SERVINGS TARGET
Berries	2
Other fruit	3
Greens and cruciferous vegetables	3
Other vegetables	3
Whole grains	3
Legumes	3*
High-fat plant foods	3

* I recommend increasing this to 4 or more serves of legumes per day for people who are relatively active, pregnant, lactating, or are sixty or older, as higher protein intake is more important for these groups (see Principle 2). You can make room for these foods by reducing your intake of whole grains.

Don't fear fruit

I am regularly asked if we should limit our fruit intake due to the naturally occurring sugars within them. I want to make it clear that as long as you're eating a balanced and varied diet, there is absolutely no scientific rationale to limit fruit intake. Fruit has been shown to be healthy at almost any amount – not just not harmful, but beneficial. When scientists had subjects consume twenty servings of fruit per day, not only did they find no adverse effects on weight, blood pressure or cholesterol, they actually saw an improvement in all these markers.[1] People who eat more whole fruit have also been shown to have a lower risk of developing type 2 diabetes.[2] Although it's true that all sugars deliver the same amount of calories whether they are in their natural or processed state, the negative health effects of eating sugars are linked to overconsumption of added sugars, not the sugars in whole fruit that are consumed alongside fibre, vitamins, minerals, water and important protective phytonutrients, which affect how that sugar is digested and ultimately how it affects our health.

The caveat to this is fruit juice. Eating a whole medium red apple is arguably healthier than downing a big glass of fresh apple juice. When we juice fruit, we separate the sugars from the fibre and create a 'natural' food product that has a low fibre to sugar ratio. Does this mean fruit juice is completely off limits? No, but I recommend sticking to whole fruits, which retain the flesh of the fruit and therefore the fibre. If you do wish to drink a glass of fruit juice, try to have it alongside a meal that contains fibre-rich food, such as a couple of slices of whole grain toast or half a cup of cooked beans.

Sweetening your food on a WFPBD

You'll be pleased to know that there are some plant-based options for adding sweetness to your food, though you should still aim to consume no more than 5% of total calories from added sugars. For the average female adult, that works out to be about 100 calories, or six teaspoons, of added sugars per day. The average Australian consumes fourteen teaspoons per day.[3]

FIGURE 10.5:
'GREEN LIGHT' AND 'ORANGE LIGHT' SWEETENERS

GREEN LIGHT	ORANGE LIGHT
Blackstrap molasses, coconut sugar, date sugar, dates, erythritol, maple syrup, monk fruit extract (calorie free), Stevia (calorie free)	Agave, aspartame, barley malt syrup, brown rice syrup, brown sugar, cane sugar, corn syrup, crystalline fructose, dextrose, fructose, fruit juice concentrate, glucose, high-fructose corn syrup, lactose, malt syrup, maltodextrin, maltose, molasses, raw sugar, rice syrup, Splenda, syrup, white sugar, xylitol

Where possible, aim for 'green light' sweeteners. 'Orange light' sweeteners are ones that I do not keep in my pantry, and would rarely eat apart from in the odd sweet treat. These ingredients are usually indicators of highly processed foods.

What about non-caloric sweeteners? First, just because certain sweeteners are calorie-free doesn't mean they are the answer to weight loss. In fact, studies show people consuming non-caloric sweeteners tend to take in the same total calories across the day compared with those consuming refined sugars; that is, they simply make up for the reduced energy in other meals.[4] However, in small doses, it appears that while these are not nutritious, certain types, such as Stevia and monk fruit extract, don't do any harm.

I sometimes add a date or two to my smoothies. These are also my preferred source of sweetness for baking and desserts as they contain a relatively high amount of micronutrients. I personally drink coffee without sweetener, but if you do want to add something to your coffee, date sugar, stevia, monk fruit extract or erythritol are the best options. I also used to add a few teaspoons of maple syrup to my porridge – one teaspoon of maple syrup is only 17 calories. Maple syrup made the oats much more enjoyable and that way I would have them almost every single day. However, as my tastebuds adjusted, I found berries provided plenty of sweetness, and they are bursting with nutrition. It's not just our tastebuds that change, but the gut too. When we reduce added sugars in our diet, sugar-craving bacteria die off and new bacteria that prefer to be fed with the new foods we've added to our diet (e.g. blueberries) proliferate.[5]

If you want to fully appreciate the natural sweetness and flavours found in whole plant foods, you're best off limiting foods that they simply cannot compete with. It's a process at first, but when you get to the other side, the new normal is the same level of bliss but from healthier foods.

Go for whole grains

As we covered in Part Two, regular consumption of whole grains, a great source of unrefined carbohydrates, is clearly associated with reduced risk of chronic disease and premature death.[6–8] Whole grains consist of three parts: the bran, the germ and the endosperm. When grains are refined, the bran and germ are removed, leaving a grain that is essentially equivalent in calories but significantly less nutritious.[9]

FIGURE 10.6:

REFINED AND UNREFINED GRAINS

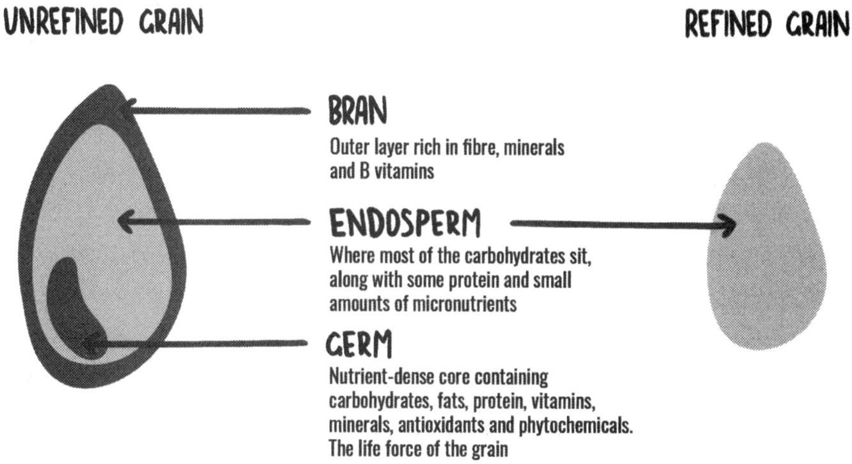

UNREFINED GRAIN

REFINED GRAIN

BRAN
Outer layer rich in fibre, minerals and B vitamins

ENDOSPERM
Where most of the carbohydrates sit, along with some protein and small amounts of micronutrients

GERM
Nutrient-dense core containing carbohydrates, fats, protein, vitamins, minerals, antioxidants and phytochemicals. The life force of the grain

Adapted from Whole Grains Council[9]

Where possible, choose whole wheat bread instead of white bread, brown rice instead of white rice, whole wheat pasta instead of white pasta, and so on. Over time, consistency with such decisions will be rewarded through better health.

FIGURE 10.7:

EXAMPLES OF WHOLE VERSUS REFINED GRAINS

REFINED GRAINS	WHOLE GRAINS
Bagel, breadcrumbs, corn flakes, corn tortillas, couscous, crackers, English muffins, flour tortillas, noodles, pasta, pie crust, pizza base, rice cakes, white bread, white flour, white pita bread, white rice	Amaranth (GF)*, barley*, brown rice (GF)*, buckwheat (GF)*, bulgur, corn (GF), farro, freekeh, millet (GF)*, oats*, quinoa (GF)*, rye*, sorghum (GF), spelt*, teff (GF)*, wheat*, whole wheat bread, whole wheat pasta, wild rice (GF)

* Also available in flour form

Note: Oats can be gluten-free. Check if the packaging specifies that they are free from gluten contamination.

Quick wins – whole rolled oats instead of boxed cereal

One of the quickest wins you can make is ditching healthy-looking boxed cereals in favour of whole rolled oats. If you find them a little bland, pair them with fresh berries, nuts and seeds for a breakfast that is incredibly nourishing and delicious. I recommend soaking your oats overnight, or cooking them, to increase the absorption of the protein and minerals (particularly iron and zinc) they contain.[10] As a bonus, oats contain beta-glucans, a prebiotic with powerful cholesterol-lowering properties. Specifically, 1.5 cups of oats contain enough beta-glucans to lower cholesterol by 5–10% after a few weeks of daily consumption.[11] If you are looking to reduce your LDL-C but don't think you could eat that many oats per day, you can also buy beta-glucans as a supplement powder.

Choosing your bread

There is a huge variety of breads available today, and it can be hard to tell those that are the healthiest from those that might offer more clever marketing or pretty packaging than health benefits.

When choosing a bread, we want one that is made from whole foods, or at least mostly whole foods. You might think this would be easy to spot but looks can be deceiving. I used to think that multigrain bread was automatically a great choice – you can literally see the grains! But most multigrain bread uses a refined flour base and thus contains less fibre, protein and micronutrients than a whole grain alternative. Just because a bread is brownish in colour, or you can see grains and seeds, or the brand uses the word 'grain' in its name doesn't necessarily mean it is made of whole-food ingredients. You'll need to review the ingredient list to know for sure. The first ingredient on the ingredient label (and therefore the major ingredient in the bread) should be something like:

- whole wheat flour
- whole wheat
- whole grain flour
- wholemeal wheat flour
- wholemeal grain.

Note that each contains the word 'whole'. Equally, you could replace 'wheat' with rye, barley, buckwheat or any other grain in the above descriptions and it would tell you that those grains have been used in their unrefined form. Some brands may even contain a blend and have two or more whole grains in the ingredient list. What we don't want to see as the first ingredient is 'wheat flour', or rye, barley or buckwheat flour, as this indicates the base ingredient is a refined flour. The other thing I like to check is that the carbohydrate to fibre ratio is 5:1 or better.[12] This means that per serve, or per 100 g, the total carbohydrates is no more than five times the amount of fibre. For example, if one serving of bread contains 20 g of total carbohydrates we are looking for at least 4 g of fibre.

When the first ingredient contains the word 'whole' and the carbohydrate to fibre ratio is 5:1 or better, you know you are truly onto a winning bread.

I tend to have two styles of bread on rotation. The first is a wholemeal sourdough that I buy locally and regularly enjoy with scrambled tofu. This is the type of bread that Sardinian centenarians eat![13] My other go-to is sprouted bread, such as Ezekiel, which is made from a blend of sprouted whole grain ingredients. Sprouting is a process that can supercharge the nutritional content of the grains – more on that later.

High-fat plant foods

I am often asked if a WFPBD needs to be low-fat in order to be health-promoting. While we certainly do want to limit saturated fats, there is insufficient science to support restriction of total fat to super low levels. While guidelines around the world differ slightly, the general recommendation is that energy from total fat should be between 15–35% of total daily calories. This lower level of 15% (in Australia, it's 20%) has been set to ensure individuals consume adequate amounts of total energy, essential fat-soluble vitamins, certain minerals found in foods rich in fat (e.g. zinc) and essential fatty acids like omega-3s and omega-6s.[14,15] In other words, if you restrict total fat too much, you may well compromise your health. What really matters more than whether we land at 15%, 25% or 35% is the type of fat we consume.

As we've seen in previous chapters, both diets very low in total fat, when part of an overall lifestyle program, and diets much higher in total fat while still being low in saturated fats, are able to lower the risk of cardiovascular disease. Further, when we look at the longest-living populations in the world, they are not all eating super low-fat diets. The Adventists following a vegan diet in the AHS-2 cohort, who are known for their incredible health and life spans, get about 30% of their total calories from fat – but, importantly, just 5% of this is from saturated fats.[16,17] So despite some of the rhetoric out there, as long as there's a strong emphasis on whole plant foods and saturated fats are kept low, people tend to greatly benefit from the inclusion of plant-based foods that are rich in unsaturated fats, such as nuts, seeds and avocado.

Figure 10.8 shows us which fats to include, reduce and exclude from our diets. Fortunately, if you follow the Plant Proof Food Pyramid, you will automatically avoid trans fats, as you will not find them in whole plant foods. You will also be greatly reducing your saturated fat consumption through the removal of meat and dairy, and, by consuming nuts, seeds, avocado and a small amount of certain oils (if that is right for you), you will be getting healthy amounts of unsaturated fats.

FIGURE 10.8:
TYPES OF FATS[18-20]

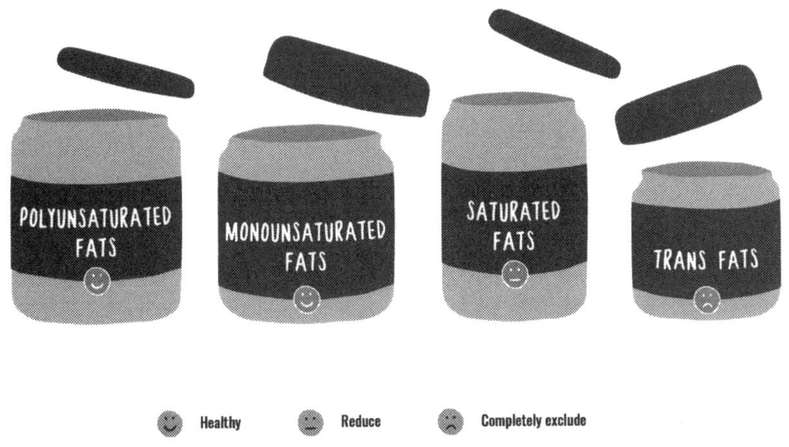

Saturated fats are not essential fats – there is no biological requirement that we consume them.[21] However, they are present in small amounts in incredibly healthy foods that we eat in order to meet our other dietary demands.[22] For example, three tablespoons of hemp seeds contains 1.4 g of saturated fats and 11 g of polyunsaturated fats. Even one can of chickpeas contains 0.5 g of saturated fats. Targeting 0 g of saturated fats is unrealistic when it comes to maintaining a healthy diet. Instead, our goal should be to avoid overconsumption of saturated fats. Generally speaking, most dietary guidelines around the world recommend minimising calories from saturated fats to no more than 7–10% of total calories.[23-25] However, the American Heart Association guidelines recommend limiting saturated fats to 5–6% of total calories for people who have or are at risk of cardiovascular disease, which, as we have seen, is a large percentage of society.[23,26] At these levels, saturated fats are perfectly healthy!

We do need to keep in mind that there are certain plant-based foods that have high saturated fat content (see Figure 10.9), and thus should be minimised in favour of the high-fat plant foods featured in the Plant Proof Food Pyramid – nuts, seeds, avocado and oils.

These plant-based foods are relatively rich in saturated fats and so are ones of which to be mindful – foods that we should try to avoid or minimise, as regular consumption will make it extremely difficult to stay within the recommended intake.

So what does a healthy level of saturated fat intake look like? Let's consider an average woman with a daily requirement of around 2000 calories. If the subject is healthy and free of chronic disease, and therefore aiming for an intake of no more than 10% of total calories from saturated fats, she should aim to limit her intake to a maximum of 200 calories per day, or around 22 g of saturated fats. If, on the other hand, she has a chronic disease or displays common risk factors such as high blood pressure, high cholesterol or BMI outside the healthy range, it would be beneficial to reduce her calories from saturated fats to 100 per day, or 11 g of saturated fats.

FIGURE 10.9:

TOP SOURCES OF SATURATED FATS IN PLANTS

FOOD	SERVING SIZE	TOTAL FAT	SATURATED FAT	% OF FAT FROM SATURATED FAT	CALORIES
Coconut milk, canned	1 cup	41.8 g	37.1 g	88.8%	406
Coconut oil	2 tbsp	27 g	22.5 g	83.3%	243
Cocoa butter	2 tbsp	27.2 g	16.2 g	59.6%	240
Coconut yoghurt	½ cup	15.5 g	14.6 g	94.2%	189
Palm oil	2 tbsp	27 g	13.3 g	49.3%	239
Fresh coconut meat	2 tbsp	13.6 g	12.1 g	89%	144
Light coconut milk, canned	1 cup	14.4 g	10.2 g	70.8%	146
Dried coconut	2 tbsp	6.5 g	5.7 g	87.7%	66

The saturated fat in cocoa butter is mostly stearic acid. Unlike animal fats, and tropical oils, it doesn't raise cholesterol

The saturated fat content of coconut yoghurt varies depending on the brand. This is an average value

Note: Coconut milk sold as a plant-based alternative to dairy milk is different to canned coconut milk. Because it is typically made with 90% or more water, it contains significantly less saturated fat

Looking at the top plant-based sources of saturated fats in Figure 10.9, it becomes clear why it's a good idea to not make a habit out of regularly consuming these foods in abundance. Just two tablespoons of coconut oil would max out the requirement for the healthy subject described above, leaving no room for saturated fats coming from other foods in their diet. Avoiding coconut products and palm oil (or having them infrequently, for example a curry with light coconut milk once a week) will make it easy to stay within the saturated fat recommendations without having to count how many grams you are consuming. This is undoubtedly one of the secret weapons of a well-planned WFPBD – unlike most other dietary patterns, if you simply stick to the food group recommendations in the Plant Proof Food Pyramid, your saturated fat intake will automatically land at a heart-healthy level.

Dark chocolate and cocoa butter

Despite being a top source of saturated fats, cocoa products have actually been shown to favourably affect cholesterol levels.[27] This is because the fat in cocoa beans, often called cocoa butter, is mostly stearic acid – a type of saturated fat that behaves very differently to the saturated fats that predominate in animal foods and tropical oils. Cocoa powder and dark chocolate also contain a high level of procyanidins, a powerful group of polyphenols with cholesterol-lowering properties.[28,29] If chocolate is your thing, look for dark chocolate that is dairy-free, 80% cocoa or more and fair trade, and stick to one serve (usually two to four squares) as a nutritious treat. Note that when recipes call for coconut oil, you can use cocoa butter instead!

What about cooking oils?

The question of whether or not you should use cooking oils if you are trying to eat the optimal diet for your health and wellbeing is one that divides a lot of people. Rather than getting into the nitty-gritty of the arguments, I want to remind you of what I said in Part Two: there is not one single optimal diet for human health. There is a set of characteristics or a theme that can be achieved through a variety of different dietary frameworks. To that point, I firmly believe that certain cooking oils may feature in some variations on this theme; that is, you can achieve peak health and wellbeing with or without them.

The science on cooking oils is somewhat nuanced, with some studies showing harm and others showing benefit. While I know as humans we like black and white answers, the simple fact is there are so many different oils, and personal circumstances, that it's impossible to have a blanket rule. What seems to be most important is the source of the oil, how it's processed, the cooking temperature it is used at, and your overall dietary pattern and health status. For example, olive oil has been repeatedly shown in RCTs to improve cardiovascular health, whereas the opposite is true for tropical oils such as coconut and palm.[30] In order to make sense of all this, I have taken the scientific literature and nutritional information about various oils and combined it into one resource: the Plant Proof Oil Pyramid.

FIGURE 10.10:

THE PLANT PROOF OIL PYRAMID[30–36]

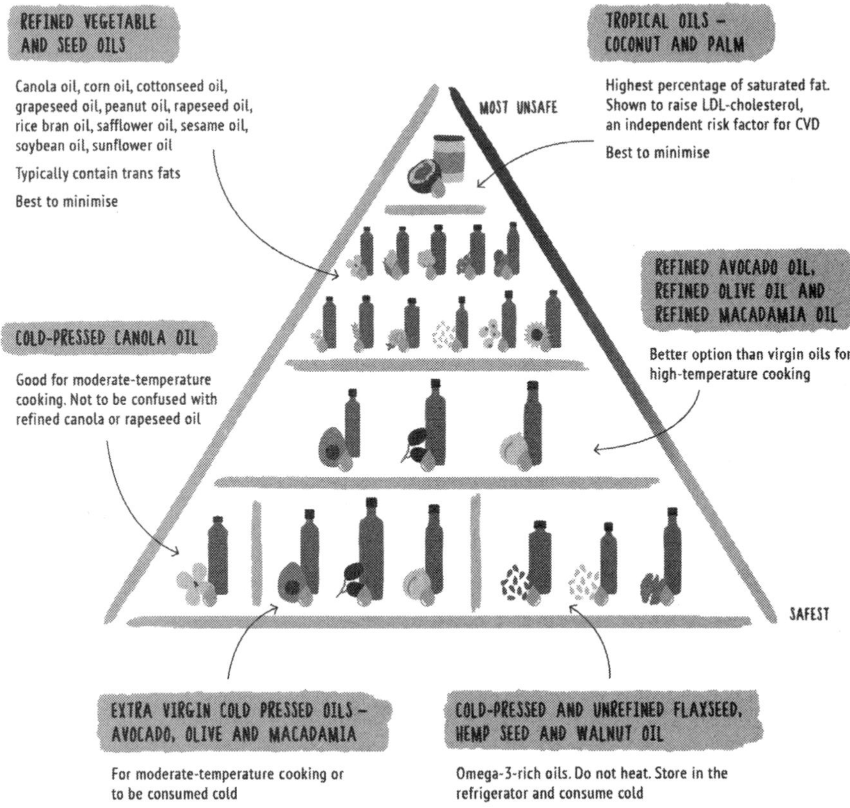
REFINED VEGETABLE AND SEED OILS
Canola oil, corn oil, cottonseed oil, grapeseed oil, peanut oil, rapeseed oil, rice bran oil, safflower oil, sesame oil, soybean oil, sunflower oil
Typically contain trans fats
Best to minimise
TROPICAL OILS – COCONUT AND PALM
Highest percentage of saturated fat. Shown to raise LDL-cholesterol, an independent risk factor for CVD
Best to minimise
MOST UNSAFE
REFINED AVOCADO OIL, REFINED OLIVE OIL AND REFINED MACADAMIA OIL
Better option than virgin oils for high-temperature cooking
COLD-PRESSED CANOLA OIL
Good for moderate-temperature cooking. Not to be confused with refined canola or rapeseed oil
SAFEST
EXTRA VIRGIN COLD PRESSED OILS – AVOCADO, OLIVE AND MACADAMIA
For moderate-temperature cooking or to be consumed cold
COLD-PRESSED AND UNREFINED FLAXSEED, HEMP SEED AND WALNUT OIL
Omega-3-rich oils. Do not heat. Store in the refrigerator and consume cold

How to use the Plant Proof Oil Pyramid

The safest oils feature at the bottom and the least safe at the top. At the top, you will find tropical oils and refined vegetable and seed oils. These are oils that I suggest minimising to the best of your ability, whether in your cooking or on your salads. The most important to minimise are tropical oils. It's true that coconut and palm oils are more stable than vegetable and seed oils during cooking, but just like animal fats, they contain a large percentage of saturated fats known to significantly raise your LDL-C and thus increase the risk of developing atherosclerosis.[31,37–41]

Refined vegetable oils are a step in the right direction, particularly oils like canola oil that have been shown to help reduce cholesterol.[30] However, while they're hardly the poison they are sometimes made out to be, there are a few reasons why I don't recommend using them for regular cooking. First, they often contain small amounts of trans fats.[34,42] In many countries, you wouldn't even know it was there, because labelling regulations allow refined vegetable and seed oil brands to declare 0 g of trans fats even when they contain small amounts (or in Australia's case, leave it off their label altogether).[43–45] Second, most of these oils also have a very high omega-6 to omega-3 ratio, which, as we'll discuss in Principle 4, can affect our bodies' ability to manufacture important long-chain omega-3s.[46] And, third, we have other options that are better.

At the bottom of the pyramid, you will find cold-pressed canola oil, extra virgin olive oil (EVOO), extra virgin avocado oil (EVAO) and extra virgin macadamia oil (EVMO). These are great options for cooking at moderate temperatures (e.g. pan frying above a medium flame). The words 'extra virgin' and 'cold-pressed' essentially mean the oil was mechanically processed rather than chemically processed, so they do not contain potentially harmful chemicals and additives. Cold-pressed canola oil should not be confused with industrially processed canola or rapeseed oil – it is a completely different product that is free from added chemicals and trans fats, is stable at high temperatures and has a very healthy fat profile.[47–49] These oils are also significantly lower in saturated fats than solid fats such as butter and coconut oil, and contain predominantly monounsaturated fats, which are stable under moderate heat.

For high temperature cooking, such as stir-frying or baking, I recommend using regular olive, avocado or macadamia oil. While these are refined oils, they are safer than the more expensive extra virgin varieties when it comes to cooking at high temperatures. You can find them positioned in the middle of the pyramid. Also included is a selection of oils that are considered safe to consume only at cold temperatures, such as to dress a salad. This is because they are extremely rich in polyunsaturated fats and are low in saturated fats. Personally, I always keep both EVOO and regular olive oil in my pantry. I tend to use EVOO for salad dressing and then regular olive oil for the majority of my cooking. This keeps things nice and simple.

How much should I use?

Most people would benefit from dramatically reducing the amount of oil they use to cook. 'A little goes a long way' is almost an understatement when it comes to oils. For example, using five tablespoons of oil during cooking will add almost 600 calories to your food. That's not so bad if you are cooking for a family of five, but if you are using that much to cook for just you, it's worth cutting back and saving those calories for more nutrient-dense whole foods. I use around half a tablespoon of oil for each person I am cooking for. So if I am making dinner for five people, I will use about 2.5 tablespoons. If I am cooking for myself, I will limit it to half a tablespoon – or, more often than not, I don't use oil and instead save those calories for more high-fat whole foods. If you simply prefer to avoid oils – that's absolutely fine – it's completely possible to cook food without oil. Ultimately, whatever method helps you eat more whole plants and leaves you feeling at your best, is the right method for you.

Who should pay particular attention to the cooking oils in their diet?

Groups that may specifically benefit from the inclusion of oils in their diet include young children, who have a higher fat requirement to support their growth and a lower appetite, and people who are trying to put on weight who are still struggling to achieve a calorie surplus.[50] Anyone who is otherwise healthy and eating according to the Plant Proof Food Pyramid and prefers to use oils in their cooking or on their salads can also use oils, preferably choosing oils from the safer options on the oil pyramid and using them in sensible amounts.

On the other hand, if you are trying to lose weight, you will likely benefit from excluding oils from your diet, at least when you're preparing your own food.

Principle 2: Be fibre-obsessed (and protein-aware)

There has been a consensus since the 1970s that fibre is a nutrient we should all be getting more of, when medical research identified diets rich in fibre to be protective against a wealth of chronic diseases.[51,52] Unfortunately, it's something almost all of us are deficient in.[53,54] The truth is that, as a society, we tend to obsess over protein when we should be obsessing over fibre!

Fibre, sometimes referred to as the fourth macronutrient, is the indigestible content of carbohydrates, meaning that instead of being broken down and absorbed in our small intestine, it passes intact through to our colon.[55,56] There are two main categories of fibre – soluble and insoluble – and both play important roles in our bodies, and are only found in plants.

Insoluble fibre acts as an intestinal cleanser by moving waste quickly through our colon, helping to keep us regular and avoid constipation. It also increases our sense of fullness after eating by absorbing water into the gut and providing bulk.[57] One of my favourite sources of insoluble fibre are whole grains – yet another reason to start the day with porridge.

Soluble fibre, along with polyphenols and a type of carbohydrate called resistant starch, are responsible for keeping the trillions of bacteria that reside within our large intestine, our microbiota, well fed and happy. Collectively, these three components of our food – soluble fibre, resistant starch and polyphenols – are known as *prebiotics*.[58,59] As the army of tiny microorganisms that make up the microbiota feed on these prebiotics, they produce compounds called *postbiotics* which provide incredible benefits both locally in the gut and throughout the body.[60] One example of a very potent postbiotic is the short-chain fatty acid butyrate, which was discussed in Chapter 6. This is one of the greatest perks of eating a WFPBD – it's a sure-fire way to up your prebiotics game, promote these microorganisms in your gut to grow stronger, and thus increase the production of these postbiotics. Feeding these microorganisms is absolutely critical to strengthening our gut lining, which in turn is linked to promoting a healthy body weight, improving blood sugar levels, helping us to think clearly, improving mood, optimising the immune system and lowering the risk of chronic disease.[61,62]

FIGURE 10.11:
SOLUBLE AND INSOLUBLE FIBRE

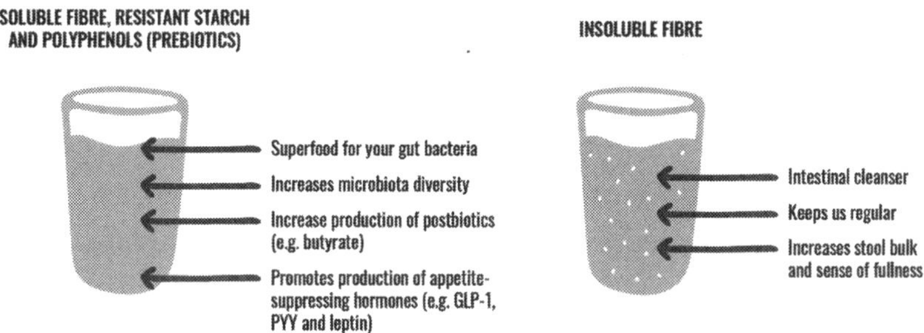
SOLUBLE FIBRE, RESISTANT STARCH AND POLYPHENOLS (PREBIOTICS)
Superfood for your gut bacteria
Increases microbiota diversity
Increase production of postbiotics (e.g. butyrate)
Promotes production of appetite-suppressing hormones (e.g. GLP-1, PYY and leptin)
INSOLUBLE FIBRE
Intestinal cleanser
Keeps us regular
Increases stool bulk and sense of fullness

Podcast highlight: Episodes 17, 70, 80, 81 and 102 with Dr B

Eating the right amount of fibre really does make for a happy gut! Just ask Dr Will Bulsiewicz, a gastroenterologist and the *New York Times*-bestselling author of *Fiber Fueled*. He is also one of my good friends and has appeared a number of times as a guest on the *Plant Proof* podcast to break down the complex science behind how nutrition affects gut health. To learn more about your gut microbes, I cannot recommend listening to these episodes enough, as well as reading his book. It's the perfect way to complement the information you're learning here.

How much fibre do we need?

In Australia, the adequate intake level for total fibre per day is 25 g for women and 30 g for men. However, this is only for promoting regular bowel movements. If you want to reap the benefits of fibre beyond this, and reduce your risk of chronic disease, the suggested daily intake is at least 28 g for women and 38 g for men.[53,63]

Given the health benefits associated with fibre are enormous, I usually consume 50–100 g of dietary fibre per day, which is in line with the amount of fibre consumed by populations with low incidence of chronic disease, and with Burkitt's hypothesis which we discussed in Chapter 6.[6,64] Unless you have a condition like ulcerative colitis, inflammatory bowel disease or irritable bowel syndrome (IBS) - which can make things trickier when it comes to adding more fibre to your diet - you will likely be fine slowly building up to consuming more than 28–38 g per day from whole foods. If you are in one of these groups, your doctor may give you more specific advice about limiting or lowering your fibre intake during what are often described as flare-ups.

FIGURE 10.12:

TOP WHOLE-FOOD SOURCES OF DIETARY FIBRE

FOOD	SERVING SIZE	DIETARY FIBRE
Split peas, cooked	½ cup	10.5 g
Navy beans, cooked	½ cup	9.5 g
Guava	1 cup	9 g
Blackberries	1 cup	7.5 g
Black beans, cooked	½ cup	7.5 g
Chia seeds	2 tbsp	7 g
Parsnip	1 cup	6.5 g
Prunes	10 prunes	6.5 g
Chickpeas, cooked	½ cup	6 g
Lentils, cooked	½ cup	6 g
Freekeh	½ cup	5.8 g
Pear	1 medium	5.5 g
Tempeh	½ cup	5.5 g
Kidney beans, cooked	½ cup	5 g
Medjool dates	3 dates	5 g
Avocado	⅓ medium	4.5 g
Pearl barley, cooked	½ cup	4.5 g
Whole wheat bread	2 slices	4.5 g
Dried figs	5 figs	4 g
Flaxseed	2 tbsp	4 g
Rolled oats	½ cup	4 g

Best sources of fibre

Both soluble and insoluble fibre are only found in plants. When you adopt a WFPBD, you will be consuming healthy amounts of both insoluble and soluble fibre at every meal and, providing you eat enough calories, will easily meet or exceed the suggested fibre target. Some of your best fibre providers are going to be legumes and whole grains.

What is protein and why do we need it?

Protein is made up of amino acids, which are often called the building blocks of life. When we consume protein, our digestive system breaks the protein molecules down into their constituent amino acids, which are then absorbed by our bodies and used to create over 30,000 different proteins, from antibodies to hormones to enzymes to transport molecules and much more, that are essential to our bodies' functioning. Proteins are defined by the amino acids that they contain and the sequence in which the acids occur.

There are two major classes of amino acids: essential amino acids (EAAs) and non-essential amino acids (NEAAs). Like essential and non-essential nutrients, NEAAs are those our bodies can manufacture on their own, and therefore we do not require them in our diet. EAAs, on the other hand, cannot be produced by our bodies, so we must obtain them from the food we eat. If we supply our body with sufficient EAAs, they will work together with the NEAAs to manufacture all of the protein molecules we require.

FIGURE 10.13:
ESSENTIAL AND NON-ESSENTIAL AMINO ACIDS

ESSENTIAL AMINO ACIDS (EAAs)	NON-ESSENTIAL AMINO ACIDS (NEAAs)
Histidine, leucine, isoleucine, lysine, methionine, phenylalanine, threonine, tryptophan, valine	Alanine, arginine, asparagine, aspartic acid, cysteine, glutamic acid, glutamine, glycine, proline, serine, tyrosine

EAAs are found in different concentrations in plant and animal foods, which leads to plant and animal foods sometimes being described as 'incomplete' and 'complete' proteins. These terms would make most people think that plant foods are missing certain EAAs, but that is not true – all plants contain all nine EAAs.[65] The term 'incomplete' only means that the quantity of one or more of the EAAs in a particular plant food is lower than what is considered optimal.[66] The problem with this narrow view of protein consumption is that, instead of looking at the overall dietary pattern, it judges a single food in isolation. The only way this could ever be a problem is if you ate a single source of protein, such as rice, or only nuts, as your sole source of calories – and even then, if you were consuming adequate calories, you would still easily be getting all EAAs in the required amounts, except lysine, which would just fall short of the daily recommendations. Fortunately, this is not how we eat and there are plenty of plant foods that are bursting with lysine – beans, lentils, tempeh and tofu, to name just a few.

You may be wondering whether this means you need to make sure you are eating 'complementary' protein sources of amino acids in each and every meal you have. Fortunately, there is no need to become hyper-focused on your amino acid intake, especially if you are eating a diverse range of plant foods. Your body has a constant pool of amino acids from the food you consume across the day. If you are eating according to the Plant Proof Food Pyramid, or even a WFPBD diet with just moderate diversity, your body will get all the EAA protein building blocks it needs.[66–68] To see this for yourself, put a day of eating according to the Plant Proof Pyramid into a nutrition tracking app. Prepare to be surprised – even foods that you may not commonly associate with protein, such as brussels sprouts, sweet potato, broccoli, mushrooms and corn, contain appreciable amounts of EAAs that add up over the day.

Is plant protein as digestible as animal protein?

While it's clear that people eating a WFPBD can easily get enough protein, the other aspect of protein quality that should be considered is its digestibility. You may have even heard someone say that plant protein is less digestible than animal protein. This belief comes from various studies that use one or both of the two main evaluation methods that rate protein digestibility, the PDCAAS and DIAAS. While these scoring systems are somewhat helpful in assessing protein quality, they are far from perfect.[69] They score proteins by looking at them in isolation, and any that are low in a particular EAA automatically lose points. But, as we touched on earlier, this would only be relevant in a real-life scenario if someone was only eating a single source of protein in their diet. For this reason, they are useful for identifying what protein sources are better in the context of limited food access to prevent malnutrition, but not so useful in the context of food abundance.

The other problem with these scoring systems is that they typically involve animals (rats and pigs) who are fed raw plant protein. However, there are many plant foods that we do not eat in their raw form, such as legumes and whole grains, and we know that when they are cooked the protein they contain becomes significantly more digestible. These animals also have different digestive systems to us. These factors combined lead to scores that underestimate the true digestibility and power of plant protein when it is properly prepared, and consumed by humans. Fortunately, as science advances we are beginning to see more precise studies conducted in humans and, so far, it seems that despite the limitations of these scoring systems, animal and plant protein digestibility only differ by a few per cent.[66,70] It's for these reasons that global protein recommendations are not any higher for vegetarians or vegans than others.[66,67]

Even if we assumed that on average plant protein was around 10% less digestible than animal protein (to play it safe), increasing our protein intake by 10% above the recommendations as an insurance policy is easily achieved on a WFPBD. For most people this is only around 5–10 g of protein more per day – equivalent to that found in two to three tablespoons of hemp seeds.

How much do we need?

The National Health and Medical Research Council (NHMRC) protein recommendations for the average adult are set out below (grams per kilogram of body weight). Men require slightly more protein than women, and the recommended dietary intake (RDI) increases slightly for people seventy and older, due to their increased risk of muscle loss and frailty.[65] Protein requirements are also higher during pregnancy and lactation to help promote healthy growth and development of a baby.[71]

FIGURE 10.14:

RECOMMENDED DIETARY INTAKE OF PROTEIN

	WOMEN (RDI)	MEN (RDI)
19–30 years	0.75 g/kg	0.84 g/kg
31–50 years	0.75 g/kg	0.84 g/kg
51–70 years	0.75 g/kg	0.84 g/kg
> 70 years	0.94 g/kg	1.07 g/kg
	PREGNANCY	
> 19 years	1 g/kg	
	LACTATION	
> 19 years	1.1 g/kg	

Adapted from NHMRC[71]

It's important to note that these recommendations are based on the amount of protein required to meet basic nutritional needs and prevent deficiency, and have not been tailored for people following a WFPBD. To illustrate what this looks like in terms of protein per day, let's go through an example using a 35-year-old woman who weighs 65 kg, spends a large percentage of their day sitting and doesn't perform intensive exercise. Working from the NHMRC protein recommendations, this woman's recommended daily protein intake is approximately 49 g (65 kg × 0.75). If we were to add an extra 10% as an insurance policy, to factor in the slightly lower digestibility of plant protein, it would increase her daily requirement to approximately 54 g. As you can see in Figure 10.15, she can easily achieve this by eating according to the Plant Proof Food Pyramid – by lunchtime, in fact.

The US Academy of Nutrition and Dietetics 2016 position paper emphasised that 'Vegetarian, including vegan, diets typically meet or exceed recommended protein intakes, when caloric intakes are adequate',[72] a finding supported by multiple studies that have analysed the protein intakes of vegetarian and vegan populations across the world.[16,73,74]

FIGURE 10.15:

EXAMPLE DAILY MEALS FOR ADEQUATE PROTEIN INTAKE

MEAL	INGREDIENTS	CALORIES	PROTEIN
Breakfast (overnight oats soaked in soy milk with fruit, nuts and seeds)	½ cup oats 1 cup soy milk ½ cup blueberries 10 walnut halves 1 tbsp ground flaxseed	439	18.1 g
Snack (hummus on whole wheat toast)	2 tbsp hummus 1 piece whole wheat toast 1 tbsp nutritional yeast	174	10.2 g
Lunch (chickpea and quinoa salad)	½ cup chickpeas 1 cup quinoa 3 tbsp almond slivers ⅓ avocado ½ cup mushrooms 1 tbsp nutritional yeast 1 cup baby spinach	608	25.4 g
Snack (chia pudding)	2 tbsp chia seeds soaked in ½ cup soy milk 2 tbsp cacao powder ½ cup strawberries	202	10.9 g
Dinner (tofu stir fry and brown rice)	100 g tofu, extra firm 1 cup brown rice ½ brown onion ½ cup mushrooms ¼ red capsicum (bell pepper) ½ cup green peas	462	25.3 g
TOTAL		1885	89.9 g

What about someone who is more physically active: how much protein do they require? There is a good amount of science to suggest that increasing protein intake is beneficial to those seeking improved muscle recovery, strength, growth and body composition. If this is you, my general recommendation is for plant-powered endurance athletes to aim for around 1.5 g per kg per day, and strength athletes to aim for around 1.8 g per kg per day, which is at a level that will maximise muscle growth and recovery while still allowing sufficient room to consume all food groups. These ranges are based on the best science available today, including a 2018 meta-analysis that looked at all of the science on optimal protein consumption for muscle repair and growth.[75–79]

FIGURE 10.16:

PROTEIN INTAKE FOR PEOPLE WHO ARE MORE PHYSICALLY ACTIVE

TRAINING TYPE	PROTEIN INTAKE
Endurance athletes	1.5 g/kg
Strength athletes	1.8 g/kg

Many of these studies looking at protein consumption and muscle growth are based on people consuming animal protein as part of an omnivorous diet. I've accounted for the slightly lower bioavailability of plant protein in my recommendations, along with the fact that there is an upper limit of protein set by the NHMRC of 25% of total calories.[71] Above this level, there is the potential for calories from protein to displace calories from other healthful food groups.

High protein and kidney health

Some of you may have heard that eating more than the RDI of protein is dangerous for our kidney health. A 2018 meta-analysis looked at twenty-eight clinical trials investigating protein intake and kidney health, which concluded that high-protein diets (1.2–2.4 g per kg per day) do not adversely affect kidney health.[80] However, that doesn't mean we should jack up our protein as high as possible. Even though there were no adverse effects on kidney health, these trials ranged from one to 104 weeks, with most being under eight weeks. So all these trials are really telling us is that in the short- to medium-term, there appears to be no harm in consuming protein above the RDI. If you have chronic kidney disease or if you have diabetes or hypertension and are therefore at risk of developing chronic kidney disease, you should not regularly consume more than the RDI of protein.[81]

Best plant-based sources of protein

While all plants contain protein, legumes are going to provide most of your protein when you eat from the Plant Proof Food Pyramid. I really cannot think of a healthier substitute for animal products! They contain all EAAs in health-promoting ratios, and are incredibly rich in fibre, vitamins, minerals and phytonutrients, while being naturally low in saturated fats and free from cholesterol. The Plant Proof Food Pyramid recommends at least three serves of legumes per day. For people who are relatively active, pregnant, lactating, or are sixty or older, I recommend increasing this to four or more serves per day, as higher protein intake is more important for these people.[65,71] You can make room for these foods by reducing your intake of whole grains.

To help you visualise how much protein is in whole plant foods, I have listed some of the most practical sources in Figure 10.17.

FIGURE 10.17:

PROTEIN CONTENT OF WHOLE PLANT FOODS

FOOD	SERVING SIZE	CALORIES	PROTEIN
Tempeh	150 g	186	22.5 g
Tofu, extra firm	150 g	166	19.9 g
Lupini beans, cooked	½ cup	100	13 g
Legume pasta, cooked	1 cup	185	11.4 g
Edamame beans, cooked	½ cup	127	11.1 g
Whole wheat bread	2 slices	181	9 g
Lentils, cooked	½ cup	115	8.9 g
Peanut butter	2 tbsp	176	7.3 g
Black beans, cooked	½ cup	120	7.1 g
Red kidney beans, cooked	½ cup	110	7.1 g
Nutritional yeast	2 tbsp	60	7 g
Hemp seeds	2 tbsp	111	6.3 g
Chickpeas, cooked	½ cup	114	5.8 g
Rolled oats	½ cup	153	5.3 g
Freekeh	½ cup	124	4.4 g
Quinoa, cooked	½ cup	111	4.1 g
Chia seeds	2 tbsp	97	3.3 g
Seitan	½ cup	138	27.5 g
Plant protein powder	1 scoop (30 g)	102	23 g

While these are technically processed foods, they can be part of a healthy diet, particularly for people who are highly active. I see these foods as tools to increase one's total protein intake without consuming animal products or ultra-processed vegan foods that are rich in saturated fat and refined sugars

Soy facts

Soy is a food demonised both for health and planetary reasons, but a lot of this is unfair, exaggerated or based on outdated information. Here are the key points to know about adding soy to your diet:

- Soy foods may protect us against certain forms of cancer. A 2018 meta-analysis of thirty observational studies, involving 266,699 subjects, suggests that soy consumption is protective against prostate cancer.[82] An overwhelming amount of evidence, including a 2020 meta-analysis of eighteen observational studies, suggests that soy is either protective against breast cancer or, at a minimum, does not have a negative effect.[83-85] Soy consumption has also been shown to reduce the risk of ovarian, colorectal, gastric and lung cancers.[86]
- Soy foods are heart-healthy. A 2019 umbrella review that combined results from over 114 meta-analyses looking at soy and health outcomes identified that people who regularly consumed soy were protected against having a stroke, developing heart disease and dying from cardiovascular disease. This protection is likely to be a result of the fact that consumption of soy foods typically shifts cholesterol, blood pressure and triglycerides to more favourable levels. In this same review, those who regularly consumed soy were also significantly less likely to be overweight or to develop type 2 diabetes, and those consuming greater amounts of isoflavones, a group of phytonutrients found in soy, had significantly better bone mineral density and cognitive function, as well as less frequent and severe hot flushes - a common symptom of menopause.[86]
- Despite all of this science, anti-soy proponents will regularly cite animal studies, where rodents, who process

soy completely differently to us, were given doses of soy, or the isoflavones found in soy, at considerably higher levels than we would ever consume in a typical day's eating.[87,88] And if they are to point to a human study, it's usually a case study involving a single male subject who consumed twelve servings of soy a day.[89] I am sure you will agree, twelve serves of any food per day is probably not the wisest idea! When we zoom back out and take a look at the highest-quality evidence we have – meaning studies that look at humans consuming soy – the evidence is clear. A 2020 meta-analysis of 41 clinical intervention studies looking at soy consumption and hormone levels concluded that soy does not negatively affect testosterone or oestrogen levels. This means that, despite what you may have heard, males consuming soy do not need to worry about developing 'man boobs'.[90]

- The only solid science in humans that supports reducing or avoiding soy consumption is for people with iodine deficiency or clinically diagnosed hypothyroidism. In these cases, the recommendation is to clear up any underlying iodine deficiency before reintroducing soy foods and, in the case of hypothyroidism, consuming soy foods at least one hour before or after taking medications, as soy can affect their absorption.[91–93]
- A common criticism of soy is that it is a GMO. It's true that the majority of soy crops are GMO – a 2017 paper reported that 82% of soybeans planted around the world in 2015 were from genetically modified seeds.[94] However, it's been estimated that 70–90% of all genetically modified food produced globally, soy included, is fed to food-producing livestock.[95] So if we want to avoid GMO soy crops and the chemical herbicides that come with them, our best bet is avoiding conventionally farmed meat. Fortunately, organic and/or

non-GMO soy products including edamame, tofu, tempeh and soy milk are now readily available in most supermarkets. Aside from the avoidance of chemical herbicides, organic soybeans also seem to have a better nutritional profile than their genetically modified counterparts.[96]

- Soy contains optimal amounts of all nine EAAs, making it a great protein source that is low in saturated fats, unlike many animal proteins. Soy is also rich in iron, calcium and potassium.[88]
- Soy products fed directly to humans have significantly lower environmental impact than animal products.[97]
- Communities traditionally consuming soy who exhibit good health tend to consume one to two serves per day – typically tofu, fermented soybeans (e.g. tempeh) or soy milk.[98] This is how I recommend including soy in your diet. Of course, if you're allergic to soy, or don't feel great after eating soy foods, not to worry – it is by no means an essential food. Just eat other legumes instead.

Principle 3: Diversity is key for gut health

More important than focusing on a handful of the best sources of fibre is eating a wide variety of fruits, vegetables, whole grains, legumes, nuts, seeds, spices and herbs. Every plant brings something to the table! This is because the unique forms of prebiotic fibre, resistant starch and polyphenols found in different plants selectively feed different species of bacteria. Just like us, the unique bacteria that reside in our gut each have their own favourite foods! And it's not until you satisfy their tastebuds that they begin to reward you. Ensuring variety in the plants we eat will promote a preponderance of healthy bacteria and a low percentage of harmful bacteria – a state of balance called *eubiosis*, where 'good' and 'bad' bacteria coexist in harmony.[99] While adding these to any dietary framework will provide benefit, it's also good to keep in mind that what you remove or limit is arguably just as important. Diets rich in animal products and/or ultra-processed foods promote a preponderance of harmful bacteria and effectively drown out the good bacteria – a state of imbalance called *dysbiosis* which, in turn, makes us more susceptible to poor health and disease.[62,100,101]

The potato hack

There is a simple hack you can use to get more bang for your buck when it comes to resistant starch. You may be doing this without even knowing! Cooking and cooling foods like pasta, potatoes and rice significantly increases the amount of available resistant starch.[102,103] One study found cooked potatoes placed in the fridge overnight almost tripled their resistant starch content.[104] They will also retain this if the food is heated back up, which is a great excuse to tuck into those leftovers.[103]

So, how many unique plants per week is best? The American Gut Project, an ongoing project headed up by famous microbiome researcher Professor Rob Knight, recently published a study that shed light on this. Rob and his team looked at microbiota samples from over 10,000 people (primarily from the United States, Australia and the United Kingdom) and found that, compared with subjects consuming fewer than ten unique plants per week, those consuming thirty or more unique plants per week had significantly more diversity in their microbiota. This is important because greater diversity within our microbiota is an indicator of a healthy gut.[61] The same study also identified that subjects eating over thirty unique plants a week had fewer antibiotic resistant genes in their microbes.[105] While this study didn't investigate why this was the case, the researchers hypothesised that those eating more plants were likely to be eating fewer animal products containing antibiotics, leading them to have a lower risk of developing antibiotic resistant infections. This is significant, as we learned in Chapter 9 that the World Health Organization (WHO) has declared antibiotic resistant infections to be 'one of the biggest threats to global health, food security, and development today'.[106]

The findings from this observational research are strengthened by an earlier RCT from 2006 involving 106 female subjects that compared a diet that had low plant diversity with a diet that had high plant diversity. Importantly, over the two-week trial, both groups consumed eight to ten servings of fruits and vegetables per day, so the only difference was the number of *unique* plants that they consumed, with subjects in one group eating large amounts of just a handful of fruits and vegetables while the other group consumed over eighteen unique plant species throughout the trial. After two weeks, those eating the diet with high plant diversity showed significantly less oxidative stress, a biomarker that is often used to assess a person's risk of developing certain chronic diseases.[107] This suggests that we are better off eating smaller amounts of many different phyto-nutrients and prebiotic fibre, rather than large amounts of fewer phytonutrients and prebiotic fibre.

One way to make sure you're getting your diversity is by tracking the number of different plants you incorporate into your weekly meals. This is a really helpful exercise both for those at the beginning of their transition to a more plant-focused diet and those who have been eating plant-based for a while but perhaps have fallen into the habit of eating the same foods every day. I recommend working your way up to forty unique plant foods per week, including room for herbs and spices for flavourful meals. Almost all herbs and spices, whether fresh or dried, are rich in polyphenols. This way, you get the benefits of the unique nutritional make-ups of thirty whole plants along with the enormous benefits of at least ten polyphenol-rich herbs and spices.

To help with this, I created the Plant Proof 40 challenge. I've found that most people get off to a flying start then begin to realise how many of the same plants they tend to incorporate in their diet day in, day out. Taking the challenge is a good way to motivate yourself to try new recipes and ingredients, and can help you switch up your supermarket shopping by taking advantage of what's in season and on special rather than relying on your old favourites. See it as a fun way to intermittently remind yourself of the importance of eating a varied diet, rather than a prescription that requires close tracking every single week. The idea being that eventually eating with variety will become effortless. I completed my own #plantproof40 to share with you as an example.

FIGURE 10.18:

SIMON'S #PLANTPROOF40

A small handful of fresh or a pinch or two of dried (→ Herbs and spices)

	PLANTS		PLANTS		PLANTS		HERBS AND SPICES (FRESH OR DRIED)
1	Apple (red)	11	Cherry tomatoes	21	Mango	31	Basil, fresh
2	Asparagus	12	Chia seeds	22	Nori	32	Black pepper
3	Avocado	13	Chickpeas	23	Oats	33	Ceylon cinnamon, ground
4	Bananas	14	Dates	24	Onion	34	Chives, fresh
5	Beetroot	15	Edamame	25	Pistachios	35	Coriander, fresh
6	Black beans	16	Garlic	26	Quinoa	36	Cumin, ground
7	Blackberries	17	Hemp seeds	27	Red lentils	37	Ginger, fresh
8	Blueberries	18	Iceberg lettuce	28	Strawberries	38	Paprika, ground
9	Brown rice	19	Kale	29	Walnuts	39	Parsley, fresh
10	Carrot	20	Leeks	30	Whole wheat bread	40	Turmeric, ground

This counts as a serve of wheat (→ Whole wheat bread)

What happens to the gut when you remove plant diversity from the diet?

A 2014 study, published in the highly prestigious *Nature* journal, was able to show that adoption of a 100% animal-based diet (yep, zero prebiotics) dramatically changed the microbiota.[101] Compared with a 100% plant-based diet, the carnivore diet increased numbers of bacteria associated with inflammatory bowel disease, decreased numbers of anti-inflammatory bacteria, increased production of a secondary bile acid called DCA (deoxycholic acid), thought to contribute to the development of liver and colon cancer, and significantly lowered short-chain fatty acid production.[108,109] All in just five days.

Handling an increase in fibre

If you're not used to consuming many vegetables, legumes and fruits, you may experience increased flatulence and bloating due to the increased activity of prebiotics in your gut. Fortunately, symptoms typically settle after a short transition period. Studies have identified that it typically takes two to three weeks for people to adjust to increased fibre.[110] During the transition, it may be helpful to:

1. Increase your fibre intake gradually, adding 2–4 g more every day (which is equal to around a quarter of a cup of lentils). As you're increasing your intake, it could be useful to substitute some foods with lower-fibre options, such as swapping brown rice for white rice, with the goal of switching back to the whole grain option in the near future.
2. Soak dry legumes for at least sixteen hours and make sure you cook them fully. This sixteen-hour soaking period

appears to be particularly important. A 2002 study showed that soaking legumes for sixteen hours was much more effective at reducing substances that may cause bloating or flatulence compared with twelve hours of soaking.[112] It also helps to skim and discard any froth that appears at the top of the pot during boiling. If using canned legumes, rinsing them thoroughly will further reduce these substances.

3. Make sure you chew well and eat slowly. Avoid straws and carbonated beverages – this will help to diminish the air you swallow while eating and improve your overall digestion.
4. Use spices like turmeric, carom, cumin, ginger and black pepper in your cooking, which have been known to counteract the production of gas and may aid with digestion.[111–115]
5. Drink plenty of water. While staying hydrated should always be on our radar, it is particularly important when consuming a higher fibre diet. The water soaked up by soluble fibre in our colon helps to soften stool, making them easier to pass.[116,117]
6. If your symptoms don't disappear after some time, there may be other causes behind your discomfort, so schedule an appointment with your doctor to rule out any gastrointestinal illnesses, such as IBS.

Prebiotics and IBS

Irritable bowel syndrome (IBS) is a condition with unexplained, recurrent abdominal discomfort that occurs with altered bowel form (constipation, diarrhoea or both), and a change in stool frequency.[118] The abdominal discomfort improves by having a bowel movement. This is a common condition, affecting around 20% of the world's population (women more so than men) and while it is primarily a gastrointestinal disorder, it does demonstrate the connection that exists between our brain and gut – compared with individuals who have healthy gut function, those with IBS are significantly more likely to demonstrate depressive symptoms.[119]

If you have been diagnosed with IBS or suspect you have it, you may have heard of the low-FODMAP diet.[118,120] A low-FODMAP diet is a low prebiotic fibre diet! When your microbiome is out of balance, in a state of dysbiosis, foods rich in prebiotic fibre can be difficult to tolerate. While it may sound like a good idea to just remove these foods for good, the low-FODMAP diet should be seen as a short-term diagnostic tool that allows those with IBS, under the strict supervision of a specialist dietitian, to identify what foods are triggering their symptoms. Once identified, they can then create a plan to strengthen their gut and move back towards a diet of greater plant diversity. This reintroduction of prebiotic-rich foods is incredibly important – following a low-FODMAP diet in the long-term may result in nutrient deficiencies and lacks the diversity required to build a thriving microbiome.[121]

This is one of the major problems with a meat-predominant diet – often people with IBS symptoms become attracted to such diets because without the prebiotic-rich foods that feed our bacteria, their symptoms settle. I understand the temptation – all of a sudden you go from bloating and abdominal pain to pain-free – but it is merely a band-aid. Over time, eating this way starves the healthy bacteria in our large intestine, leading to greater dysbiosis, lower short-chain fatty acid production, breakdown of the gut lining, inflammatory molecules entering the blood, and more risk of negative health consequences downstream such as increased risk of colorectal cancer, type 2 diabetes and cardiovascular disease.[6,122,123]

Gluten, lectins and gut health

Gluten and lectins are proteins that have suffered from some negative press in recent years, which led some people to remove them from their diet over fears of gut damage. I think that, for the most part, they have been the victims of poor science or negative marketing.

Let's start with gluten. There is a certain group of people, about 1% of the global population, who should categorically avoid gluten, primarily people with the autoimmune conditions coeliac disease or gluten ataxia.[124–126] However, nearly three out of every four people who are eliminating gluten from their diet are doing so with no symptoms.[125] Furthermore, a large percentage of the one in four who do have symptoms do not actually have an issue with gluten when challenged under strict testing protocols.[127] So how should you navigate gluten?

- Avoid eliminating gluten-containing whole foods unless you have coeliac disease or gluten ataxia, or have been recommended to do so by a health professional who fully understands your history and has conducted a gluten challenge test.
- One condition that causes many people to remove gluten is non-coeliac gluten sensitivity (NCGS). However, recent clinical trials suggest that it's mostly not gluten that is triggering symptoms but a specific FODMAP in wheat called fructans.[128–130] Rather than avoiding wheat and gluten for life, it's better to address the source of the problem with a health professional.[131]
- If you do eliminate gluten, be aware that often this leads to reduced plant diversity in the diet and increased consumption of gluten-free ultra-processed foods, which are often disguised as health foods. Instead, swap gluten-containing whole grains for gluten-free whole grains (see Figure 10.7) to ensure adequate fibre intake and

> plenty of prebiotics for the health-promoting microbes in your gut. Eliminating gluten doesn't automatically mean your diet becomes less healthy, but if you remove it and do not replace it with gluten-free whole grains, large amounts of science suggest you will be at increased risk of developing several chronic diseases, including cardiovascular disease and type 2 diabetes.[132–135]

What about lectins? These are a group of proteins that bind to sugar molecules and are most prevalent in foods such as legumes, whole grains, nuts, potatoes and nightshade vegetables (such as capsicum, eggplant and tomato). They pass through our gut undigested and can reduce the absorption of nutrients. This effect on nutrient absorption has seen them classified as an *anti-nutrient*. A few studies exist that show humans became quickly sick after consuming legumes, but it needs to be noted that in these studies the legumes were eaten raw or improperly prepared.[136,137] Despite this, certain people will have you believe lectins are the root of all evil and should be avoided. Specifically, they claim that lectins damage the gut wall and lead to leaky gut, bloating, diarrhoea and a bunch of other gut health issues. That sounds scary and may have you questioning whether it's healthy to consume the foods richest in lectins.

The problem with this theory is that first, what you won't hear from those generating fear about lectins is that even at a mechanistic level (petri dish), there is significantly more science demonstrating the potential benefits of lectins, particularly for destroying cancer cells.[138] Second, and most importantly, as we discussed in Part One, good science looks at converging lines from multiple types of studies from across the world. When we do that, it's clear from large observational studies and controlled clinical trials that consuming lectins in whole plant foods (such as legumes) leads to better health outcomes time and time again.[139–142] For example, a study looking at dietary predictors of survival across five cohorts found that for every 20 g of legumes consumed per day, subjects reduced their risk of premature death by 7–8%.[141] When you prepare lectin-rich foods as you would to eat them (e.g. cooking beans or grains), you destroy the majority of lectins.

If we take a step back, it makes complete sense. Lectins are a natural insecticide – they protect the growing plant from being attacked by insects. Humans worked out how to bypass this protective system by harvesting the plant and preparing it in a way that allowed for an enjoyable eating experience, easier digestion and promotion of health.

One way to put the whole lectin fear into context is by looking at oxygen, a molecule that I am sure we all agree is healthy. Did you know if you consume 100% oxygen (air is only 21% oxygen) beyond forty-eight hours, you would experience tissue damage and eventually death?[143] Yet we don't think of oxygen as dangerous – it's essential, in the right dose. Anti-nutrients like lectins are similar.

Should I take prebiotic and probiotic supplements?

It's really important to understand that the most important aspect of our diet is the diversity of whole plants. It's like the foundations of a house – you simply cannot trade diversity of plants for anything else, including a supplement, and expect better results. However, there are scenarios where taking a prebiotic or probiotic supplement may be useful to help nourish your microbiome and get you to a point where you can handle more plant diversity.

Until there is further science that fills a bunch of knowledge gaps, the current scientific consensus is as follows.

Prebiotic supplements

Taking prebiotic supplements derived from plants (such as acacia fibre, artichoke fibre, beta-glucans, guar gum, psyllium husk or green banana fibre), either on a rotational basis or as a blend, is a good way to nourish a diverse microbiome.[58] I personally use a prebiotic blend daily when travelling, due to more inconsistent eating habits, and on an ad-hoc basis when at home – at least a few times a week, usually in smoothies. Multiple studies have shown that prebiotic supplementation significantly reduces the chance of developing travellers' diarrhoea – a worthy investment to maximise time for sightseeing![58]

The other great thing about prebiotic supplements is that they can help you strengthen your gut. If you are struggling to include a wide variety of plants in your diet due to bloating, gas, abdominal pain or related problems, a prebiotic supplement can be a way to gently nourish your microbiota and promote the growth of probiotics to a point where you can handle more plant diversity.[144] In this instance, it's best to start with one type of prebiotic supplement rather than a blend, and increase the dose and varieties as your toleration increases. This increased tolerance will reflect an increase in your microbiota diversity, the eventual goal being that you will be able to slowly reintroduce more whole foods and eventually consume a diet rich in plant diversity without symptoms or the need for a supplement.

Probiotic supplements

Despite being marketed as a panacea, most of the buzz surrounding probiotics is overhyped. If you have a healthy gut without any digestive symptoms, you are far better off focusing on the diversity of plants in your diet.

Some studies found benefits for particular probiotics for subjects with gastrointestinal conditions, such as ulcerative colitis and IBS, but the 2020 clinical guidelines from the American

Gastroenterological Association clearly state that such evidence is very low and there is insufficient data to make specific recommendations.[145] Rather than this meaning that probiotics never work, a more accurate interpretation would be that probiotics are not a one-size-fits-all solution. The problem is currently specificity. Most of us have thousands of strains of bacteria in our gut. These strains, and the number of them, vary greatly between individuals, so much so that our microbiota is not too dissimilar to our fingerprints.[146] That means our weak points, and therefore where our gut needs support, are likely to be vastly different to the next person's. A probiotic supplement is lucky to contain a handful of strains, and whether those are going to be helpful depends on the unique microbiome composition of the person taking them.

Fortunately, probiotics appear to be quite safe, although more studies are needed, particularly on subjects who are immune compromised.[147,148] Because probiotics are low risk, my advice is that adding them to your gut-health regime, pending approval from your doctor, requires a trial-and-error approach.[149] If you think your microbiome could do with some extra hands on deck and want to try your luck, take a multi-strain probiotic that contains over 25 billion bacteria and is shelf stable at room temperature, for a period of at least eight weeks.[131,150] It may help, it may not – whether you want to go down this route of trial and error largely boils down to whether you can justify the cost.

What about after a course of antibiotics – should we take probiotics to replenish the healthy bacteria that gets wiped out? While once upon a time it was common practice to take probiotics during and after a course of antibiotics, recent science suggests that although probiotic supplementation can help reduce antibiotic-associated diarrhoea, it may actually impair the recovery of your microbiota after antibiotics.[148,151] A more evidence-based approach seems to be to focus on the diversity of plants in your diet and take a prebiotic supplement to support the healthy bacteria that remain so they can proliferate after their numbers have been reduced by antibiotics.[152]

Fermented foods

I love fermented foods. Not only do they taste delicious but they are nutritional powerhouses! While fermentation was historically used to preserve foods, giving them a longer shelf life, what has become increasingly understood and appreciated is the way that fermentation can upgrade the nutritional quality of food.[153] Some of the more popular fermented foods you are likely to be familiar with are sauerkraut, kimchi, kefir, tempeh, miso, natto, sourdough and kombucha.

Here are a few examples of how fermentation can upgrade the properties of our food:

- Fermentation produces probiotic bacteria strains which, despite being transient just like probiotic supplements, can compete with pathogenic bacteria and produce beneficial metabolites in our gut.[152] One single serving of sauerkraut has been shown to contain up to twenty-eight strains of probiotics.[154]
- Fermentation can increase the vitamin, mineral and antioxidant content of food.[155,156]
- Fermentation can increase the availability of nutrients in our food, particularly minerals, by breaking down anti-nutrients such as phytic acid and lectins by up to 95%. A prime example of this is fermented soybeans (natto, miso and tempeh).[157-159]
- Fermentation has the ability to convert inactive molecules in our food, such as polyphenols, into active molecules.[160,161] This is particularly important if we have compromised gut health, as we may not have the required

bacteria to carry this out for us in our colon. We can use fermented foods to do some of the heavy lifting that our gut is currently not equipped to do. This is one of the reasons that I recommend anyone with IBS try to include small amounts of sauerkraut (red cabbage form, as it is lower in FODMAPs) in their diet.

- Fermentation has been shown to lower FODMAPs in several foods, such as tempeh and whole grain sourdough.[162,163]

My recommendation with fermented foods, particularly for those rich in salt such as kimchi and miso, is to stick to just a few serves per day within the context of a well-diversified WFPBD. Where possible, it's also best to opt for low-salt or low-sodium versions.

Principle 4: Consider nutrients of focus

All dietary patterns, whether they include animal products or not, have certain micronutrients in abundance and certain micronutrients that require a bit of thought in order to consume them in adequate quantities. I call the latter *nutrients of focus.* The fact that we need to put a bit more effort into acquiring these nutrients is nothing to be alarmed by – we just need to be aware that removing animal products doesn't guarantee instant success. Poorly executed diets can lead to poor health outcomes, so you must be aware of what to focus on ahead of time. Before you know it, it will become a routine part of your lifestyle, and you'll enjoy the benefits of these essential nutrients without any of the baggage that comes with consuming animal products or ultra-processed foods.

When you are eating a WFPBD, the nutrients you will be consuming an abundance of are dietary fibre, omega-3 polyunsaturated fats, monounsaturated fats, folate, vitamin C, vitamin E, iron and potassium, while minimising sodium and saturated fats.[73,164,165] The fact that these nutrients are plentiful in a WFPBD can often be overlooked because naysayers focus instead on the nutrients that a WFPBD tends to be lower in, such as calcium, vitamin D, vitamin B_{12}, zinc, iodine and selenium.[163–172] It is these nutrients, along with iron and omega-3 fats, that are the eight essential nutrients of focus I want to discuss here as part of a Plant Proof diet.

Of course, there are a host of other nutrients obtained through our diet that contribute to good health, but rest assured that a WFPBD like the one described in the Plant Proof Food Pyramid will have you covered for those. The eight nutrients in this section are simply those that you might need to pay a bit more attention to, especially when you first make the shift.

Blood tests

There tends to be mixed advice when it comes to whether you should undertake some routine blood tests before making changes to your diet. I don't advocate overdoing it, but I do think blood tests are important when it comes to optimising your diet, and they are particularly useful to determine a baseline before you make changes to the food you eat. For example, before switching to a WFPBD, you might perform a baseline blood test and notice your iron is moderately low. Then, six months after making dietary changes, you test again and it's now only slightly low. If you didn't do the baseline test, you could wrongly think that your slightly low iron levels are a negative impact of your dietary changes, when in fact they have improved! With that in mind, I recommend a baseline test to see where everything is at, and then re-tests at six months and twelve months to see how you are tracking. Thereafter, if everything is normal, I would recommend yearly tests, particularly if you are over the age of thirty-five, for peace of mind. If your results are consistently normal, it's unnecessary to be testing more frequently than this.

1. Omega-3s

Omega-3 and omega-6 are both types of fat called polyunsaturated fats. These are *essential fatty acids*, meaning that, unlike saturated and monounsaturated fats, our bodies cannot produce them and it's important we consume them in adequate amounts to avoid health complications. Omega-3s are in particularly high concentrations in the brain and retina, and play a key role in maintaining healthy cell membrane function and gene expression.[173] Omega-6s have traditionally been thought of as inflammatory, but this is a misinterpretation of the science – they are also extremely healthful and have also been shown to reduce the risk of cardiovascular disease and decrease insulin resistance when consumed instead of saturated fats.[19,174–176]

However, it is important to ensure that we do not overconsume omega-6 fats, as this can affect our ability to maintain omega-3 levels. Both omega-3s and omega-6s come in two forms: short-chain fatty acids and long-chain fatty acids. The short-chain form of omega-3s are called alpha linoleic acid (ALA), and the short-chain form of omega-6s are called linoleic acid (LA). These are precursors to the long-chain forms because when ALA and LA are absorbed by the body, they are converted into the long-chain forms, which are the biologically active forms.[177,178] Specifically, ALA is converted into long-chain omega-3s called docosahexaenoic acid (DHA), eicosapentaenoic acid (EPA) and docosapentaenoic acid (DPA), while LA is converted into a long-chain omega-6 called arachidonic acid (AA).

The conversion of ALA to DHA, EPA and DPA in our bodies is not particularly efficient, and it can be even lower in the presence of high amounts of LA, which compete with ALA for the same conversion enzymes.[173,179–181] If you are eating a WFPBD that does not supply a direct source of EPA and DHA, and is rich in LA, which can happen when you are consuming a lot of refined seed oils, you could end up with inadequate concentrations of these important long-chain omega-3s.[179] So, in order to ensure adequate consumption of omega-3s and omega-6s in the right ratio, minimise refined seed oils in your diet by avoiding ultra-processed vegan junk foods, and consume whole plant foods rich in omega-3s each day. The best sources of omega-3s are shown in Figure 10.19, and the serving size that would be required in order to achieve the daily requirement is in Figure 10.20. Importantly, when creating these recommendations I factored in findings from studies which suggest that if you are not consuming DHA and EPA directly, you should double your daily intake of ALA.[173,179] You'll notice that just one to two tablespoons of ground flaxseeds or chia seeds provides enough short-chain omega-3s for an adult consuming a WFPBD to ensure adequate levels of DHA and EPA without requiring omega-3 supplementation. And as long as you have sufficient levels of DHA, it appears our bodies can produce adequate amounts of DPA.[182]

Where possible, try to consume these foods in the whole forms as the oil forms are less nutrient-dense. If you do opt for an oil, it's best to choose a cold-pressed unrefined oil, per the Plant Proof Oil Pyramid. And remember, these omega-3-rich oils should be stored in the refrigerator and consumed cold.

FIGURE 10.19:

THE BEST SOURCES FOR YOUR DAILY DOSE OF ALA OMEGA-3 FATS

	LA (Omega-6)	ALA (Omega-3)	SATURATED FAT*
Chia seeds (1 tbsp)	0.6 g	1.8 g	0.4 g
Walnuts (9 halves)	6.9 g	1.7 g	1.1 g
Ground flaxseeds (1 tbsp)	0.4 g	1.6 g	0.3 g
Hulled hemp seeds (1 tbsp)	2.9 g	0.9 g	0.5 g

* Included to show how low in saturated fats these foods are.

FIGURE 10.20:

DAILY SERVING SIZE OF OMEGA-3-RICH FOODS REQUIRED TO CONVERT ENOUGH DHA AND EPA FROM ALA (IF NOT SUPPLEMENTING) TO MEET DAILY RECOMMENDATIONS[173]

	WOMEN (SERVING SIZE TO EXCEED 1.6 g/DAY OF ALA)	MEN (SERVING SIZE TO EXCEED 2.6 g/DAY OF ALA)
Ground flaxseeds*	1 tbsp	2 tbsp
Chia seeds	1 tbsp	2 tbsp
Hulled hemp seeds	2 tbsp	3 tbsp
Walnuts (halves)	9 halves	14 halves

* It's best not to consume whole flaxseeds, as your body is unlikely to absorb the fats and other nutrients they contain – often you will see they pass right through! The best way to consume them is by buying them as whole seeds and then gently grinding a single serving into powder just before consuming.

While consuming omega-3-rich plant foods on a daily basis will ensure that adequate amounts of these long-chain omega-3s are produced for essential functions, a case can be made for taking a DHA and EPA omega-3 supplement. Emerging evidence suggests that supplementation to levels above what would likely be achieved by eating omega-rich plant foods is a heart-healthy move.[183–185] In 2019, results from the VITAL study, a five-year RCT looking at over 25,000 subjects without cardiovascular disease, identified that supplementation of DHA and EPA (840 mg per day) was beneficial. While there wasn't a decrease in the risk of experiencing a major cardiovascular event when these were analysed as a group (i.e. stroke, heart attack or death from any cardiovascular event combined), which is what the researchers were most interested in, when these events were looked at separately, there was a 28% reduction in the risk of having a heart attack, and a 50% reduction in the risk of a fatal heart attack.[186] The reduction in risk was even greater for people who consumed fewer than 1.5 serves of fish per week. This is an important point – the reason many previous omega-3 trials have failed to show benefit may be because subjects had a high baseline intake of fish, and thus because their long-chain omega-3 needs were already met, there was no additional benefit to be obtained from supplementation. A similar seven-year RCT out of the United Kingdom involving over 15,000 people living with diabetes, the ASCEND trial, found that the exact same dose of DHA and EPA significantly reduced the risk of dying from cardiovascular disease by 19%.[187] But remember that multiple meta-analyses show us that vegetarians, including vegans, already have significantly lower risk of dying from heart disease without optimising omega-3 intake. This is one of the powerful advantages of a WFPBD.[188,189] If we were to add a direct source of DHA and EPA to such diets, it's possible the results would be even better![173] Until we have a study that sets out to precisely investigate this, it seems like a reasonable insurance policy if you can justify the cost of the supplement – particularly for those who may be somewhat inconsistent in their consumption of ALA-rich plant foods.

As we spoke about in Chapter 7, a direct source of these long-chain omega-3s may also give you greater protection against cognitive decline, and additional research shows that their inclusion during pregnancy may improve outcomes.[191]

If you are wanting to take an omega-3 supplement, the recommended dose depends on your individual circumstances. If you are otherwise healthy, I recommend taking 840–1000 mg per day. If you have cardiovascular disease, diabetes or high triglycerides and are taking a statin medication, there is evidence to support supplementation of a specific type of omega-3 supplement at 4 g per day; however, this requires a prescription and therefore needs to be discussed with your doctor.[190] And if you're pregnant, findings from a 2018 meta-analysis of seventy RCTs looking at omega-3 supplementation during pregnancy found that daily supplementation of 500–1000 mg of long-chain omega-3s (providing at least 500 mg of DHA) from twelve weeks of pregnancy onwards significantly reduced the risk of premature birth and having a baby with low birth weight.[191]

When it comes to choosing an omega-3 supplement, we should be aware that, despite the prevalence of fish oil, fish are not the original source of these essential fats. The original source is microalgae. Fish feed on microalgae and accumulate omega-3s in their body over time. Fortunately, today we can now supplement DHA and EPA without having to buy in to a practice that exploits trillions of fish, and without the associated risk of ingesting heavy metals and microplastics, by going straight to the source. For peace of mind, it's good to know that algae oil omega-3 supplements have been shown to be just as if not more effective than fish oil, krill oil, and fish themselves in raising levels of long-chain omega-3s in the body.[192–194] I take a daily algae oil supplement that provides 850 mg of DHA and EPA, which is equivalent to eating around three pieces of salmon per week.

2. Vitamin B_{12}

Vitamin B_{12}, also known as cobalamin, is a water-soluble vitamin that has many important roles in the body, including DNA synthesis, cellular energy production, promotion of growth in infants and children and the synthesis of myelin, a lipid-rich sleeve that wraps around our nerves to form a protective layer.[195,196] Because the active form of vitamin B_{12} is only found in animal products, it receives a lot of attention in discussions about WFPBDs. However, B_{12} isn't just a nutrient of focus for vegans – a large study of 3000 American adults from the general population found that 39% were low or deficient in B_{12}![73,197] Signs of B_{12} deficiency include fatigue, impaired immune function, cardiovascular issues, infertility, visual disturbances, cognitive decline, and numbness or tingling in the hands and feet.[195,198,199] Deficiencies in B_{12} have also been linked to developmental defects in unborn children.[200–202]

FIGURE 10.21:

RECOMMENDED DIETARY INTAKE OF VITAMIN B_{12}

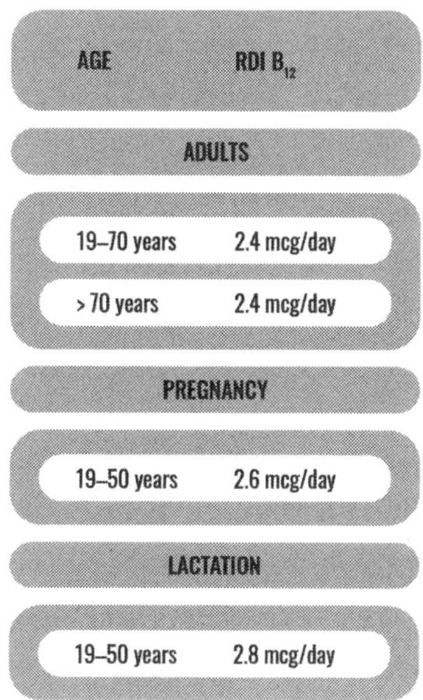

AGE	RDI B_{12}
ADULTS	
19–70 years	2.4 mcg/day
> 70 years	2.4 mcg/day
PREGNANCY	
19–50 years	2.6 mcg/day
LACTATION	
19–50 years	2.8 mcg/day

Adapted from NHMRC[203]

How can we ensure adequate B_{12} intake?

There are essentially three options for people following a WFPBD to reach the RDI and maintain healthy B_{12} levels:

FIGURE 10.22:

OPTIONS FOR MAINTAINING HEALTHY B_{12} LEVELS ON A WFPBD

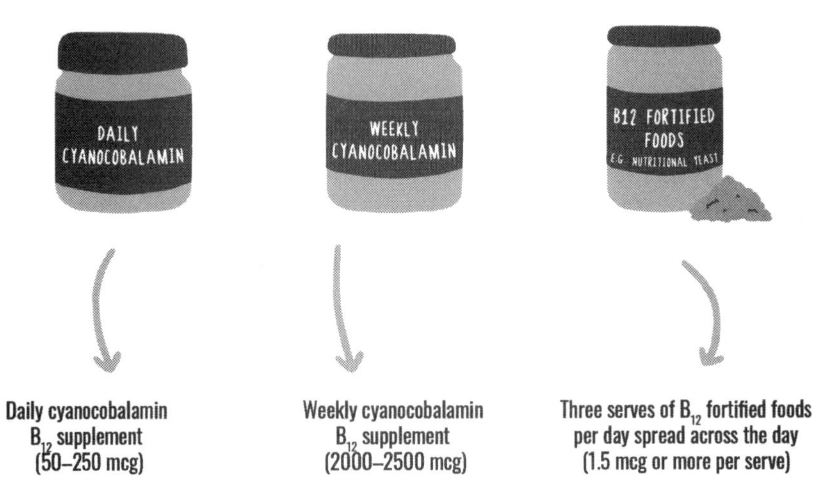

The great thing is that in studies where vegans have taken a B_{12} supplement or eaten B_{12}-fortified foods, their B_{12} levels are completely normal.[73] In fact, these sources of B_{12} are actually more effective than consuming animal foods for maintaining healthy B_{12} status![197]

How is this possible? The first reason is that B_{12} in animal tissue is bound to protein and requires digestive enzymes and stomach acid to detach it for absorption – a process that becomes less efficient as we age, irrespective of the diet we follow, and can be impaired in people with certain digestive issues.[204,205] Second, the B_{12}-producing bacteria in ruminant animals rely on cobalt, a mineral found in soil that in many parts of the world has become less abundant as a result of our intensive farming practices.[206] A farmed animal grazing on degrading pasture is not the same as a wild animal roaming around on truly thriving soil and drinking out of cobalt-containing streams.

As a result, it seems that for those who do choose to eat meat, the safer option for ensuring adequate B_{12} intake, although no doubt worse for overall human health and animal welfare, is factory farmed meat. This is in fact where 90% of the world's B_{12} supplements go – they are fed to livestock to prevent them developing B_{12} deficiency as a result of being confined to an area away from cobalt-containing soil.[207] To put it another way, the most reliable source of B_{12} in our diets is taking a supplement ourselves, or consuming animal products sourced from animals that we know were supplemented with B_{12}.

So, while a tiny bit of planning is required to ensure optimal B_{12} status on a WFPBD, this is not a nutrient about which to be concerned. In fact, the National Academy of Medicine in the United States recommends everyone over fifty years old meet the B_{12} RDI with a supplement or fortified foods, even if they eat animal foods.[205]

You might be wondering, if the RDI is 2.4 mcg, why are the supplement dosages so high? The simple answer is that we do not absorb all of the B_{12} we consume, and studies have shown that as the dosage increases, the percentage that is absorbed drops dramatically. If you are eating animal products or B_{12}-fortified foods three times per day, you do not need to be consuming a huge amount of B_{12} in order to reach the recommendations. At these small doses, we absorb 56%.[208] However, let's say for convenience we want to take a supplement once a day or even once a week and absorb enough to maintain healthy B_{12} status. As the dosage increases from 1 mcg of B_{12}, the absorption rate drops. So much so that at 1000 mcg you are only absorbing around 1.3%. This is why a daily supplement of 50–250 mcg, or weekly supplement of 2000–2500 mcg, is recommended – manufacturers take these absorption rates into account when producing B_{12} supplements.

There are only a few circumstances where I would recommend taking a form of B_{12} other than those depicted in Figure 10.22. If you have kidney disease or are a smoker, the methylcobalamin and adenosylcobalamin forms (taken together) would be more sensible.[209,210] However, until further studies are published, it is difficult to make recommendations about the dosage for these other forms of B_{12} to prevent or reverse deficiency, so it is best to discuss this with your doctor and perform periodic blood tests to ensure the dose you are taking is adequate to achieve healthy B_{12} status.

3. Vitamin D

Vitamin D is a fat-soluble vitamin that plays an important role in calcium absorption and healthy bone formation and mineralisation (hardening).[211] It's often called the *sunshine vitamin*, because our bodies can synthesise vitamin D_3 when exposed to sunlight.[212] Vitamin D is also found in certain foods, in two forms: D_3 and D_2. Vitamin D_3 is found in various animal products including oily fish, liver, meat and egg yolk, and is often added to dairy and other foods via fortification.[213,214] More recently, a vegan form of D_3 has been discovered in lichen, an algae-like plant. Vitamin D_2 is another vegan-friendly form of vitamin D which is found in certain sun-exposed mushrooms.[215]

Despite these various sources, more than half of the global population has vitamin D insufficiency, and an estimated 1 billion people have clinical vitamin D deficiency, largely due to lifestyle factors (spending more time indoors and wearing more sunscreen) and environmental factors (such as pollution) that decrease our exposure to sunlight.[212,216] Even in sunny Australia, around one-third of adults are deficient in vitamin D.[217] Insufficient vitamin D can lead to a weakened musculoskeletal system, compromised immune and respiratory health and vascular stiffness, a known risk factor for cardiovascular disease.[216,218] Recent research has also linked low vitamin D levels to the development of various cancers, type 1 diabetes and other autoimmune conditions, as well as cognitive decline and symptoms of depression.[219–221]

With over 90% of vitamin D derived from sun exposure, you wouldn't expect that people eating fewer animal products would be at higher risk of deficiency.[217] Findings from large population studies show us that while vegetarians and vegans tend to have a lower vitamin D status than meat-eaters, they are typically within the healthy range.[222,223] Where someone adopting a vegan diet is most likely to run into issues is if they are from northern latitudes where UVB rays are limited or if they purposefully avoid the sun, and do not take a vitamin D supplement, particularly in winter.[224,225]

FIGURE 10.23:
ADEQUATE INTAKE OF VITAMIN D

AGE	AI VITAMIN D	UPPER LIMIT
ADULTS		
19–50 years	5 mcg/day (200 IU/day)	80 mcg/day (3280 IU/day)
51–70 years	10 mcg/day (400 IU/day)	80 mcg/day (3280 IU/day)
> 70 years	15 mcg/day (600 IU/day)	80 mcg/day (3280 IU/day)
PREGNANCY AND LACTATION		
19–50 years	5 mcg/day (200 IU/day)	80 mcg/day (3280 IU/day)

Adapted from NHMRC[226]

How can we ensure adequate vitamin D intake?

Direct exposure to sunlight is the primary way to obtain vitamin D. Specifically, it's the sun's UVB rays that kickstart vitamin D synthesis in our skin. During the summer months, you should aim for five to twenty minutes of sun exposure daily to the face and lower arms and hands. Given the need to balance the risk of skin cancer from sun exposure, especially for Australians, with the need to maintain vitamin D levels, it is advisable to limit sun exposure to the mid-morning or mid-afternoon, outside of peak UV times.[227–229] There's also a general rule of thumb to keep in mind that it takes about half the time in direct sunlight for your body to produce adequate amounts of vitamin D as it does for your skin to burn. So while five to twenty minutes may be sufficient time for someone with fair skin, someone with darker skin will require more time in the sun to produce the same amount of vitamin D. In the winter months, you would need to spend considerably more time in the sun to achieve the same level of vitamin D, but the same rule of thumb applies – about half the time in the sun that it would take for your skin to start burning should ensure sufficient vitamin D.

Vitamin D levels can be supplemented through dietary intake, but in Australia there are few products on the market that have been fortified with vitamin D, and so the overall recommendation is to adopt a routine consisting of healthy sun exposure and/or take a dietary supplement in order to reverse or prevent deficiency of this vitamin.[214] There are bound to be more vitamin D–fortified products hitting the shelves, such as plant-based milks, making it easier to maintain vitamin D levels in this way.

The easiest and most reliable way to increase vitamin D levels for anyone who has low levels and cannot increase their sun exposure is through a supplement. Vitamin D supplements are usually expressed in international units (IU), where 40 international units equals 1 microgram (mcg). Typically, you will find supplements ranging from 12.5 mcg (500 IU) to 125 mcg (5000 IU) per serve. Supplements may contain either vitamin D_2 or D_3; however, it's worth keeping in mind that there is some evidence to suggest that vitamin D_3 may be more bioavailable than vitamin D_2 at doses above 1000 IU.[230,231] So if you are vegan, look for a vitamin D_3 supplement that clearly states the supplement is vegan or derived from lichen.

Despite the adequate intake (AI) levels shown in Figure 10.23, several studies have shown 25–50 mcg per day (1000–2000 IU per day) to be an effective and safe dosage for the average person to maintain healthy vitamin D levels.[232–235] Additional studies have shown that this dose should be slightly higher again for people who are overweight or elderly, as shown in Figure 10.24.[236,237]

FIGURE 10.24:

RECOMMENDED SUPPLEMENTAL DOSAGE OF VITAMIN D FOR VARIOUS GROUPS[232–237]

VITAMIN D SUPPLEMENT DOSAGE	
Average person	25–50 mcg/day (1000–2000 IU/day)
Overweight/obese	75 mcg/day (3000 IU/day)
> 70 years	100 mcg/day (4000 IU/day)

How you choose to maintain adequate vitamin D status really comes down to your personal circumstances – your age, where you live, your skin type, whether you or a family member has had skin cancer before, and your lifestyle. Personally, I supplement with a daily dose of 1000 IU of vitamin D_3 from lichen all year round as an insurance policy, which, based on my skin tone and level of sun exposure, results in healthy vitamin D status throughout all seasons.

Getting the most from your minerals

It's important to understand a little bit about mineral bioavailability and how we can increase the absorption of these key nutrients from the plants that we eat.

The best way to think about minerals in plants is that in their natural state, they are locked, and it is best to unlock them before we consume them. In whole grains, legumes, nuts and seeds, minerals such as zinc, iron and calcium bind to phosphorus to form what are known as *phytates*. In other foods, such as spinach, rhubarb and beetroot, these same minerals bind to oxalic acid to form what is known as *oxalates*. This is why you may have heard people recommending low-oxalate greens such as kale, collard greens and bok choy instead of spinach for people looking to increase their calcium absorption.

Because phytates and oxalates make minerals less available to use, they are often referred to as anti-nutrients. However, through standard preparation techniques such as soaking, sprouting, blending, leavening, cooking and fermentation, we can significantly increase the mineral availability in these foods.[158,238-242] This is why it's a good idea to soak, or 'activate', your nuts and seeds in water, for example. It's also why I prefer fermented whole wheat sourdough bread to a traditional bread – up to 90% of phytates are broken down during the fermentation of sourdough.[158] In fact, even though spinach gets a bad rap, one study showed that boiling reduced oxalates in spinach by 87% while steaming spinach reduced oxalates by 42%.[243] So if you're looking to bump up your calcium absorption, you'll want to cook your spinach – just make sure you drain away the water, as that's where the oxalates end up!

4. Calcium

When you think about calcium, the most abundant mineral in our bodies, you will probably immediately think about our bones and teeth, and osteoporosis, a chronic disease that affects almost 1 million Australians and is a major cause of disability and premature death.[244] Typically, osteoporosis is a disease that affects people aged sixty-five and over, and more women than men. One in three women aged fifty years and over and one in five men will experience an osteoporotic fracture in their lifetime.[245] The main reason women are more affected by the disease than men is because women typically experience 2% bone density loss every year after menopause, due to a decrease in oestrogen levels.[246,247]

Many of us have an oversimplified understanding of what's required to keep our bones strong. While it's true that dairy is rich in calcium, and calcium is an important structural component of our bones and teeth, we now understand that vitamin B_{12}, vitamin C, vitamin D, vitamin K, potassium and protein are also essential to bone formation and integrity.[248–250]

Vitamin K and bone health

In the past few decades, vitamin K has become recognised as an important nutrient for bone health. Vitamin K has two forms, known as vitamin K_1 and vitamin K_2. K_1 is found in abundance in plant foods, particularly dark leafy greens – just half a cup of kale will provide you with around eight times the NHMRC's adequate vitamin K intake level. In fact, the top ten foods richest in vitamin K_1 are plants, so it's highly likely that those following a WFPBD consume significantly more K_1 than the general population. Vitamin K_2, on the other hand, is produced by bacteria in our own intestines, or in the intestines of animals. There is no evidence that we need to consume K_2 from our food, which is why a daily recommended intake has not been set.[251] There are only a few specific circumstances, generally identified by a health professional, where someone following a WFPBD may need to consider directly consuming K_2 – a common instance is after extensive antibiotic therapy, where the antibiotics have reduced the numbers of the bacteria responsible for producing K_2.[252] There is also some evidence that postmenopausal women with low bone density may benefit from supplementing K_2.[253,254]

Calcium also has important functions in the heart, blood vessels, muscles and nervous system. So important that when dietary calcium intake is below a certain threshold, our bodies draw on the calcium stores in our bones and, if this continues over time, bone density will gradually decline, leaving us at risk of developing osteopaenia (slight bone density loss), osteoporosis (significant bone density loss) and fractures. Think of it like your bank account – if you keep drawing on what's there without topping it back up, you'll find yourself in trouble!

How much do we need?

Doctors, nutrition scientists, dietitians and nutritionists continue to debate what is an adequate intake level for calcium. For example, the National Health Service in the United Kingdom recommends 700 mg per day, the Institute of Medicine in the United States recommends 1000–1200 mg per day and both the WHO and Australia's NHMRC recommend 1000–1300 mg per day (shown in Figure 10.26).[255–258] Taking all of this into account, how much should we aim for?

First, we need to recognise that there are many other nutrients and lifestyle factors that affect bone health. Looking at absolute calcium intake on its own is not a very good way of predicting whether certain populations are at higher risk of osteoporosis or not.

The fact that countries consuming the highest amounts of milk (a very rich and convenient source of calcium) tend to have the highest rates of hip fractures is evidence of this.[259] It's widely thought that, despite their high calcium intake, these milk-guzzling populations have lower vitamin D status as a result of their geographical location and lifestyles – as we know, vitamin D is incredibly important for calcium absorption and building strong bones. Building strong bones is a team effort – we can consume all the calcium in the world, but if other aspects of our diet or lifestyle are letting us down, we will be at more risk of a fracture.[260]

FIGURE 10.25:

BUILDING STRONG BONES IS A TEAM EFFORT[248,261-236]

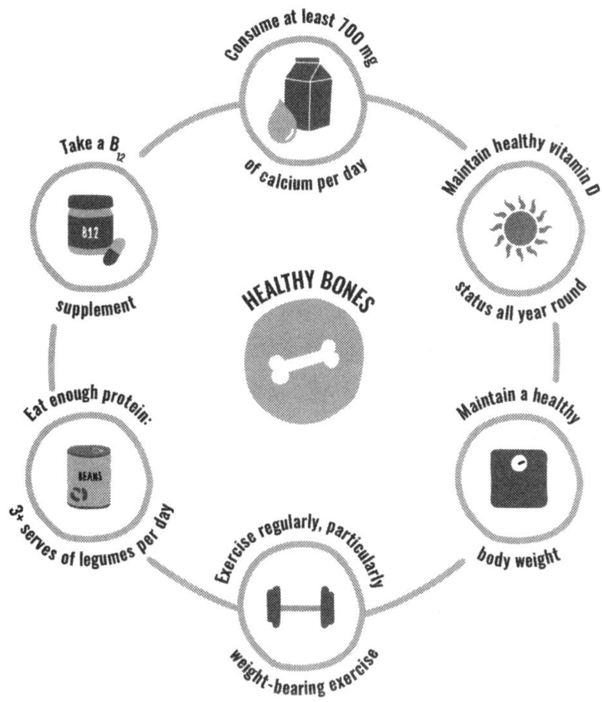

In saying that, there definitely seems to be a minimum level of calcium intake that we want to avoid falling under. The WHO states that intakes lower than 400–500 mg[264] do in fact put one at increased risk of fracture for the general population eating the standard Western diet, and it extends to people following a WFPBD too. Findings from 34,696 subjects in the EPIC-Oxford cohort clearly show that if people following a WFPBD consume over 525 mg per day, their risk of fracture is the same as omnivores, whereas vegans who consumed less than 525 mg per day had higher risk of fracture.[265] This tells us that the calcium in a balanced WFPBD is perfectly bioavailable to build strong bones – you just have to consume enough.

In 2020, researchers published an updated study on this EPIC-Oxford cohort, this time concluding that vegans were at risk of twenty more fractures per 1000 persons over a ten-year period.[266] This increased risk was only observed for vegans with a low BMI and for postmenopausal women. Importantly, the researchers stated that this risk existed even when protein and calcium were adjusted for. This means that even when they compared vegans and meat-eaters who had the same calcium and protein intake, the vegans still had increased risk of fractures, suggesting that perhaps there is another aspect of the vegan diet that contributes to weak bones.

While this reported risk is only modest, it created headlines globally and of course was a study I wanted to really get to the bottom of. The first thing I noticed is that the vegans in this study were not exactly following a Plant Proof diet. We know this because their average fibre intake was 26 g per day – a fair bit lower than would be expected if they were eating a healthy WFPBD. That aside, it's not until you dive into the methodology that it becomes clear why, despite the headlines, this study does not tell us that a plant-exclusive diet is inherently bad for bone health. One of the major limitations was that the study failed to account for the vitamin D status of the participants. As only 51% of vegans in this study were taking supplements (these were subjects recruited in the 1990s and early 2000s, before we had a lot of the nutrition information we have today), and they had previously been shown to suffer from vitamin D deficiency during winter, it's very possible that this at least partly explains the small increase in fractures observed.[222,266] This is a problem with education, not with a vegan diet – vegans living in the United Kingdom, where this cohort is from, who are not getting regular sun exposure should be supplementing with vitamin D.

Another major limitation was the study's statistical adjustment for BMI. The idea with adjusting for BMI is that we can compare vegans and omnivores with the same BMI and identify if there was a difference in their fracture rates. If so, we would know it was their diet, not their body weight, creating the difference in risk. Large amounts of data have established that, as BMI falls, the risk of fracture increases rapidly.[261] When a person weighs less, they have less weight going through their bones, and increased stress going through bones creates greater bone density. Additionally, when lighter people fall over, they have less 'padding' to provide a cushioning effect and therefore a higher chance of bone damage. In this study there were many vegans with a low BMI, so when the researchers simply compared all people with a BMI under 18.5, rather than at specific levels below 18.5, it's likely they were comparing omnivores who were closer to a BMI of 18.5 and vegans who were considerably lower. Thus, again the increased risk of fracture is likely to be partly explained by BMI, rather than being an inherent problem with a vegan diet.[266,267] This is supported by the fact that when we look at other groups of vegans, who have a more comparable BMI to the omnivores in the same population, we do not see any differences in bone mineral density and fracture risk.[268]

With all of this in mind, and findings from other populations, including a 2011 study looking at fracture risk in over 60,000 Swedish women,[262] I do still think it's a good idea to play it safe and aim to exceed 700 mg per day as a bare minimum calcium target to reduce your risk of osteoporosis, and then to optimise your diet to give yourself the best chance of reaching the Australian RDI, which is likely to be a more optimal intake. (Keep in mind that, for the purposes of building strong bones, once you have reached this minimum recommended level of calcium intake, whether your overall diet and lifestyle are conducive to bone health is going to be more significant than whether you consume 850 mg per day or 1000 mg per day.) Consuming this amount of calcium on a plant-based diet is entirely possible – for example, various studies show us that vegans in the AHS-2 cohort average 1150 mg per day, Spanish vegans average just over 1000 mg per day, and Swiss vegans a little over 800 mg per day.[16,73,269]

FIGURE 10.26:

RECOMMENDED DIETARY INTAKE OF CALCIUM

AGE	RDI CALCIUM	UPPER LIMIT
	ADULTS	
19–50 years (women)	1000 mg/day	2500 mg/day
> 50 years (women)	1300 mg/day	2500 mg/day
19–70 years (men)	1000 mg/day	2500 mg/day
> 70 years (men)	1300 mg/day	2500 mg/day
	PREGNANCY AND LACTATION	
19–50 years	1000 mg/day	2500 mg/day

Adapted from NHMRC[257]

How can we ensure adequate calcium intake?

You can get enough calcium via a balanced plant-based diet from whole foods alone, but it is undoubtedly easier to achieve with the help of fortified foods, such as calcium-fortified plant-based milk and calcium-set tofu. Just half a cup of each daily can provide a combined total of almost 500 mg of calcium. Building these fortified foods into your routine can be particularly helpful if you are finding the food volume associated with getting all of your daily calcium from whole plant foods a little too much to handle.

FIGURE 10.27:

EXAMPLE OF A DAILY EATING PLAN TO ENSURE ADEQUATE CALCIUM INTAKE

MEAL	INGREDIENTS	CALCIUM
Breakfast	½ cup oats 1 cup fortified plant milk 2 tbsp almonds Fruit	364.8 mg
Lunch	½ cup kidney beans 1 medium sweet potato 1 cup steamed bok choy Dressing with 1 tbsp tahini	333.6 mg
Dinner	½ cup calcium-set tofu, firm 1 cup cooked quinoa 1 cup cooked broccoli 1 tbsp toasted sesame seeds	425.6 mg
TOTAL		1124 mg

While the bioavailability of calcium does indeed vary from food to food, in most cases the percentage of absorbable calcium in plants is as good as milk if not better (e.g. around 30% of calcium in milk, fortified plant-based milk and calcium-set tofu is absorbed, and around 60% of calcium in broccoli is absorbed).[270–273] Most importantly, the calcium RDIs are based on the assumption that on average, about 30% of dietary calcium is absorbed from a diet that includes a wide range of foods.[270] That means, rather than worrying about which foods contain more bioavailable calcium than others, all you have to focus on is regularly including a variety of calcium-rich plant foods in your diet.

FIGURE 10.28:

GOOD SOURCES OF CALCIUM IN A WFPBD

FOOD	SERVING SIZE	CALCIUM	FOOD	SERVING SIZE	CALCIUM
Orange juice, calcium fortified	1 cup	350 mg	Brazil nuts	5 nuts	38 mg
Calcium-set tofu, firm	½ cup	326 mg	Bok choy, raw	½ cup	37 mg
Plant based milk, calcium fortified	1 cup	300 mg	Chickpeas, cooked	½ cup	37 mg
Moringa powder	2 tbsp	280 mg	Flaxseed	2 tbsp	36 mg
Soy yoghurt, calcium fortified	½ cup	173 mg	Kiwifruit	1 medium	36 mg
Tahini	2 tbsp	128 mg	Mustard greens, raw	½ cup	32 mg
Blackstrap molasses	1 tbsp	100 mg	Cocoa powder	2 tbsp	28 mg
White beans, cooked	½ cup	96 mg	Cabbage, raw	½ cup	26 mg
Dried figs	5 figs	68 mg	Broccoli, raw	½ cup	21 mg
Almonds	20 nuts	66 mg	Chickpea flour	½ cup	21 mg
Navy beans, cooked	½ cup	63 mg	Brussels sprouts, raw	½ cup	19 mg
Kale, raw	1 cup	53 mg	Pumpkin, cooked	½ cup	18 mg
Kidney beans, cooked	½ cup	50 mg	Sunflower seeds	2 tbsp	14 mg
Collard greens, raw	½ cup	42 mg	Cauliflower, raw	½ cup	12 mg
Tomatoes, canned	½ cup	40 mg	Goji berries	2 tbsp	12 mg

One of my favourite sources of calcium is unhulled tahini, a creamy paste made from whole sesame seeds that is perfect to drizzle over your favourite meal, blend into a smoothie or mix with chickpeas, garlic and lemon juice to make a delicious home-made hummus. It contains 64 mg of calcium per tablespoon and is a good source of unsaturated fats. Some of the other whole-food sources of calcium I recommend making friends with are white beans, broccoli and dark leafy greens. All of these are staples in my home.

Choosing the best plant-based milk

Because of the food volume associated with getting all of your daily calcium from whole plant foods, it's a good idea to replace dairy milk with a calcium-fortified plant-based milk as a straight swap that offers the same convenience and an equivalent amount of total and bioavailable calcium per serve.[273] With so many plant-based milks on the market today, it can be helpful to understand some of the basic differences between the most common options.

The first thing I want to see in any plant-based milk is that they are not adding sugars or artificial flavouring. You can do this by checking their ingredient list and looking out for 'orange light' sweeteners from Figure 10.5. Fortunately, most brands now offer sweetened and unsweetened versions. Although the unsweetened versions may taste slightly bland at first, your tastebuds will adjust over time. I also recommend choosing plant-based milks that are free from carrageenan, a thickening agent. There is enough evidence to be cautious about consuming this compound until we better understand whether it's safe.[274-278]

Next, check the nutritional information to see that it has been fortified with calcium. Then, think about the purpose of the plant-based milk. If you are substituting for cow's milk and want something that's relatively high in protein, a non-GMO soy milk is going to be a good option (both soy and cow's milk provide about 8 g of protein per serve). There are also new forms of protein-rich plant milks still emerging. In the United States, pea milk is becoming more widely available, and some brands offer the same amount of protein as cow's milk, as well as 50% more calcium, vitamin B_{12}, vitamin D and omega-3s.

If you feel as though you are already getting sufficient protein in your diet, then my recommendation is oat milk, which has the lowest environmental footprint of the common plant-based milks.

FIGURE 10.29:

ENVIRONMENTAL IMPACT OF ONE GLASS (200 ML) OF DIFFERENT MILKS[97]

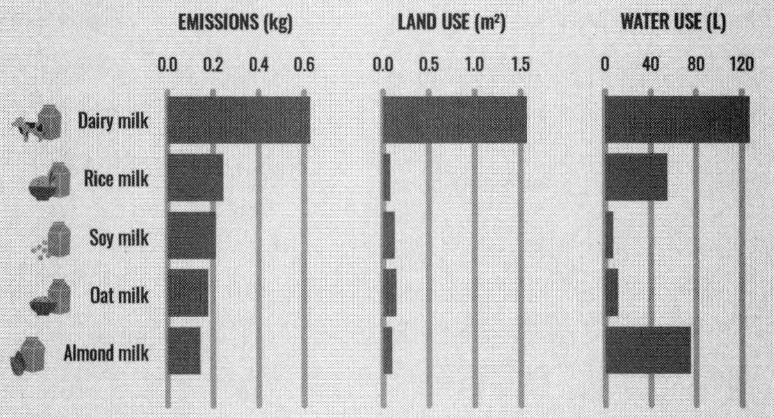

I recommend consuming 1.5 cups of a fortified plant-based milk per day that offers around 100 mg of calcium per 100 ml. In doing this, you will supplement your diet with 375 mg of calcium.

If you cannot access calcium-fortified plant-based milk or prefer to make your own plant-based milk, you can fortify the milk yourself with calcium powder. I use a completely natural red algae calcium powder and add 1000 mg to a litre.

My favourite plant-based milks to make are hemp (rich in protein and omega-3s), macadamia (super creamy) or oat. Whichever option you choose, always shake your milk before consuming to evenly distribute the calcium, as it tends to settle at the bottom.

If you do not want to consume fortified foods, you can either increase the portion sizes and/or frequency of calcium-rich plant foods or consider supplementation. If you have osteopaenia or osteoporosis, supplementing is definitely recommended. I suggest a red algae-derived calcium supplement, as emerging data suggests that this may be better for bone health than calcium carbonate, the most common synthetic form of calcium.[279–281] Calcium citrate is the most well absorbed of the synthetic calcium supplements.[282] It's recommended not to exceed 500 mg per day from supplements (including fortified foods), to avoid the risk of kidney stones and increased risk of heart disease.[283–285]

5. Iodine

Iodine is often forgotten in conversations about mineral intake, possibly because we only need trace amounts of it. However, given it's not uncommon for people to have mild iodine deficiency, and the number of people with an iodine deficiency is on the rise,[286] it should be given more attention, particularly for those eating a WFPBD, as numerous studies have shown that vegetarians and vegans are most at risk of developing this deficiency if not eating an appropriately planned diet.[73,168,287–289]

When we have insufficient iodine in our diet, our bodies make fewer thyroid hormones.[290] One of the most common symptoms of iodine deficiency is weight gain, caused by a condition known as hypothyroidism that results in the slowing of a person's metabolism. Other symptoms include hair loss, dry skin, lethargy, impaired fertility, elevated LDL-C, cognitive impairment, an enlarged thyroid gland (known as a goitre) and a number of other conditions that affect the heart, liver, muscles, kidneys and developing foetuses, and are collectively known as iodine deficiency disorders.[291,292] Because iodine is associated with foetal development and linked to stillbirth, anyone who is considering becoming pregnant should pay extra attention to their iodine levels, regardless of the dietary pattern they follow.[292–294]

FIGURE 10.30:

RECOMMENDED DIETARY INTAKE OF IODINE

AGE	RDI IODINE	UPPER LIMIT
ADULTS		
19–70+ years	150 mcg/day	1100 mcg/day
PREGNANCY		
19–50 years	220 mcg/day	1100 mcg/day
LACTATION		
19–50 years	270 mcg/day	1100 mcg/day

Adapted from NHMRC[295]

How can we ensure adequate iodine intake?

The majority of iodine on Earth is stored in the ocean, with some making its way into coastal soil and far less reaching inland soil. For this reason, the iodine content of produce is hugely variable, making it incredibly difficult to know how much you are actually getting per serve.[296] The most iodine-rich plant-based food sources are sea vegetables such as nori, wakame, dulse and kelp (kombu). However, because the amount of iodine they contain varies, some are safer sources than others. In order to avoid iodine toxicity, my recommendation is to stick with nori, dulse or wakame, as just slight variations in the iodine content of kelp or a slightly increased serving size can quickly see you exceeding the recommended upper limit of iodine intake.

FIGURE 10.31:

RECOMMENDED SOURCES OF IODINE

FOOD	SERVING SIZE TO SUPPLY 150 mcg
Dulse flakes	2 tsp
Nori	3 tsp or 2 sheets
Wakame	2 tsp
Iodised salt	½ tsp
Fortified bread	6 slices

Always read the label as iodine content can vary from brand to brand

Nori sheets can be eaten by themselves, used to make sushi rolls or mixed with ginger to make a flavourful tofu scramble. Wakame is delicious in soup and dulse flakes are great for sprinkling on top of any savoury meal in place of salt. My recommendations take into account that, depending on their source, these seaweeds may in fact be less rich in iodine. These serving sizes are essentially an insurance policy, ensuring adequate intake while placing you at no risk of exceeding the upper limit.

As an alternative to sea vegetables, you will often hear of iodised salt and supplements as methods of providing a more consistent dietary intake of iodine. Iodised table salt was first introduced in the United States in the 1900s as a way of preventing iodine deficiency, and has since been introduced globally.[297] Other fortified foods are now available too.

Based on what we saw about sodium intake in Part Two, you may be thinking that you should avoid table salt, but this is not necessarily true. In the right context, sodium can actually be very healthy! If you are eating a WFBPD and minimising or avoiding ultra-processed foods, half a teaspoon of iodised salt (which typically contains around 1150 mg of sodium and 150 mcg of iodine but can vary from brand to brand) a day is a healthy move to avoid iodine deficiency, unless you have specifically been told by a medical professional to go on a low-salt diet. In this specific circumstance, an iodine supplement is definitely the preferred option. For those who do choose to supplement, my recommendation is to opt for a potassium-iodine based supplement or a kelp supplement, preferably from a company that tests for iodine concentration and for the presence of arsenic, a known carcinogen that has been found in some kelp supplements.[298,299]

6. Iron

Iron is a mineral crucial to the transportation of oxygen around our bodies in the blood and muscle tissue. Iron deficiency is the most prevalent nutrient deficiency worldwide, affecting approximately 1 to 1.2 billion people.[300–302] Insufficient iron affects the body's ability to produce normal red blood cells and can result in iron deficiency anaemia, a condition that affects women more than men. Symptoms of iron deficiency anaemia include fatigue, impaired cognitive function, paleness, dizziness, reduced immunity, adverse pregnancy outcomes, infertility and reduced quality of life.[303,304] This is typically caused by insufficient dietary intake, impaired absorption, chronic blood loss (e.g. from menstruation, surgery, childbirth) or a combination of the three.[300] In addition, conditions such as inflammatory bowel disease, chronic heart failure, colon cancer and chronic kidney disease increase our risk of developing iron deficiency.[303] Populations who are at higher risk of developing low or deficient iron levels include people who menstruate, pregnant people, children, female athletes, people who are overweight or obese, and anyone experiencing heavy or prolonged bleeding.[302,305,306]

Because red meat and other animal products are rich in iron, it is often assumed that people reducing their animal-based food consumption, vegetarians and vegans in particular, are at higher risk of developing iron deficiency. While Western vegetarians and vegans do typically have lower iron stores than omnivores, iron deficiency is no more prevalent in these populations.[73,307,308] Furthermore, having lower iron stores does not seem to affect how a person feels, or functions, as long as they are consuming enough iron in their diet to replace what their body is losing. If anything, lower iron stores may in fact be protective against certain chronic diseases, such as type 2 diabetes.[309] Nonetheless, given that it is the most prevalent nutrient deficiency worldwide, iron is a nutrient we should all be conscious of, particularly women.

How much do we need?

How much dietary iron we need depends on the types of food we're eating. Iron comes in two forms: heme iron (from animals) and non-heme iron (which can come from animals and plants).[166,303] Heme iron and non-heme iron are absorbed by the body at different rates, so it is recommended that vegetarians and vegans consume 1.8 times the normal RDI for iron.[304,310] This means that, according to NHMRC guidelines, a woman of childbearing age who is following a vegetarian or vegan diet should be aiming for 32.4 mg of iron per day. While at first glance this may seem like quite a lot, it's important to understand that these recommendations are based on single-meal and short-term studies, so do not take into consideration adaptive changes that occur over time – specifically, increased absorption of non-heme iron when someone has low iron stores.[308] Additionally, they do not consider the fact that iron absorption can be enhanced or inhibited by a number of other dietary factors. When studies have looked at iron absorption from multiple meals that contain both inhibitors and enhancers, the net absorption of non-heme iron is much greater than if you look at a single food in isolation.[311] There is a lot more at play when it comes to healthy iron levels than the absolute amount we consume, so rather than obsessing over the absolute amount of iron you consume, my recommendation is to include good amounts of iron-rich whole plant foods consistently in your diet and to optimise for absorption.

FIGURE 10.32:
RECOMMENDED DIETARY INTAKE OF IRON

AGE	RDI IRON	RDI FOR VEGANS AND VEGETARIANS
	ADULTS	
19–50 years (women)	18 mg/day	32.4 mg/day
51–70+ years (women)	8 mg/day	14.4 mg/day
19–70+ years (men)	8 mg/day	14.4 mg/day
	PREGNANCY	
19–50 years	27 mg/day	48.6 mg
	LACTATION	
19–50 years	9 mg/day	16.2 mg

Adapted from NHMRC[304]

As you can see, the daily requirement for men is much lower than for women of reproductive age. The human body is quite good at recycling iron and may require as little as 10% of our iron to be topped up from our dietary intake, but women require a higher intake to make up for iron lost during their menstrual period.[312] This is the major reason why studies have found vegetarian and vegan men have a much lower risk of developing iron deficiency anaemia compared with women.[74,313]

Even though the recommendations for vegans and vegetarians are likely to be overstated, the following example meal plan gives you an idea of how you can source the RDI of iron from plant-based sources.

FIGURE 10.33:

EXAMPLE OF 33.5 MG OF IRON FOR A WOMAN EATING A VEGETARIAN OR VEGAN DIET

MEAL	INGREDIENTS	IRON
Breakfast	½ cup rolled oats 1 ½ cups fortified almond milk 1 tbsp chia seeds ½ cup raspberries 2 tbsp pumpkin seeds	6.2 mg
Lunch	2 slices whole wheat bread 1 cup chickpeas, mashed 2 tbsp tahini 1 cup boiled spinach	12.6 mg
Dinner	1 cup cooked quinoa 1 medium baked potato ½ cup tofu, extra firm 1 cup broccoli 2 tbsp sliced almonds	9.2 mg
Snacks	½ cup cashews 6 dried figs	5.4 mg
TOTAL		33.4 mg

How can we ensure adequate iron intake?

When it comes to the best sources of non-heme iron, legumes and whole grains are two of the best food groups, as you can see in Figure 10.34.

FIGURE 10.34:

PLANT-BASED FOOD SOURCES OF IRON

Varies slightly from brand to brand (Iron-fortified cereal)

FOOD	SERVING SIZE	IRON	FOOD	SERVING SIZE	IRON	FOOD	SERVING SIZE	IRON
Chlorella	1 tbsp	9.1 mg	Tempeh	½ cup	2.2 mg	Quinoa, cooked	½ cup	1.4 mg
Iron-fortified cereal	1 cup	7.5 mg	Cashews	15 nuts	2 mg	Kidney beans, cooked	½ cup	1.3 mg
Spinach, cooked	1 cup	6.4 mg	Black beans, cooked	½ cup	1.9 mg	Tahini, unhulled	1 tbsp	1.3 mg
White beans, cooked	½ cup	3.9 mg	Chickpeas, cooked	½ cup	1.9 mg	Yellow split peas, cooked	½ cup	1.3 mg
Whole wheat or grain bread	2 slices	3.5 mg	Peas, cooked	½ cup	1.9 mg	Pumpkin seeds	2 tbsp	1.2 mg
Tofu, extra firm	½ cup	3.4 mg	Bok choy, cooked	1 cup	1.8 mg	Broccoli, cooked	1 cup	1 mg
Chia seeds	2 tbsp	3.3 mg	Nutritional yeast	2 tbsp	1.8 mg	Kale, cooked	1 cup	1 mg
Lentils, cooked	½ cup	3.3 mg	Pak choi, cooked	1 cup	1.8 mg	Dried apricots	10 halves	0.9 mg
Beet greens, cooked	1 cup	2.8 mg	Soy beans, cooked	½ cup	1.8 mg	Dried figs	5 figs	0.9 mg
Blackstrap molasses	1 tbsp	2.8 mg	Rolled oats	½ cup	1.7 mg	Millet, cooked	½ cup	0.8 mg
Amaranth, cooked	½ cup	2.6 mg	Sweet potato	1 cup	1.6 mg			
Silverbeet/collard greens, cooked	1 cup	2.2mg	Mung beans, cooked	½ cup	1.4 mg			

Interestingly, even though spinach is sometimes described as a poor source of bioavailable iron, because it is so rich in iron the net amount absorbed (in milligrams) is around four times greater per serve than kale.[314]

A sprinkle of chlorella

This high-protein, high-iron seaweed has been shown in multiple RCTs to lower cholesterol.[315] I like to add a few teaspoons to my smoothies. But it doesn't stop there - not only will chlorella boost your iron stores, but it may even have an effect on your mood! Just under one teaspoon of chlorella per day has been shown to reduce symptoms of depression and anxiety.[316] This is not to be confused with spirulina, also a form of algae rich in protein and iron, which testing has revealed often contains appreciable amounts of neurotoxins.[317,318]

When looking to improve your iron levels, it's important to consider absorption enhancers and inhibitors, especially for women of reproductive age and other at-risk groups.

FIGURE 10.35:

COMPOUNDS THAT ENHANCE AND INHIBIT IRON ABSORPTION[319-325]

COMPOUND	BIOAVAILABILITY EFFECT ON IRON	FOOD EXAMPLES
Vitamin C	Enhances	Capsicum (bell pepper), guava, orange, broccoli, kiwifruit, strawberries, papaya, cauliflower, pineapple, lemon juice
Beta-carotene (precursor to vitamin A)	Enhances	Carrot, sweet potato, kale, spinach, cantaloupe (rockmelon), apricot, peas, broccoli
Alliums	Enhances	Onion, garlic
Tannins	Inhibits	Tea, coffee, nuts
Calcium	Inhibits	Dairy, fortified plant-based milks, calcium supplements*
Phytates**	Inhibits	Legumes, nuts, whole grains
Polyphenols	Inhibits	Tea, coffee, cocoa

* Calcium supplements are best to have one hour or more either side of iron-rich meals for optimal iron absorption.

** These are significantly reduced by soaking, cooking and sprouting, and can be offset by the presence of vitamin C.

With this in mind, anyone who has low iron levels should try to eat foods that are rich in vitamin C, the best enhancer of iron absorption, at the same time as eating foods rich in non-heme iron. Just 100 mg of vitamin C, around the amount found in one large orange, has been shown to increase the absorption of non-heme iron by up to four times.[326,327] Additionally, to further maximise absorption, foods and beverages such as coffee, tea and chocolate, which contain tannins and polyphenols (both inhibitors), should not be consumed for at least an hour either side of a meal, as opposed to with meals.

FIGURE 10.36:

PLANT-BASED FOOD SOURCES OF VITAMIN C

FOOD	SERVING SIZE	VITAMIN C	FOOD	SERVING SIZE	VITAMIN C
Guava	1 cup	377 mg	Chilli pepper	1 medium	65 mg
Capsicum (bell pepper), yellow	1 large	341 mg	Cauliflower	1 cup	52 mg
Blackcurrants	1 cup	300 mg	Red cabbage	1 cup	51 mg
Capsicum (bell pepper), red	1 large	209 mg	Potato, with skin	1 medium	42 mg
Papaya	1 cup	158 mg	Brussels sprouts	½ cup	37 mg
Lychees	1 cup	136 mg	Lemon	1 medium	31 mg
Capsicum (bell pepper), green	1 large	132 mg	Broccoli sprouts	1 cup	24 mg
Kiwifruit	1 medium	98 mg	Kale, raw	1 cup	20 mg
Orange	1 large	98 mg	Tomato	1 medium	17 mg
Strawberries	1 cup	89 mg	Parsley	2 tbsp	10 mg
Broccoli	1 cup	81 mg	Spinach	1 cup	8 mg
Pineapple	1 cup	79 mg	Thyme	2 tbsp	8 mg
Grapefruit	1 cup	72 mg			

Here are a bunch of my favourite food combinations to improve iron absorption:

- Dried apricots and strawberries
- Green smoothie with strawberries, chlorella, chia seeds, overnight-soaked oats and frozen spinach (blanched)
- Bean dip with added garlic
- Stir-fry with beans, broccoli, mixed capsicum, garlic, onion and lemon juice
- Quinoa, broccoli, legumes and a glass of homemade orange or grapefruit juice with pulp
- Overnight-soaked oats with chia seeds, cashews, tahini and strawberries
- Tofu and lime coconut curry with onion, yellow capsicum and brown rice.

Sulphoraphane and broccoli sprouts

Cruciferous vegetables such as rocket, cabbage and cauliflower are not only good sources of vitamin C, but also contain phytonutrients that act as precursors to compounds that researchers believe prevent healthy cells from becoming cancerous.[328-331] Just three to five servings of cruciferous vegetables a week may lower the risk of developing cancer by around 30-40%.[332] Being precursors means that these molecules need to be activated in order for humans to reap the rewards of their cancer-fighting properties.[333] Through a complex sequence of events, the phytonutrients are activated by an enzyme called myrosinase, and sulphoraphane is produced – the most well studied and potent of these anti-cancer molecules.[333,334] Why is this relevant to you? Because myrosinase is deactivated during cooking, resulting in food with minimal to no sulphoraphane. So if you're taking the broccoli out of your fridge, chopping it up and steaming it straightaway, chances are you are missing out on your daily dose of sulphoraphane. Thankfully, there are a few tips and tricks you can use to maximise the amount of sulphoraphane available in your cruciferous vegetables:

- **Raw**: Enjoy cruciferous vegetables like broccoli and cauliflower raw rather than cooked. Simply chewing raw broccoli is enough to activate myrosinase and stimulate the sulphoraphane precursors to turn into sulphoraphane!
- **Chop**: The enzyme myrosinase is essentially dormant unless the plant undergoes damage. If cooking, chopping your cruciferous vegetables before heating sends a signal to the enzyme myrosinase to start working. Forty minutes later, sulphoraphane will have been produced. Sulphoraphane is heat stable, unlike the enzyme, so after forty minutes, you can cook these chopped foods and the sulphoraphane will remain!
- **Mustard seed powder**: Don't have forty minutes to wait? Simply cook your cruciferous vegetables as you desire and add mustard seed powder when serving. The precursor molecules are also heat stable and mustard seed powder, which is rich in myrosinase, will get to work and bring that sulphoraphane to life.[335,336] This little trick even works for frozen cruciferous vegetables. Because they are flash cooked and then frozen, the enzyme in frozen broccoli, for example, is deactivated, but can be reactivated by adding mustard seed powder after cooking. Just 1 g of mustard seed powder has been shown to increase the available sulphoraphane in cooked cruciferous vegetables by over 400%! Alternatives to mustard seed powder that are also rich in myrosinase are radishes and wasabi, so use whatever you prefer.[337]
- **Sprout:** While all cruciferous vegetables are incredibly healthy in their own right, gram for gram, broccoli sprouts

contain between twenty and fifty times the amount of sulphoraphane as broccoli – just a small handful of broccoli sprouts provides the same amount as an entire mature broccoli head![338] And you can dial up the sulphoraphane content of broccoli sprouts even more by freezing them.[339] For this reason, I have about half a cup per day – usually blended into a smoothie. Today, broccoli sprout seeds are widely available in supermarkets and online and you require just minimal equipment to get started. While broccoli sprouts are also available in a more concentrated supplement form, my recommendation is to consume them in their whole-food form – at least until there is science suggesting that doses above what would naturally be found in a typical serving of sprouts is safe and beneficial.

Anyone diagnosed with iron deficiency anaemia will likely be advised to take an oral iron supplement (usually the ferrous forms, as they tend to be better absorbed) or have a series of injections until their iron levels return to normal.[300,340] As with vitamin C-rich foods, combining a vitamin C supplement with an oral iron supplement may enhance absorption.[341] It's also best to consume iron supplements away from meals on an empty stomach to increase absorption – ideally at least one hour prior to a meal or two hours after. High doses of iron supplementation can come with a number of side effects, including constipation, nausea and increased free radicals in the body (unstable molecules that can cause damage to the body), so it is generally recommended not to rely on these long-term.[300,342]

If you have low iron levels without deficiency, my recommendation is to simply review the foods you are eating and ways to improve iron absorption before considering supplementation.

7. Selenium

Like iodine, selenium is crucial for healthy thyroid hormone production, and is also incredibly important for DNA synthesis, reproduction, immunity, reducing inflammation and for cardiovascular health.[343] Deficiency of this mineral can result in cognitive decline, depressed mood, anxiety, muscle weakness, reproductive issues, inflammation, cardiomyopathy in children and young women, impaired growth, impaired immunity and impaired thyroid function.[344] Around 1 billion people globally are estimated to be selenium deficient.[345] Like many nutrients, selenium is found in soil and absorbed by plants as they grow, so selenium deficiency is expected to increase in the not-too-distant future, regardless of your dietary pattern, due to climate change and soil depletion.[345] As a result, countries are looking at a fertilisation program that was implemented with good results in Finland to improve the selenium content of their soils.[346,347]

FIGURE 10.37:
RECOMMENDED DIETARY INTAKE OF SELENIUM

AGE	RDI SELENIUM	UPPER LIMIT
ADULTS		
19–70+ years (men)	70 mcg/day	400 mcg/day
19–70+ years (women)	60 mcg/day	400 mcg/day
PREGNANCY		
19–50 years	65 mcg/day	400 mcg/day
LACTATION		
19–50 years	75 mcg/day	400 mcg/day

Most government recommendations also set an upper limit of selenium intake at 400 mcg per day for adults, as an excess of selenium can cause selenium toxicity, or selenosis, which may result in hair loss, nausea, vomiting, diarrhoea, abdominal pain, nerve damage, cardiovascular disease and/or kidney failure.[348–350] This is very rare, typically only occurring in parts of the world with soil that is abnormally rich in selenium, or through incorrect use of supplements.

How can we ensure adequate selenium intake?

The easiest way to get a healthy daily dose of selenium is by consuming whole plant foods and having adequate diversity in your diet. As an insurance policy, in the Plant Proof Food Pyramid, I recommend a single brazil nut per day, as long as you are not allergic to tree nuts, which typically contains around 90 mcg of selenium. If you know you live in an area with selenium-poor soil, two nuts per day could be a sensible amount, while still being very unlikely to put you over the 400 mcg limit. In fact, an RCT involving fifty-nine adults in New Zealand found that two brazil nuts per day was as good as a 100 mcg selenium supplement at raising selenium levels in the blood.[351] Regardless of where you live, think of brazil nuts as a selenium supplement rather than a snack – you wouldn't want to eat a handful of them in case it put you close to selenium toxicity territory.

If brazil nuts are not accessible to you, or you are allergic, there are plenty of other plant-based sources of selenium that will help you easily reach your daily requirement.

FIGURE 10.38:

PLANT-BASED FOOD SOURCES OF SELENIUM

FOOD	SERVING SIZE	SELENIUM
Brazil nuts	1 nut	≈90 mcg
Whole wheat pasta, cooked	1 cup	51 mcg
Whole wheat flour	½ cup	37 mcg
Wheat bran, raw	½ cup	23 mcg
Tofu, extra firm	½ cup	22 mcg
Whole wheat bread	2 slices	19 mcg
Rolled oats	½ cup	12 mcg
Chia seeds	2 tbsp	11 mcg
Barley, cooked	½ cup	10 mcg
Tahini	2 tbsp	10 mcg
Sunflower seeds	2 tbsp	9 mcg
Cashews	15 nuts	6 mcg
Mushrooms	½ cup	5 mcg
Chickpea flour	½ cup	4 mcg
Peanut butter	2 tbsp	3 mcg
Couscous, cooked	½ cup	3 mcg
Pumpkin seeds	2 tbsp	2 mcg

Given selenium can be sufficiently obtained from foods that are fairly accessible globally, most people following a WFPBD do not need to consider supplementing this nutrient. In the case where you cannot access selenium-rich foods, daily supplements and selenium-fortified foods are available, but keep in mind the

400 mcg upper limit. I would not recommend a supplement of more than 200 mcg per day, given that you will still be getting selenium from your diet. When it comes to selenium supplements, there are quite a few different types. Studies show the organic selenium supplements, such as selenomethionine, are better retained and utilised by the body than inorganic selenium supplements such as sodium selenite.[352]

A stickler for smoothies

At this point in the book I'm sure it's clear that I enjoy my fair share of smoothies! I fell in love with them when I first started transitioning to a WFPBD due to the fact that back then I really didn't love eating dark leafy greens. If they were blended into a smoothie, however, I didn't even realise they were there. While I no longer need to mask my dark leafy greens with other flavours in order to enjoy them, my love for smoothies is just as strong as ever. I probably average one a day. For me a typical smoothie contains 3–4 servings of fruits and vegetables (e.g. frozen banana, berries, cauliflower and various greens), calcium-fortified plant-based milk, a few tablespoons of chia or flaxseeds, and a brazil nut. If it's a training day, I'll also add 30 g or so of a plant-based protein powder. A convenient and tasty way to fuel my body with nutritious plants.

As smoothies can make it very easy to consume a lot of calories in a short period of time, if weight loss is your goal, I recommend using low-calorie-density ingredients such as frozen cauliflower and frozen berries as your base. (See Figure 10.44 in Principle 7 for more on calorie density.)

8. Zinc

Zinc has many crucial functions in the body, including maintenance of a healthy immune system, testosterone regulation, healthy thyroid function, promotion of healthy growth beginning from the foetal stage, DNA synthesis, cell division and wound healing.[353,354] Typical symptoms of deficiency include loss of appetite, loss of taste, stunted growth, impaired immune response, diarrhoea, hair loss, male infertility, and mood disorders such as depression.[354–359] In developed countries, the prevalence of zinc deficiency is reported as very low; however, because it is hard to detect with laboratory tests, it's highly probable that many cases of mild deficiency go undiagnosed.[360] Populations at greater risk of zinc deficiency include children, pregnant and lactating women, the elderly and people who eat fewer animal products.[73,167,355]

FIGURE 10.39:

RECOMMENDED DIETARY INTAKE OF ZINC FOR ADULTS

AGE	RDI ZINC	RDI FOR VEGANS	UPPER LIMIT
ADULTS			
19–70+ years (men)	14 mg/day	21 mg/day	40 mg/day
19–70+ years (women)	8 mg/day	12 mg/day	40 mg/day
PREGNANCY			
19–50 years	11 mg/day	16.5 mg/day	40 mg/day
LACTATION			
19–50 years	12 mg/day	18 mg/day	40 mg/day

Adapted from NHMRC[361]

While the daily zinc recommendations for those following a WFPBD may seem high, these are based on the average bioavailability of zinc in a typical person following a single meal.[362] This does not take into account food preparation methods that increase bioavailability, or the fact that our bodies can adapt to lower levels of zinc in our diet by increasing its absorption rate.[362] For example, one study found that when subjects consumed less than 11 mg of zinc per day, their bodies increased absorption by up to 92%.[363] Pretty nifty if you ask me.

How can we ensure adequate zinc intake?

In order to ensure adequate zinc intake from a WFPBD, you should consider making sure you are eating adequate servings of zinc-rich foods, particularly nuts and legumes, and also increasing the bioavailability of zinc in those foods. Methods we have already seen, such as soaking, heating, sprouting, fermenting and leavening, have all been shown to unlock zinc from its bond with phytate and increase zinc bioavailability.[362] This is why, for example, the zinc in fermented sourdough bread or yeast-leavened wholemeal breads is far more bioavailable than other breads.[364] It's also why activating your nuts and seeds through soaking is really important.[365] One of my favourite recipes that is bursting with zinc is cashew cheese.

FIGURE 10.40:

BEST PLANT-BASED SOURCES OF ZINC

FOOD	SERVING SIZE	ZINC
Hemp seeds	2 tbsp	2 mg
Tofu, extra firm	½ cup	1.8 mg
Cashews	15 nuts	1.7 mg
Tahini, unhulled	2 tbsp	1.4 mg
Chickpeas, cooked	½ cup	1.3 mg
Sesame seeds	2 tbsp	1.3 mg
Lupini beans, cooked	½ cup	1.1 mg
Pumpkin seeds	2 tbsp	1.1 mg
Pecans	15 halves	1 mg
Quinoa, cooked	½ cup	1 mg
Peanuts	30 nuts	0.8 mg
Pine nuts	2 tbsp	0.7 mg
Flaxseeds	2 tbsp	0.6 mg

Does cooking affect vitamins and minerals?

Although it's true that excessive heat can decrease the vitamin and mineral content of our food, I am certainly not an advocate for a completely raw vegan diet. While technically it's possible to consume a healthy raw vegan diet, it is considerably more time-consuming and difficult for the average person to achieve adequate intake of calories and all of the nutrients they require. Furthermore, heating some foods, such as tomatoes, carrots and spinach, actually makes certain nutrients more available for absorption![243,366,367] For example, while moderately heating tomatoes for thirty minutes decreases vitamin C content by 29%, it increases their antioxidant content by 62%.[367] This is true of most foods – heating increases the availability of some nutrients and decreases the availability of others. We also know from a 2019 study conducted at Harvard University, led by microbiome expert Peter Turnbaugh PhD, that while cooking certain foods, such as potatoes, is better for our gut health, it's less important for other foods, such as raw beetroot.[368] The short answer is that there is no clear winner or one-size-fits-all answer when it comes to whether we should heat our food. So, rather than making life unnecessarily tough for ourselves, I recommend consuming a diet that contains good amounts of both raw and cooked foods so you get the best of both worlds and can adopt a diet that is highly nutritious and at the same time easy to adhere to. Fortunately, the dietary guidelines and recommended nutrient intakes have taken this into account – assuming that the average person consumes certain foods cooked, and others raw.

Various studies have examined how different cooking methods affect the nutrient value of vegetables. Typically, steaming is the best cooking method for preserving nutrients, while boiling results in the greatest nutrient loss. Other methods such as microwaving, baking and roasting tend to fall somewhere in the middle. Ultimately, though, the best cooking method is the one that results in you eating more whole plant foods.[369–371]

In addition to these preparation strategies, zinc absorption can be increased by up to 160% by adding onion and/or garlic to your meals.[324] Adding a single clove of garlic or about half an onion to an average size meal will greatly increase the zinc that will be available for absorption. Both of these vegetables are also excellent sources of prebiotic fibre, so you'll be feeding your friendly gut microbes at the same time as improving your zinc intake. That's a win worth celebrating!

Get more out of garlic with the crush-and-wait technique

Garlic also contains heart-healthy and anti-cancer phytonutrients, which are greatly reduced in number under heat. To maximise the full potential of your garlic, there are two ways around this: add garlic to your meals raw or, after cutting or crushing, let the garlic sit for ten minutes before cooking to give the phytonutrients time to form.[372,373]

The majority of people following a diverse WFPBD that provides sufficient calories will achieve perfectly healthy zinc levels without requiring supplements. Supplementation is most beneficial for someone with a low appetite who is eating fewer calories, as we can often see in elderly people. If supplements are required, keep in mind that the upper limit to avoid zinc toxicity is 40 mg per day. Because you will still inevitably get zinc from your diet, it's generally recommended supplements should not exceed 25 mg per day unless directed by a qualified health professional.

Iron supplements and zinc

Iron supplements have been shown to reduce the absorption of zinc, but iron-rich plant-based foods such as legumes do not interfere with zinc absorption.[374] If you're taking an iron supplement, it's best to take it an hour before meals, or two hours afterwards if possible.

Sodium

We saw in Part Two that most Australians consume nearly twice as much as the recommended amount of sodium. As sodium is a molecule found in salt, this can lead some people to be wary of the salt shaker. However, like sugar, it's the dose that's the poison! Sodium is actually an essential mineral which is crucial for hydration and fluid balance in the body, and just as too much of this mineral can cause health issues, so can too little. The excessive sodium intake seen in those adopting Western diets comes from eating too many animal products and ultra-processed foods. If you eat according to the Plant Proof Food Pyramid, your sodium intake will automatically fall to a healthy level, decreasing your risk of cardiovascular disease and premature death.[375,376]

I'm often asked if I personally add salt to my food. The simple answer is that yes, most of the time, I do add a small amount – a few twists of the salt mill – to increase the sodium content of my meals. This is because my diet is mostly made up of whole or minimally processed plant foods that are naturally low in salt, and I exercise vigorously every day. When you sweat, you excrete sodium, so I need to ensure that I am replacing that through my diet. If you are eating a WFPBD and do not have high blood pressure, there's nothing wrong with adding a little salt to your food, especially if you exercise regularly. I use iodised salt, because iodine is a nutrient of focus and, despite the hype surrounding pink salt, you're better off saving your money – a 2020 study out of Australia, which analysed thirty-one different brands of pink salt, concluded that you'd need to consume five times more pink salt than daily sodium recommendations permit in order to see any benefit from the marginally higher concentrations of certain minerals that it contains.[377]

For anyone who does have high blood pressure, or who has been advised by their doctor to adopt a low-salt diet (usually 1500 mg per day or less), here are a few tips to help you make sure your sodium intake doesn't creep up.[378]

1. Be careful of ultra-processed vegan foods sneaking into your diet. Like all ultra-processed foods, they can often contain appreciable amounts of salt. A 2019 review of 564 'meat alternatives' in Australia – foods like tofu, falafel, plant-based burgers, plant-based sausages and plant-based bacon – identified that on average these products contained 333 mg of salt per serve – around 17% of the maximum daily level recommended for an adult.[379]
2. Buy non-marinated plant-based foods, such as tofu and tempeh, and flavour them at home with spices, as the marinated products usually contain appreciable amounts of sodium.
3. Rinse and drain canned legumes, or buy low-sodium options. Alternatively, you can cook dried beans at home.
4. Take an iodine supplement rather than obtaining your iodine requirement through iodised salt.

Tracking your salt intake

If you want to track your sodium intake, you can put information about a day of eating into a food tracking app. In Australia, the suggested daily target for sodium is 2000 mg, or around 5 g of salt. For every hour of vigorous exercise, add around 300–600 mg of sodium (0.75–1.5 g salt) to your daily target, aiming for the higher end of the range if you sweat more heavily.[380]

Supplements

If you're worried that maintaining a healthy WFPBD sounds like a lot of supplements, remember that taking supplements to complement our diet and ensure nutritional adequacy is nothing new, nor is it exclusive to vegans or vegetarians. Today's omnivores get a lot of their vitamin D from fortified milk, and folate and iodine from fortified bread or iodised salt. Not to mention that non-vegetarians regularly take supplements such as multivitamins, fish oil, folate, calcium and iron, and are recommended to take vitamin B_{12} when over the age of fifty.[381,382] One of the greatest fortification success stories here in Australia is that of folic acid. To reduce the incidence of neural tube defects in babies, the Australian government introduced mandatory folic acid fortification of flour in 2009. After just two years, rates of these birth defects dropped by around 15%.[383] The billion-dollar supplement industry, including the fortification of food, is certainly not propped up by folks following a WFPBD.[382,384]

Still, often I am asked whether taking supplements such as vitamin B_{12} is *natural*. Well, if your definition of natural is obtaining nutrients from only food, no. But there are many parts of our lives – such as taking antibiotics, wearing clothes, developing chronic diseases in our midlife, or hoping to live a healthy life into our eighties or nineties – that would not be considered *natural* by the standards of most of human history. I think it's more important to look at hard outcomes. People eating more plants and fewer animal products typically experience better health for longer. It's also a way of eating that is more environmentally friendly and kinder to the sentient beings with whom we share the planet. If you are better able to achieve this by taking a few specific supplements, with known efficacy, I see no problem with that.

A case for creatine

You may have heard of creatine before. A non-essential molecule that our bodies produce that can be further boosted via supplementation and/or eating animal products. I've been taking 5 g of creatine monohydrate (the most studied form) daily for years, well before I removed animal products from my diet, because even when eating meat (which provides about 1 g of creatine per day for the typical person), our creatine stores only reach approximately 60–80% saturation.[385] The science looking at its safety and effectiveness at improving strength and muscle mass is very compelling.[385,386] And it turns out that creatine may have extra benefits beyond improving strength.[385] Those I am most impressed by are for brain health, with creatine supplementation being shown to improve memory and intelligence, and reduce mental fatigue.[387–389] In other words, creatine is not just good at strengthening our muscles, but also our minds.

Summary

Figure 10.41 summarises my recommendations about the nutrients of focus at a glance.

FIGURE 10.41:

SUMMARY OF THE EIGHT NUTRIENTS OF FOCUS

NUTRIENT OF FOCUS	BEST PLANT-BASED FOOD SOURCES	TIPS FOR ACHIEVING HEALTHY INTAKE
Omega-3s	Chia seeds, ground flaxseeds, hemp seeds, walnuts, microalgae	1 tbsp of ground flaxseeds or chia seeds per day (2 tbsp for men) Consider supplementing with a DHA/EPA omega-3 algae oil (840–1000 mg daily)
Vitamin B_{12}	Fortified foods (e.g. fortified nutritional yeast) or a supplement	Consume B_{12} fortified foods 3 times per day (> 1.5 mcg per serve) Or supplement with cyanocobalamin once per day (50–250 mcg) or once per week (2000–2500 mcg)
Vitamin D	Sun, fortified plant-based milk or a supplement	Aim for 1000 IU through fortified foods and/or a supplement per day, particularly if not getting regular sun exposure If overweight, supplement with 3000 IU per day If over 70 years of age, supplement with 4000 IU per day
Calcium	Calcium-set firm tofu, fortified foods (orange juice, plant-based milk, etc.), tahini (unhulled), almonds, cruciferous vegetables, kale, bok choy	Aim for at least 700 mg per day. Use fortified foods and supplements as required Use fortified foods or supplements to help you reach your RDI (1000–1300 mg)
Iodine	Dulse, nori, wakame, iodised salt, supplement	2 tsp of dulse or wakame flakes per day, or 2 sheets of nori Alternatively, ½ tsp of iodised salt per day or a supplement
Iron	Chlorella, legumes (incl. tofu and tempeh), whole grains, spinach, nutritional yeast, cashews, pumpkin seeds, dried apricots, blackstrap molasses	Meet RDI by consuming whole plant foods Consider enhancers and inhibitors to increase absorption if you have low iron levels Supplement if you are diagnosed with iron deficiency anaemia
Selenium	Brazil nuts, chickpea flour, wheat bran (raw), whole wheat flour, whole grain bread, chia seeds, cashews, pasta (cooked), Weet-Bix, tahini, tofu (firm), barley (cooked), mushrooms, peanut butter, couscous (cooked), pumpkin seeds, rolled oats, sunflower seeds	Meet RDI by consuming whole plant foods Have one brazil nut per day (if you are not allergic to tree nuts)
Zinc	Hemp seeds, pumpkin seeds, tofu (firm), cashews, sesame seeds, tahini, pine nuts, lupin flakes, pecans, chickpeas (cooked), peanuts, flaxseeds, quinoa (cooked)	Meet RDI by consuming whole plant foods Cook with garlic and onion to increase absorption

Aside from vitamins B_{12} and D, the majority of people following a WFPBD can get all of these nutrients in adequate amounts from whole plant foods with or without the addition of fortified foods. Whether you decide to supplement more of these nutrients will come down to your personal circumstances and should be guided by a health professional, ideally a nutritionist or dietitian who can assess your nutrient intake, laboratory test results and how you're feeling to work with you to devise a plan based on your goals.

Considering oysters and mussels

A case can be made for certain individuals to add oysters and mussels to an otherwise plant-exclusive diet, particularly those who are forgetful with important supplements such as vitamin B_{12}.

In terms of human health, if these bivalves were not such nutrient powerhouses, there would be little point entertaining the idea of their inclusion in your diet. However, they are jam-packed with nutrients that are often low or deficient in people eating poorly planned vegan diets, including iron, zinc, selenium, iodine, vitamin B_{12}, vitamin D and DHA/EPA omega-3s. They also contain much lower levels of heavy metals and environmental contaminants compared with many species of fish.[390,391] And, in terms of planetary health, it turns out that farming oysters and mussels is incredibly sustainable, even more so than the production of many plant foods.[392]

FIGURE 10.42:

NUTRIENT CONTENT OF OYSTERS AND MUSSELS

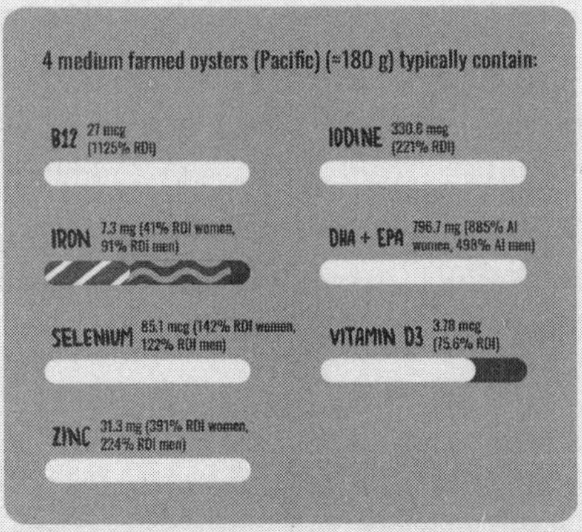

4 medium farmed oysters (Pacific) (≈180 g) typically contain:
B12 27 mcg (1125% RDI)
IODINE 330.6 mcg (221% RDI)
IRON 7.3 mg (41% RDI women, 91% RDI men)
DHA + EPA 796.7 mg (885% AI women, 498% AI men)
SELENIUM 85.1 mcg (142% RDI women, 122% RDI men)
VITAMIN D3 3.78 mcg (75.6% RDI)
ZINC 31.3 mg (391% RDI women, 224% RDI men)

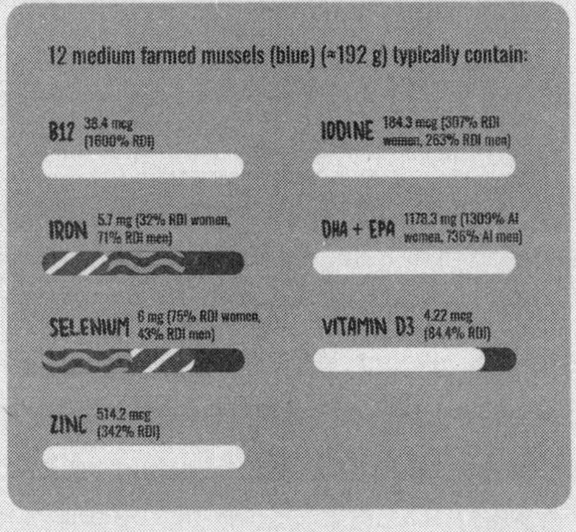

12 medium farmed mussels (blue) (≈192 g) typically contain:
B12 38.4 mcg (1600% RDI)
IODINE 184.3 mcg (307% RDI women, 263% RDI men)
IRON 5.7 mg (32% RDI women, 71% RDI men)
DHA + EPA 1178.3 mg (1309% AI women, 736% AI men)
SELENIUM 6 mg (75% RDI women, 43% RDI men)
VITAMIN D3 4.22 mcg (84.4% RDI)
ZINC 514.2 mcg (342% RDI)

RDI | % OF RDI ACHIEVED FOR MEN & WOMEN | % OF RDI ACHIEVED FOR WOMEN | % OF RDI ACHIEVED FOR MEN

They tick the human and planetary health boxes, but what about animal welfare? Clearly they are animals – but is it cruel to consume them?

Oysters, mussels, clams and scallops are a group of shellfish called bivalve molluscs. Bivalves, despite having a peripheral nerve network, have no head, face or central nervous system. Because they have no brain, it is widely believed that they do not have thoughts, have no experiences and cannot feel pain. In this respect, bivalves are more like plants or fungi than sentient creatures. Beyond this, we have even more reason to believe that oysters and mussels in particular cannot feel pain.[393] Both are considered *sessile* bivalves, meaning they cannot move or swim on their own. It would make little sense for a living animal to feel pain if it couldn't move away from its threat. So, although eating oysters and mussels does not fall into certain definitions of veganism that eliminate the consumption of all animal products, it doesn't mean that consuming them will cause more suffering in the world. It's from this idea that the label 'ostrovegan' was born, for a person adopting a vegan diet who believes reducing pain is what matters, and consumes oysters and mussels.[393]

If this sounds like something for you, my recommendation would be to seek out oysters or mussels sourced from farms, as unfortunately those that are wild-caught can result in a tremendous amount of bycatch. It's also worth noting that, unlike the farming of fish, farming oysters and mussels does not involve the use of antibiotics.[394-396]

Principle 5: When we eat matters

We know *what* humans should be eating for optimal health, but emerging science suggests *when* we eat is also incredibly important. The area of research exploring how meal timing affects our health is called *chrononutrition*.

Each of our cells is under the influence of a biological clock, predominantly regulated by cues such as light and food, which affects the way that our body temperature, heart rate, blood pressure, hormone levels, alertness, metabolism and other important processes fluctuate across the day. It is these fluctuations that are often referred to as our circadian rhythms, which optimise our body to make the most of our waking and sleeping hours. An example of this is the way that the hormone melatonin naturally rises close to bedtime, to help send us into a deep restful sleep, and falls in the morning as cortisol, another hormone, rises to help us become alert for the day ahead.[397,398] If we think about this from an ancestral point of view, it's these rhythms that enabled *Homo sapiens* to be alert and energetic during daylight hours, allowing them to source and consume calories, and tired during the dark hours so that their bodies could utilise stored energy for rest and repair, and to prepare for when food next became available.

When we can sync our meals with these natural circadian rhythms, there are health benefits up for grabs. On the flip side, when we eat erratically without routine, and expose ourselves to unnatural amounts of light, we can disrupt these natural rhythms and place ourselves at higher risk of gaining weight and developing chronic diseases such as cardiovascular disease and type 2 diabetes.[398]

So how can we achieve this? There is a rapidly growing body of evidence that suggests that avoiding late-night meals and having more of our calories in the first half of the day offers benefits, particularly for promoting a healthy body weight. A 2020

RCT conducted by a group of researchers from Johns Hopkins University investigated how a 6 pm dinner versus a 10 pm dinner differentially affected metabolism in twenty healthy subjects. By keeping all other meals and sleep the same, they were able to identify that the late-night meal resulted in impaired ability to utilise carbohydrates and fats, favouring fat storage over fat usage.[399] While this was only a short-term study, it does help shed some light on why observational research has identified that people who regularly eat late-night meals are more likely to be obese.[400] Researchers put this down to circadian rhythms, which influence how effectively we are utilising nutrients at various times of the day.[398,401] Specifically, when our melatonin levels are high (which is late at night and first thing in the morning), we are more likely to store the energy in our food as body fat.[398]

This gives us good reason, where possible, to not eat at these times. A general rule of thumb is to allow a few hours with no food before going to sleep, and the same for a few hours after waking. Additional research has also shown that it is beneficial to eat more of our calories in the first half of our day, when we are usually more active.[402] Not only does starting the day with a hearty breakfast typically lead to less snacking and fewer total calories across any given day, but when researchers have compared people eating a good sized breakfast versus an equivalent sized dinner, with total calories for the day matched, they identified that the former results in greater weight loss. It seems that in the morning, our bodies use more energy to absorb and utilise the nutrients we eat – about 2.5 times as much as we do compared with having the same meal at night.[402]

At different times of the day, your body interprets the same food completely differently. From a few hours after you wake until the early evening, you're better at digesting and burning calories, and late at night, you're better at rest and repair. Taken together, this area of nutrition science creates a strong case for *circadian rhythm eating*. Simply put, this means eating within a ten to twelve hour window close to the rise and fall of the sun (e.g. 8 am – 8 pm or 9 am – 7 pm) – an eating window which has been shown by several studies, with male and female subjects, to safely promote weight loss, improve sleep and improve biomarkers of disease and ageing.[*] [398,403–407] While you may think this sounds like a normal eating pattern, unfortunately most of us eat for fifteen or more hours per day, and less than 10% of us have at least twelve hours per day in a fasted state.[403] If you have your first calories at 6 am (e.g. a latte) and last food at 9 pm (snacking after dinner), that's fifteen hours of consuming calories. Combine that with staring at a bright screen until right before bed and it's easy to see how we can totally confuse our bodies and cause chronic circadian disruption, in turn increasing our risk of weight gain, anxiety, depression, fatigue, loss of concentration, gastrointestinal symptoms (bloating, constipation, abdominal pain, diarrhoea), chronic disease and a shorter life span.[403,408–410] This is certainly quite an underrated and often forgotten aspect of our health that truly deserves our attention. Many of us have experienced the crummy feeling that comes with jet lag. That's a perfect example of acute circadian disruption. When we eat erratically and expose ourselves to an unnatural amount of light, we are essentially creating chronic jet lag.[408] So if you're lacking energy, experiencing brain fog, feeling bloated, troubled by your mood or having problems sleeping, look at how you can better optimise your meal timing and sleep routine.

---

* It's worth noting that this conclusion is based on relatively short-term trials, which typically lasted from a few weeks to three months. Because narrowing your eating window can reduce your overall caloric intake, it's not recommended for people who are pregnant or lactating, or people who have a history of disordered eating. While there is evidence in favour of eating in sync with our circadian rhythms, if you intend to make changes to the timing of your meals you should do so under the guidance and observation of a doctor, nutritionist and/or dietitian.

FIGURE 10.43:
MEAL TIMING AND YOUR HEALTH[398,399,402-407,409-411]

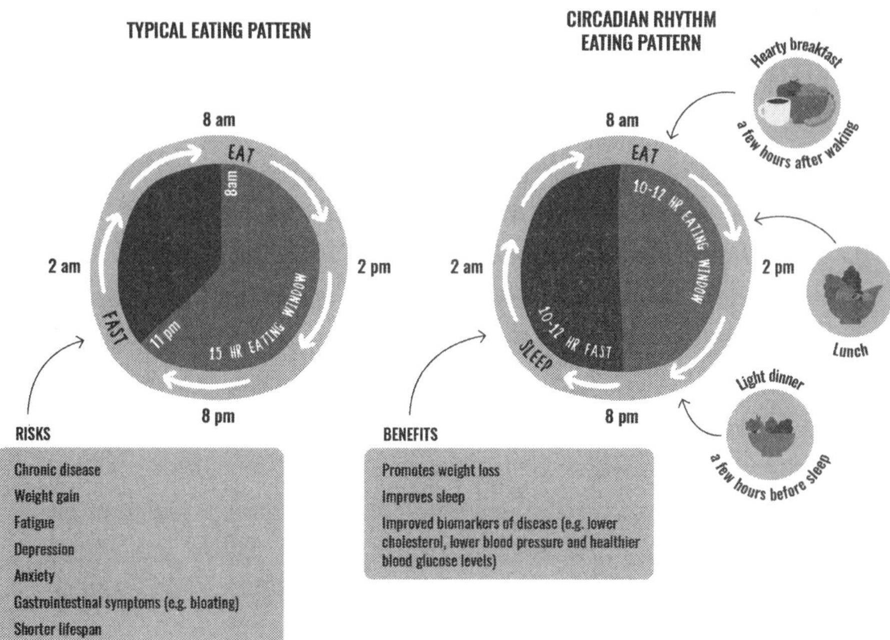

I personally eat this way on as many days as possible. However, when life throws a curveball, or I have a fun dinner planned with friends, I'm certainly very flexible. I see it as a tool rather than a strict rule, and I probably get it right 80% of the time. However, the more I do it, the better I feel, so if I am feeling run-down and stressed, it's one of the first things I come back to.

Principle 6: Drink water for thirst

One of the most indisputable facts about what we consume in our diet is that when it comes to beverages, nothing beats water for thirst. This is why dietary guidelines recommend eight to ten 250 ml cups per day, although this is the recommendation for an average person, and your specific requirement will vary based on your body weight and activity levels.[412] The best indicator really is the colour of your urine. If it's clear to a light straw colour, you're doing good; any darker means you are not hydrated enough. With just a bit of tracking, you will easily be able to determine how much you personally need to drink to maintain adequate hydration all day.

One of the most overlooked sources of water is our food – particularly fruits and vegetables, which should take up half of your plate. Whole plant foods such as celery, cucumber, watermelon, broccoli, spinach, carrots, lettuce and strawberries are over 80% water by weight.[413] Chances are, when you transition to a WFPBD you will be eating more water!

As discussed in Chapter 8, I'm an advocate of both coffee and tea for everyone except people who are highly caffeine-sensitive. With more than one thousand different active plant compounds, including various polyphenols, coffee has been repeatedly shown by large meta-analyses to reduce risk of type 2 diabetes, cancer and cardiovascular disease, and premature death.[414,415] The optimal dose of coffee is around four cups per day and the findings are similar for tea, with three or more cups of tea per day shown to reduce the risk of both cardiovascular disease and premature death.[416,417] My favourites are green tea and hibiscus tea, the latter having been shown to help lower blood pressure. The hibiscus plant does contain heavy metals, though, so it's recommended not to have more than four cups per day.[418]

There is a caveat, however. What you add to your cup of coffee or tea could quickly offset the benefits. If you're someone who likes to add milk, ideally you will have your calcium-fortified plant-based milk at hand, as the fortification will offset the decrease in calcium absorption that is associated with coffee consumption.[419] And if you have a sweet tooth, try to stick to 'green light' sweeteners (as seen in Figure 10.5). If you are pregnant or breastfeeding, it's recommended to restrict your caffeine intake to 200 mg a day, which is around three cups of coffee or six cups of tea.[420,421]

Finally, when it comes to drinks, try to avoid soft drink, whether diet or not, drinks that contain refined sugars, and fruit juices with their fibre removed. If you like kombucha, while most in-store brands are significantly better than soft drink, brewing your own at home means you can control how much sugar is added.

Principle 7: Customisation is key

Science tells us that increasing our plant intake promotes health, but when it comes to the specific plants on our plate there is no one-size-fits-all approach. While I am sharing the best available evidence to optimise a WFPBD, I encourage you to personalise the specifics of your own dietary pattern to suit your unique preferences.

The Plant Proof Food Pyramid is a guide to the food groups you want to focus on, but just how your shopping list and meals specifically look will differ from the next person. Listen to your body and understand your own goals. For example, someone wanting to lose weight is likely to focus on slightly different foods than someone wanting to build muscle. Someone living with diabetes, who gets real-time objective feedback in the form of blood sugar readings, may find they have better blood glucose control when they get their fat intake super low, and thus may avoid cooking oils and instead eat nuts, seeds and avocado in modest amounts. Someone may feel better eating lentils than chickpeas. The point is, I want you to adapt to a WFPBD that works for *you*.

In the future, as the field of personalised nutrition becomes more advanced, we may even have diagnostic tools that help us identify specific foods that are best for our unique microbiome and genetic make-up.[422]

Changing your body on a WFPBD

There are a number of different ways that someone might want to change their body. As we saw in Chapter 4, when it comes to losing weight, we must achieve a calorie deficit by using more energy than we are consuming. In contrast, to gain weight you must use less energy than you are consuming, creating a calorie surplus. This energy balance principle is simple on paper but may be more difficult when applied to real life. However, there are various strategies we can put in place to make it easier to reach the energy balance that will help us get closer to our goal. I've focused on two common scenarios here and outlined some strategies that you can put in place to help improve your results when following a WFPBD.

Key to this is the idea of *calorie density* – the amount of calories in a specific volume of food. A simple way of thinking of it is *calories per bite*. Typically, the more calorie-dense a food is, the easier it will be to overconsume. On the flip side, foods that are less calorie-dense are much harder to overconsume. This is one of the major reasons why people moving from a standard omnivorous diet to a WFPBD lose weight – overall, animal products and ultra-processed foods tend to be far more calorie-dense than plants. Given two-thirds of Australians are obese or overweight, this is pretty handy![423]

That said, there are relatively high-calorie and low-calorie plants. For example, compare cashews and broccoli. One handful of cashews is around 160 calories. To get the same number of calories from chopped broccoli, you would need to eat five cups. Essentially, for a given number of calories, you can consume a larger portion of food that is relatively lower in energy, as can be seen in Figure 10.44.

FIGURE 10.44:
CALORIE DENSITY OF PLANT-BASED FOODS PER 100 G

LOW CALORIE DENSITY (0–99 kcal)

Cucumber	Asparagus	Mango	Orange	Sweet potato
Spinach	Cauliflower	Strawberries	Apple	Capsicum
Mushrooms	Tomato	Pear	Peach	Eggplant
Banana	Broccoli	Blueberries	Kiwifruit	Corn
Artichoke	Brussels sprouts	Grapes	Papaya	Green peas
Kale	Grapefruit	Raspberries	Zucchini	Tofu, silken
Watermelon	Potato	Nectarine	Lettuce	Plant-based yogurt
Cabbage	Carrot	Blackberries	Pumpkin	Plant-based milks

These high-volume, nutrient-rich, low-calorie-density foods are a great way to increase the bulk in your meals when trying to lose weight while still feeling satisfied

Plant-based yogurt: Soy, almond and cashew (not coconut)

Plant-based milks: Oat, soy, almond, macadamia, coconut (not canned), cashew and hemp

MEDIUM CALORIE DENSITY (100–299 kcal)

Avocado	Quinoa	Chickpeas	Tofu	Millet
Dates	Polenta	Lentils	Barley	Buckwheat
White rice	Whole wheat bread	Red kidney beans	Tempeh	Chestnuts
Pasta	White bread	Black beans	Oats	Edamame
Brown rice	White beans			

HIGH CALORIE DENSITY (300–699 kcal)

Dried fruit	Walnuts	Dried coconut	Tahini	Hazelnuts
Peanuts	Pumpkin seeds	Pecans	Dark chocolate	Pistachios
Almonds	Hemp seeds	Brazil nuts	Chia seeds	Cashews
Rice cakes	Flax seeds	Sesame seeds	Granola	Nut butters

Nut butters: Almond, hazelnut, peanut, etc.

VERY HIGH CALORIE DENSITY (700+ kcal)

Cooking oils	Macadamia nuts

This by no means is a categorisation of how healthy these foods are: they are all healthy. Understanding calorie density is a great tool to help manipulate your energy balance and, depending on your goals, promote weight loss or gain.

Strategies to customise for promoting fat loss

Of course, there are also people who transition to a WFPBD and do not lose weight, while others might experience initial weight loss then plateau. This is usually because your energy requirements have changed after losing weight (when you are lighter, you require less energy) but your food intake has not, so you are no longer naturally achieving a calorie deficit.

If this happens and you are still looking to lower your body fat, the first thing I recommend is to go back to the Plant Proof Food Pyramid and assess your current diet. Are you actually eating the recommended serves of greens, other vegetables, whole grains, legumes, etc? Or have ultra-processed vegan foods, takeaway meals and more generous amounts of cooking oils made their way into your diet? A few days of monitoring should show you where you might be getting off track.

If your food selection is in line with the pyramid, next see if you can make shifts from higher-calorie-density foods to lower-calorie-density foods, such as switching a snack of dried fruits to fresh berries, or replacing a serving of granola and plant-based milk with a serving of whole oats and plant-based milk topped with fruit. This will allow you to eat the same volume of food while hopefully creating a calorie deficit. Keep in mind that we only need to create a deficit of 300–500 calories per day to achieve sustainable weight loss.

In addition to looking at calorie density, also compare the frequency and portion size of what you are eating with those recommended on the pyramid. Are you eating a cup of nuts as a single serve rather than a small handful? Could you swap a whole avocado for half an avocado? Despite the temptation for immediate results, it's best to make these smaller changes than to do something drastic like adopting a diet that consists of less than 1000 calories per day. When it comes to successful, safe weight loss, slow and steady wins the race. You should be looking to reduce your weight by no more than 0.5 kg per week. If you want to keep track of your weight loss, I recommend weighing yourself upon waking, after you go to the toilet, with no clothes, at the same time each day and using the same set of scales. Record your weight each day and take an average once a week. This will help even out day to day fluctuations from changes in hormone activity, fluid intake, etc. It's also good to keep in mind that while weighing ourselves can help keep us motivated, there are arguably many more important measures of success. How are you feeling mentally? Are you less tired? Are you sleeping better? Are you recovering better from your workouts? How do your clothes fit?

In addition to modifying the calorie density of your diet, here are some extra tips to help you achieve a calorie deficit.

1. Include protein-rich whole plant foods such as tofu or lentils at every main meal. Similar to fibre, protein is very satiating and the body burns quite a bit of energy to process it.[424]
2. Drink a few glasses of water thirty to sixty minutes before your main meals to increase the feeling of fullness.[425]
3. Aim to stop eating when you are 80% full, to allow your body time to process the food and signal that it is full.
4. You know the saying 'out of sight, out of mind'? Well that applies to ultra-processed foods. Protecting your calorie deficit starts at the supermarket. If it doesn't end up in your fridge or pantry, you won't consume it.
5. Be mindful of liquid calories. It's easy to consume a lot of

calories from fruit juices, smoothies, alcohol and sugar-sweetened beverages.[426]

6. If you are feeling stressed or emotional, take a twenty-minute break to relax before eating. When you can eat mindfully you are far less likely to overconsume.[427]
7. Eat more home-cooked meals where possible. A 2014 study looking at almost 10,000 adults identified that, compared with people who rarely or never cooked at home, people who cooked dinner six to seven times per week consumed around 1000 fewer calories over the week. Over a year, that's equivalent to the calories from 7 kg of butter![428]

Nuts and portion size

Nuts are incredibly health-promoting but also very calorie dense. For some of us (me), it can be beneficial to consume nuts as part of a meal rather than as a snack. As you may have experienced first-hand, it's quite easy to snack away on an entire bag of nuts without too much thought. When we use nuts to top our oats or salad, or within a smoothie, we are better able to control the portion size.

Strategies to customise for promoting muscle gain

Any bodybuilder, whether they are a professional or recreational lifter, will tell you that gaining muscle is incredibly rewarding. Our body is an adaptive machine, and consistent training equals constant adaptation. For this reason, those who are able to build a lifestyle around their nutrition and training generally see the best results.

Coupled with high-volume resistance training, involving progressive overload (where you are constantly performing challenging exercises), here are my top nutrition tips for anyone who wants to optimise a WFPBD to promote muscle gain. First, to build appreciable amounts of muscle it's beneficial to be consuming more energy than you are burning – a calorie surplus of around 300–500 calories per day.[429] For most people, this is quite easy to achieve – it's essentially an additional meal or a few extra snacks per day beyond what you would eat to maintain your current weight. For those with a low appetite who are struggling to achieve a calorie surplus, look at Figure 10.44 and increase the calorie-dense foods such as tahini, avocado, nuts and seeds in your diet. In addition to this, as mentioned earlier, you should aim for a protein intake of around 1.8 g per kg per day, evenly distributed across your food intake for the entire day – meaning that if your target is 120 g of protein, you should have four meals containing around 30 g of protein throughout the day, with one meal being soon after a workout.[430–435] Protein timing matters, at least to those pumping iron. Consuming a huge amount of protein in a single meal isn't a way to fast-track your results. You are better off spacing it out. For most of us, this is about as complex as it needs to be to build lean muscle and increase our strength.

FIGURE 10.45:

SUBOPTIMAL VERSUS OPTIMAL PROTEIN DISTRIBUTION FOR A PERSON WHO WEIGHS 67 KG TARGETING 120 G OF DAILY PROTEIN INTAKE

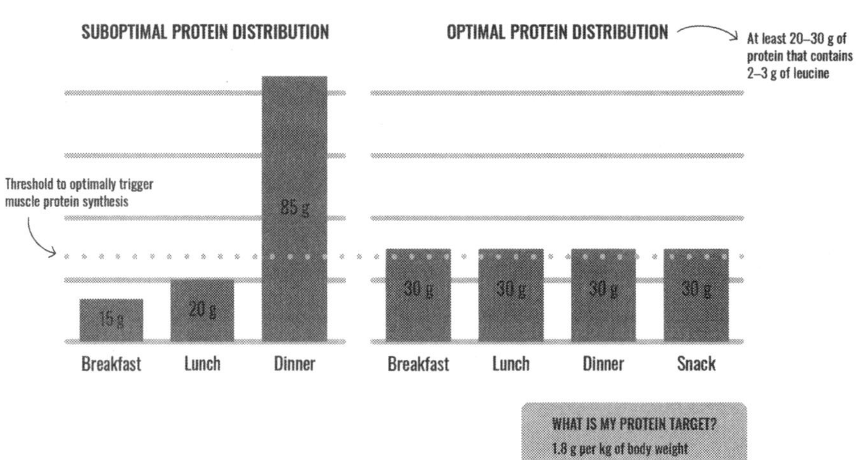

For the very small percentage of people who are looking to absolutely maximise muscle growth, it would also be beneficial to ensure each of your main meals contains 2–3 g of the amino acid leucine, the amount required to maximally trigger muscle protein synthesis, the physiological process responsible for our muscles growing stronger and bigger in response to stress.[436,437]

FIGURE 10.46:

TOP PLANT-BASED SOURCES OF LEUCINE

FOOD	SERVING SIZE	LEUCINE
Tofu, extra firm	½ cup	1.3 g
Tempeh	½ cup	1.2 g
Edamame beans	½ cup	0.6 g
Lentils, cooked	½ cup	0.6 g
Red kidney beans, cooked	½ cup	0.6 g
Baked beans	½ cup	0.5 g
Fava (broad) beans, cooked	½ cup	0.5 g
Almonds	20 nuts	0.4 g
Cashews	15 nuts	0.4 g
Peanuts	30 nuts	0.4 g
Rolled oats	½ cup	0.4 g
Walnuts	15 halves	0.4 g
Sunflower seeds	2 tbsp	0.3 g
Baked potato	1 cup	0.2 g
Broccoli	1 cup	0.2 g
Brown rice, cooked	½ cup	0.2 g
Corn	½ cup	0.2 g
Green peas	½ cup	0.2 g

FIGURE 10.47:

AN EXAMPLE OF A WFPB MEAL RICH IN BOTH PROTEIN AND LEUCINE

FOOD	CALORIES	PROTEIN	LEUCINE
120 g tofu, extra firm	132	15.9 g	1.3 g
¾ cup cooked lentils	172	13.4 g	1 g
2 tbsp pumpkin seeds	85	4.4 g	0.4 g
½ cup cooked quinoa	111	4.1 g	0.2 g
1 cup spinach	7	0.9 g	0.1 g
½ cup mushrooms	11	1.5 g	0.1 g
TOTAL	518	40.2 g	3.1 g

While it's certainly not impossible to achieve this by focusing on eating leucine-rich plant-based foods, it is made easier with the addition of a plant protein powder or essential amino acid powder that contains 2–3 g of leucine per serve. If the label doesn't clearly show the leucine content, look for another brand. For protein powder, I recommend brown rice protein or pea protein – both typically have over 2 g of leucine per serve, and recent clinical trials have shown them to be just as effective as whey protein (considered the gold standard of protein powders) at increasing lean muscle mass and strength.[438–440] Importantly, these studies used the same 24 g serving for plant protein and whey protein. As long as you can reach your protein target and consume 2–3 g of leucine per meal, it doesn't seem to matter where the protein comes from. I personally have a blend of brown rice and pea protein – one serving on a typical day and two servings on more intensive training days.[439] Multiple clinical trials have also shown that soy protein is as effective as whey protein at improving body composition and strength.[441,442] Other plant protein powders that have excellent amino acid profiles, which I am hopeful will become more widely available in the coming years, are potato and corn protein. Corn protein, for example, contains a higher percentage of leucine per gram of protein than both whey and egg protein.[443]

To remove the guesswork and ensure your diet is consistently providing your body with the necessary building blocks, you could track your calories and macronutrients closely using an app like Cronometer, or you could track your protein as the primary goal and eat intuitively. The former is going to be more precise and the latter will be easier on your lifestyle. Personally, I started by using an app and now keep a loose track of the protein that I am eating over the day and know how many total meals I am targeting to eat sufficient calories. If you are putting on more than around half a kilogram per week and gaining excessive body fat, you are probably underestimating the amount of calories you are eating, overestimating how much exercise you are doing, or a combination of the two. And vice versa if you are struggling to gain weight, improve your strength and build muscle.

Principle 8: Don't let perfection be the enemy of good

Shifting to a WFPBD can seem like a daunting process but it doesn't have to be. Rather than placing enormous pressure on yourself and thinking you have to do everything perfectly, I want you to take a step back and think of the big picture – long-term adherence to this new way of eating. You don't need to feel guilty if you stray from the guidelines. In fact, a little bit of straying from the guidelines is expected, and can be good for you. I want you to enjoy your food and to not feel guilt or shame when you veer off course. For example, sometimes going out and enjoying a plant-based pizza or burger with friends is better for your overall health than restricting yourself from that experience. And while I suggest brown rice, I'm not going to pretend that I don't have the odd bowl of white rice too. I don't recommend cooking with coconut oil, but I'm not averse to an occasional vegan doughnut, or other vegan treats that no doubt contain appreciable amounts of this. And I enjoy every mouthful. Practising flexibility doesn't make you a failure – it's smart. By doing this, I guarantee you will be happier, healthier and create a more sustainable lifestyle.

There are no extra brownie points for following the pyramid down to a tee – consistently good is better than occasionally perfect! In fact, if anything, the extra brownie points are for those who take the principles onboard, upgrade their diet and health, and integrate it into their lifestyle while still maintaining a healthy relationship with food and enjoying the many other aspects of life that extend beyond what we feed ourselves three or more times per day.

Orthorexia

If a person never feels 'cleansed' and always feels like they need to eat better, is constantly thinking about food and judging others for not eating correctly, these could be signs of a medical condition called *orthorexia*. This is an obsession with eating foods they deem to be healthy while avoiding foods considered to be harmful at all costs. This is something we all want to avoid, and you should seek out professional help if you experience any of these feelings or symptoms.

Making the shift simple – tips to get you started

Essentials for a well-stocked plant-based kitchen

Besides fresh fruits, vegetables and herbs, here are some pantry staples that are super handy to keep in stock within your household.

FIGURE 10.48:
KITCHEN ESSENTIALS[444-447]

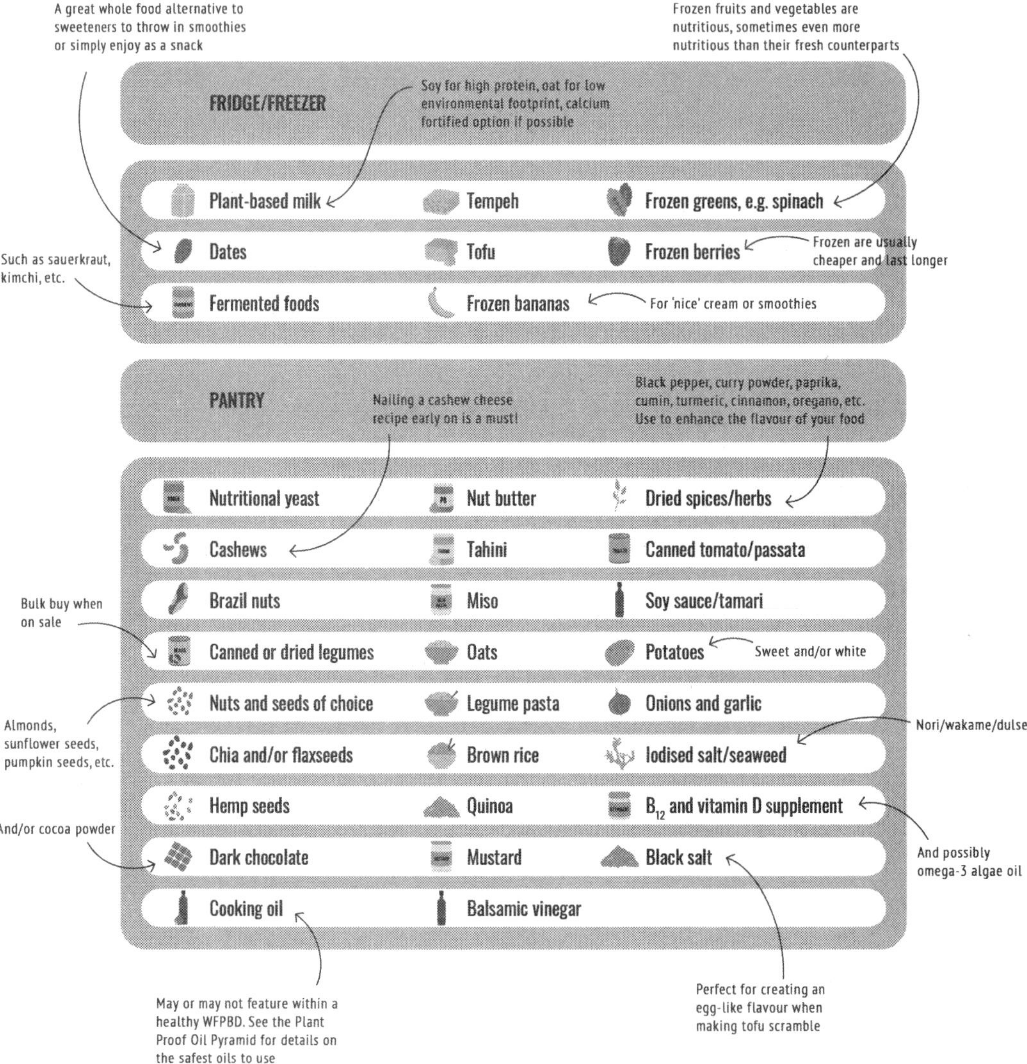
A great whole food alternative to sweeteners to throw in smoothies or simply enjoy as a snack
Frozen fruits and vegetables are nutritious, sometimes even more nutritious than their fresh counterparts
FRIDGE/FREEZER
Soy for high protein, oat for low environmental footprint, calcium fortified option if possible
Plant-based milk
Tempeh
Frozen greens, e.g. spinach
Dates
Tofu
Frozen berries
Frozen are usually cheaper and last longer
Such as sauerkraut, kimchi, etc.
Fermented foods
Frozen bananas
For 'nice' cream or smoothies
PANTRY
Nailing a cashew cheese recipe early on is a must!
Black pepper, curry powder, paprika, cumin, turmeric, cinnamon, oregano, etc. Use to enhance the flavour of your food
Nutritional yeast
Nut butter
Dried spices/herbs
Cashews
Tahini
Canned tomato/passata
Brazil nuts
Miso
Soy sauce/tamari
Bulk buy when on sale
Canned or dried legumes
Oats
Potatoes
Sweet and/or white
Nuts and seeds of choice
Legume pasta
Onions and garlic
Almonds, sunflower seeds, pumpkin seeds, etc.
Chia and/or flaxseeds
Brown rice
Iodised salt/seaweed
Nori/wakame/dulse
Hemp seeds
Quinoa
B_{12} and vitamin D supplement
And possibly omega-3 algae oil
And/or cocoa powder
Dark chocolate
Mustard
Black salt
Cooking oil
Balsamic vinegar
May or may not feature within a healthy WFPBD. See the Plant Proof Oil Pyramid for details on the safest oils to use
Perfect for creating an egg-like flavour when making tofu scramble

Sustainability tips

If you find yourself with too much fresh produce and are concerned it's going to spoil, chop it up and store in the freezer. When it comes to vegetables, if they are only going to be frozen for a few weeks, freezing them in their fresh form is perfectly fine, but if they are likely to be frozen for a longer period, it's better to blanch them first. (This means to briefly submerge them in boiling water until they just start to soften, and then plunge them in an ice bath to stop the cooking process.) Fruit, on the other hand, can always be frozen fresh. I also recommend eating as much of your plants as possible. For example, why peel potatoes and carrots when the skin offers so much nutrition? This goes for the majority of fruits and vegetables we eat - their outer layer is jam-packed with fibre, vitamins, minerals and antioxidants. You can even eat banana peels - give them a good wash, then chop them up and throw them into your favourite curry, or shred them with a fork and marinate to create 'pulled pork'. Finally, where possible, return the nutrients in the inedible parts of your food to soil by composting - at home for your own garden, or through an external service in your area. Remember, food waste is a significant driver of greenhouse gas emissions and planetary harm - the less food that ends up in the bin, the better.

Making it stick

Go at your own pace and do what feels best for you. Here are a few things that helped me, or have helped others that I know to make their transition stick!

- **DO IT IN STAGES AND START SMALL.** Rather than making the shift overnight, you may find it easier to transition over an eight- to twelve-week period – for example, starting with one meal a day (breakfast is usually easiest) and then gradually progressing to two (see 'Vegan before 6 pm' below) then three meals a day as you build confidence. Like many things in life, the hardest part is simply starting. So start small, get some success and build momentum from there bit by bit.
- **FOCUS ON EASY SWAPS.** Simple swaps implemented gradually can be very useful, such as swapping cow's milk for plant-based milk, red meat for lentils, butter for olive oil and chicken for tofu or tempeh. You will often find that just these single swaps instantly turn a favourite dish of yours into a whole food plant-based meal (or at least very close). In fact, adjusting your favourite recipes is one of the best places to start. For example, mastering a scrambled tofu to replace scrambled eggs. Focusing on the swap and what you will be adding to your diet, rather than what you're removing, is a more positive way to frame these changes (see Figure 10.49). While I certainly do not advocate regular consumption of ultra-processed plant-based meat products (because, let's face it, beans are healthier), it's comforting to know that in a sixteen-week RCT conducted in 2020, consuming plant-based meat products improved several cardiovascular risk factors when compared with organic animal-based meats.[448] This makes them a good option during a transition to a WFPBD, and a healthier alternative to animal products on the odd occasion (e.g. when you're at a barbecue with friends or family). Despite these very much being 'once in a while' foods, it's still worth trying to find products that contain around 5 g or less saturated fat, 400 mg or less sodium and around 5 g or more fibre per serving.

- **SET UP YOUR FRIDGE AND PANTRY FOR SUCCESS.** Prepare for success by having the foods you need on hand. This will help you stay on track!
- **SEASON YOUR MEALS.** By itself, tofu is about as bland as chicken, yet most of the world has no problems eating chicken on the regular. It's all in the seasoning – herbs, spices and condiments. That's what really gets our tastebuds dancing, not the animal foods. Want to make plant-based sushi? Work in wasabi, ginger and tamari. By taking your favourite flavour combinations and replacing animal protein with a source of plant protein that provides a similar texture, you'll enjoy your new meals so much more. You'll have the same experience, or even better, minus the health trade-offs.
- **USE LISTS.** When you aren't used to cooking plant-based meals, it can be overwhelming if you head to the supermarket without a plan. When I first transitioned, I selected a handful of easy recipes and used those to create ingredient lists to guide my shopping.
- **EAT ENOUGH.** Remember, plant foods are typically much less calorie-dense than animal and ultra-processed foods. That means your plate needs to look fuller or you will likely be consuming fewer calories than you are used to and may notice a drop in energy. Over time, you will get used to eating higher volume meals.
- **BATCH COOK.** If you are the type of person that feels overwhelmed by a lot of changes, you may find batch cooking removes a bit of the pressure. That way you can cook something new (e.g. lentil lasagne) and enjoy it for multiple meals. This can also help you with eating on the go.
- **RESEARCH.** If you are eating out with friends, in the early days where you may feel a little awkward or embarrassed

asking the waiter about vegan options (the more common term used at restaurants to identify dishes without animal products), prepare ahead of time by checking out their menu online or giving them a quick call. Additionally, apps like Happy Cow can be really helpful for identifying vegan-friendly restaurants.

- **TRACK, IF YOU WISH.** Sometimes, you may benefit from using a tracking app like Cronometer so you can see how many calories you're consuming as well as your intake of nutrients of focus. Early on during your transition this, along with the Plant Proof Food Pyramid, can help you work out if there are any foods or food groups that you need to focus on a little more.
- **SHARE YOUR TRANSITION.** While it is by no means necessary, having a partner or friend to share your transition with can often make it easier. That way, you can learn and progress together. You can also share your journey with the Plant Proof Community group on Facebook.
- **BE PATIENT AND ENJOY YOURSELF.** It can be tempting to be hard on ourselves during a transition away from animal products and ultra-processed foods. Remember, we are changing habits that many of us have had for decades, so be patient and understand it's not a race. You're going to make mistakes along the way, so rather than chasing the perfect transition, it's best to understand that this is going to involve some trial and error.
- **DON'T JUDGE.** Try to avoid judging others and instead lead the way by setting a good example. Just because you have made the decision to change your diet doesn't mean everyone else is ready. Certainly give them information but remember they'll ultimately make changes when the time is right for them.

FIGURE 10.49:

SIMPLE SWAPS FOR A SIMPLE SHIFT

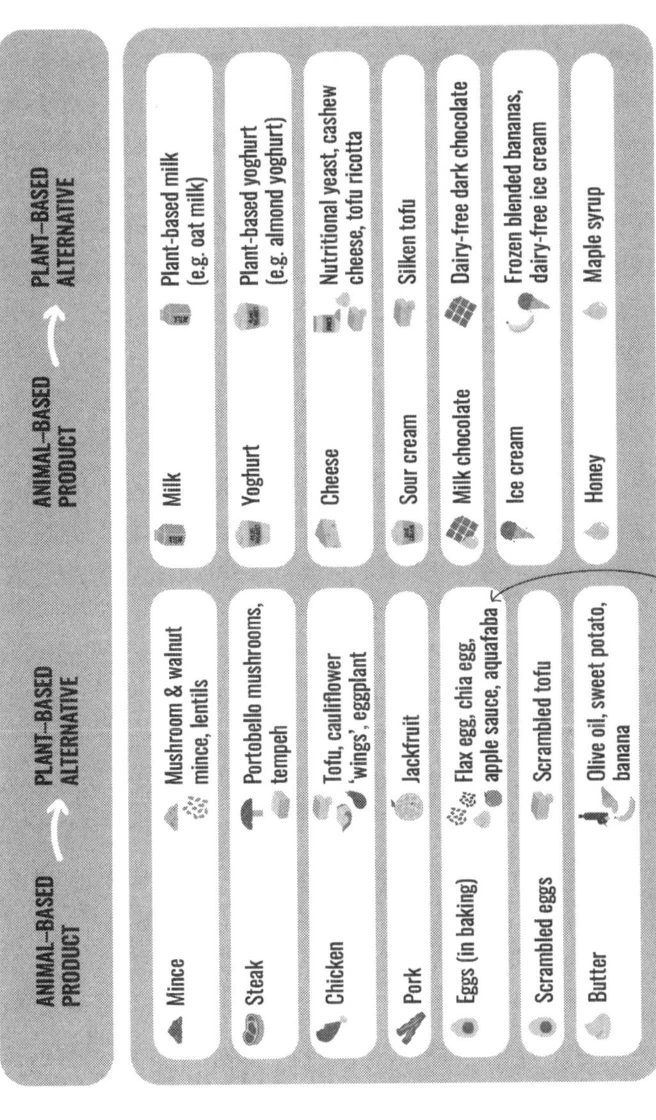

ANIMAL-BASED PRODUCT
PLANT-BASED ALTERNATIVE
Mince
Mushroom & walnut mince, lentils
Steak
Portobello mushrooms, tempeh
Chicken
Tofu, cauliflower 'wings', eggplant
Pork
Jackfruit
Eggs (in baking)
Flax egg, chia egg, apple sauce, aquafaba
Scrambled eggs
Scrambled tofu
Butter
Olive oil, sweet potato, banana
Liquid from canned chickpeas – behaves like egg white
ANIMAL-BASED PRODUCT
PLANT-BASED ALTERNATIVE
Milk
Plant-based milk (e.g. oat milk)
Yoghurt
Plant-based yoghurt (e.g. almond yoghurt)
Cheese
Nutritional yeast, cashew cheese, tofu ricotta
Sour cream
Silken tofu
Milk chocolate
Dairy-free dark chocolate
Ice cream
Frozen blended bananas, dairy-free ice cream
Honey
Maple syrup

'Vegan before 6 pm' – a flexitarian approach

If you are not ready to adopt a 100% WFPBD but still want to eat more plants and reduce the number of animal products you consume, a flexitarian approach may be for you. Remember, I'm in your corner no matter the extent of the changes you make! Anyone moving in this direction is part of the solution, not the problem. In this instance, I suggest aiming for a diet that contains at least 85% of calories from plants in order to achieve the health and environmental benefits we saw in Part Two. So, practically speaking, what does an 85% plant-based diet look like, and what is the most healthy and sustainable way to do it?

We've already seen some dietary patterns that do this, such as a pro-vegetarian Mediterranean diet or the EAT-*Lancet* planetary health diet. Another approach that is easy to keep track of is to eat two meals and all of your snacks in a day that are 100% plant-based, and just one meal a day that contains animal products. American food journalist Mark Bittman has dubbed this approach 'vegan before 6 pm'.[449]

FIGURE 10.50:
VEGAN BEFORE 6 PM

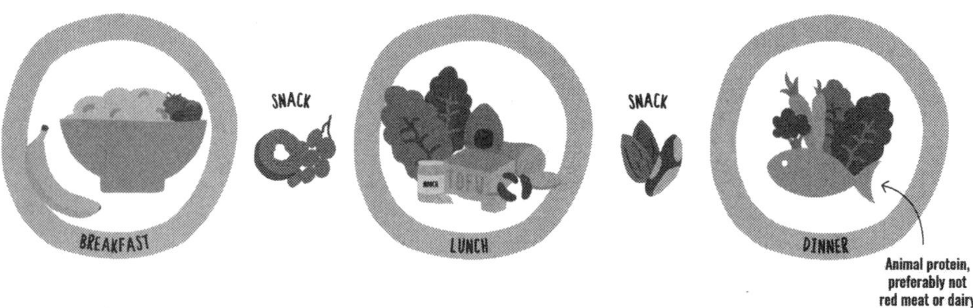

A study published in 2020 by a team from Johns Hopkins University, looking at data from over 140 countries, identified that this type of flexitarian diet can be better for the environment than a typical vegetarian diet, largely due to the fact that vegetarian diets often contain a lot of dairy, which has a large GHG footprint.[450,451] While transitioning from a standard Australian diet to a vegetarian diet would reduce the average Australian's GHG emissions by around 50%, a vegan before 6 pm diet would reduce GHG emissions by around 65%, and a vegan diet by around 90%.[450]

FIGURE 10.51:

THE GHG FOOTPRINT OF DIFFERENT DIETARY PATTERNS IN AUSTRALIA[450]

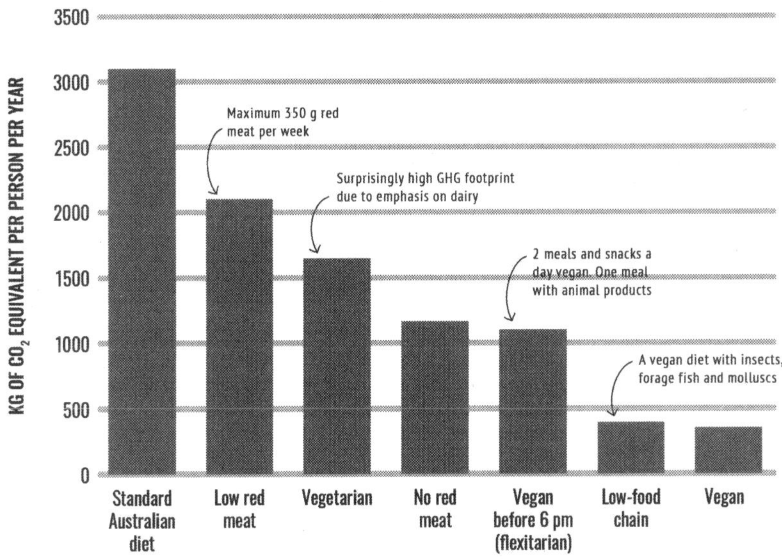

If this sounds like the best approach for you, I would encourage you to avoid red meat and dairy, the two biggest contributors to environmental harm in our food system, and instead stick to oysters, mussels, clams, scallops, eggs, chicken or small fatty fish like sardines, anchovies and mackerel in the meals that include animal products.[451,452]

Other than those additions, I would still suggest eating according to the Plant Proof Food Pyramid. I know many people who have adopted 'vegan before 6 pm' as an entry point to a plant-focused diet with great success. While some have continued with it long-term, others have progressively removed animal products until arriving at a plant-exclusive diet, as their health and confidence went from strength to strength.

The Plant Proof Audit

I'm a big believer in living life to its fullest, and getting bogged down in calorie-counting and nutrients of focus on a daily basis can rob us of some of the enjoyment that food offers us. But there's no arguing that, from time to time, we need to come back to the principles and conduct a mini audit to see where things are at. To help us achieve that, I have developed the Plant Proof Audit, which is a one-week tracking tool to give you an indication as to how Plant Proof your diet really is. I recommend doing this every three to four months, particularly during your transition from a more Western-style eating pattern. In this week, you will track:

1. How many unique plants you consumed (1 point per unique plant)
2. Whether or not your diet or supplement regime included sufficient amounts of the eight nutrients of focus (4 points per nutrient)
3. How many days a week you stuck to the circadian rhythm eating pattern (4 points per successful day).

At the end of the week, you add up your score to give you a total out of 100. The idea here is not to be on your best behaviour and score 100, but rather to get a genuine score that reflects how you have naturally been eating.

- 80–100: That's as Plant Proof as it gets. You should probably consider sharing some of that wisdom.

(Note: I've purposely created a large range for this top tier because the goal is not perfection. A score of 80 is just as good as 95.)

- 70–80: While this is certainly above average, you can probably tweak a few little things to optimise your health even further.
- 60–70: Looks like you have a lot of the basics down pat but could do with some extra planning to be more consistent and take things up a notch. You'll feel better for it.
- <60: Take some time to reread through the eight principles and identify areas of your life that may be impeding you from creating a Plant Proof lifestyle.

The Plant Proof resources

Anybody who knows me knows I have a lot to say! It was impossible to cover everything in a single book. But I still want to share all of that information that I so desperately wanted to fit in, so I have created a set of bonus resources for you to explore in your own time.

Just visit plantproof.com/book and you will find, available to download:

- Plant Proof Food Pyramid
- Plant Proof Oil Pyramid
- the weekly #plantproof40 checklist (And be sure to share your journey with the hashtag #plantproof40. I'd love to cheer you on as you add more plant diversity to your diet!)
- the Plant Proof Audit template
- a guide to laboratory and blood tests
- a guide to nutritional supplements
- deep dives into the science (including choline and brain health, myths about plant protein, and vitamin A on a WFPBD)

- a bunch of social media assets for you to share about the amazing benefits of a WFPBD.

I also encourage you to sign up to my newsletter at plantproof.com (I will only email you when I have something worthwhile to share!), follow me on Instagram and Twitter (@plant_proof) and tune in to the *Plant Proof* podcast.

I'm dedicated to providing the Plant Proof community with ongoing information and am always around to answer questions.

You have the power and the proof to optimise your life

The eight principles and the tips and tricks to get you started are my best recommendations for making the switch to a WFPBD. Consider them your trusty compass and road map, together guiding you towards a diet that is as plant-exclusive as possible, a way of eating that will help radically transform your health.

I know it's easy to get overwhelmed, confused and distracted – there are many voices of confusion and they have a vested interest in keeping you in the ultra-processed food aisles and at the butcher rather than with the fresh veg. But remember that the scientific consensus is clear and plants offer us amazing protective potential. And most importantly, remember that *you* have the power to decide what you put on your plate. Every step you take towards a plant-exclusive diet is a step towards improving your health now and for your future.

What your specific transition looks like will be unique to you – we all have different life circumstances and embark on this journey with our own unique dietary habits. You may make the shift quicker than others, or more slowly, and that's completely okay. The most important thing is that you get started – hopefully today. Start with just one meal, or one small healthy swap.

No matter how you start, have a clear goal in mind. Why is it important to you that you make changes to the foods on your plate? For me, it was because I'd seen what my dad endured when he had his heart attack in his early forties – not only was this something I wanted to avoid but, alongside my brother, I also wanted to set a good example for my friends and family to follow. Over the years, this is one of my greatest learnings. If making the shift is truly important to you, you will invest your time in making your new habits stick. It's really as simple as that.

I'm not asking you to do a six- or eight-week challenge, but rather adopt a whole new way of looking at your food choices. For that to be sustainable for you, there needs to be a deeper level of meaning behind the changes you make. So when you go searching for a new plant-based recipe to make or experiment with different fruits and veggies, you'll be bolstered by that goal, whatever it is for you.

Rest assured, the lifestyle change you're embarking on won't date – in one, five or even ten or twenty years, the Plant Proof principles will still stand true, and the benefits they will bring to your life are always compounding. So much so that you will see a healthy return on investment for the remainder of your life. While new science continues to be published at a rapid pace, it takes a long time for scientific consensus, which is based on converging lines from multiple levels of evidence, to change. If anything, based on the strength of science we have today on human and planetary health, I predict the case for adopting a plant-based diet will only become stronger as more and more research is conducted.

Most of all, I want you to know you've got this. I certainly believe in you. The very fact that you picked this book out of all the nutrition and diet books out there, and you've made it this far, tells me that you are on a mission for the truth and are looking for a permanent lifestyle change. You're not here for a quick fix or a magic pill. With that mindset, I trust that you will have connected with the information in this book, and should you put it into practice you will only go from strength to strength – physically, mentally and spiritually – never looking back.

With every plant-based meal you consume, you are doing your part to make yourself healthier, to make our planet less vulnerable and to reduce the cruelty inflicted on our fellow animals. At times, you may feel your individual impact is small, but don't underestimate your power. There is definitely magic to be found in this world, but we don't need magic to make it a better place – what we need is enough people like you, willing to cut through the noise and uncertainty and to make the shift, however slowly or imperfectly you do it. And together, our individual actions can and will transform the world.

References

To make it easier for you to review any of the 1000-plus scientific references in this book, I have listed them online. Simply visit **plantproof.com/bookreferences**, select the chapter and reference number you are interested in reading and you will find the citation or hyperlinked resource.

Further reading

To further expand your knowledge on the impact of our food choices, and build on many things in this book, I also recommend checking out the following.

Books

Fiber Fueled by Will Bulsiewicz, MD
Nourish by Reshma Shah, MD MPH, and Brenda Davis, RD
Mastering Diabetes by Cyrus Khambatta, PhD, and Robby Barbaro, MPH
The Plant-Based Baby and Toddler by Whitney English, MS RDN and Alexandra Caspero, MA RDN
The 30-Day Alzheimer's Solution by Dean Sherzai, MD and Ayesha Sherzai, MD
Proteinaholic by Garth Davis, MD
We Are the Weather by Jonathan Safran Foer
Why We Love Dogs, Eat Pigs and Wear Cows by Melanie Joy
The Plant-Based Diet Revolution by Dr Alan Desmond and Rob Andrews
The Plant Power Doctor by Dr Gemma Newman

Recipe books*

The Blue Zones Kitchen by Dan Buettner
Forks Over Knives: The cookbook by Del Sroufe
Vegan One-Pot Wonders by Jessica Prescott
The Happy Health Plan by David Flynn and Stephen Flynn
BOSH!: Simple recipes, amazing food, all plants by Henry Firth and Ian Theasby
More Plants Less Waste by Max la Manna
Minimalist Baker's Everyday Cooking by Dana Schultz
The Global Vegan by Ellie Bullen
Plants Only Kitchen by Gaz Oakley

* Note: I encourage you to tweak recipes based on the information in this book. For example, if a recipe calls for coconut oil, try using cocoa butter or olive oil instead.

Podcasts

The Plant Proof Podcast with Simon Hill
The Rich Roll Podcast with Rich Roll
The Brain Health and Beyond Podcast with Team Sherzai, MD
The Disclosure Podcast by Earthling Ed

Documentaries

Dominion
Seaspiracy
David Attenborough: A Life on Our Planet

YouTube

Nutrition Made Simple! by Gil Carvalho, MD PhD

Gratitudes

There are many people I would like to thank for helping me bring this book into the world.

First, my biggest inspiration – my family.

To my dad, Michael. There's no doubt about it, this book is a tribute to you. You were lucky to get a second chance (and you've definitely made the most of it!), but many are not. You've dedicated your life to science, and along with your research, I hope this book is another way in which your life will change this world for the better. Your curiosity, love of science and endless positive encouragement has, and will, always give me the confidence to do my best at whatever I set out to achieve. And the making of this book is no exception.

To my mother, Mary. You are such a sweet person. Thank you for your ongoing interest in what I do and for saying you like my writing (even though I know you would never say otherwise!). You've taught me the importance of active listening and that to be compassionate and kind is to be strong.

To Jeff and Luanne. Having two 'bonus' parents has been a dream. Thank you for your love, support and guidance.

To my partner, Tanya. Thank you for believing in me and always cheering me on.

To my furry friends, Gnocchi and Giuseppe. Thank you for the endless kisses and for being the best distractions ever.

To my brother, James, and sister-in-law, Lauren. You are living proof of how powerful it is to lead by example. Without each of you, I would have never put pen to paper.

To Will Dalton. Thank you for your words of wisdom. The conversations we had about life, writing and communication are ones I will never forget. You were a brilliant author and had a profound effect on my life and this book. Although you can't be here to read the final product, I know you would be extremely proud.

To all who helped me craft the 90,000 or so words in this book. Thank you for helping me communicate my message and encourage people to eat more plants. To the entire team at Penguin Random House Australia, especially Isabelle Yates and Kathryn Knight. We did it. I will be forever grateful that we had the opportunity to work together on this project. You are both so incredible at what you do. Colleen Martell, thank you for coming in at the eleventh hour and working your magic! Katherine Annessi, Nicholas Carter, Janina Gelbke, Dr Matthew Nagra, Dr Will Bulsiewicz, Dr Cyrus Khambatta, Dr Ayesha Sherzai and Dr Dean Sherzai – each of you played a tremendously important role in bringing this book to life. My great friends Jeremy Butler and Drew Harrisberg, I love our 'workshops'. As you will read, many of the outcomes from these daily conversations are found throughout these pages.

To Chloe Gordon for your wonderful creative direction and illustrations. Your special touch made the information in this book much more accessible.

To each of my podcast guests. Our time spent together provided me with the necessary energy and optimism to show up daily and conduct the research that went into creating this book. Your wisdom is sprinkled throughout.

To all of my friends, my extended family and the entire Plant Proof community. My dad's experience planted the seed for this book, but it was your interest and engagement that fuelled me during the long days of writing. This is *our* book, and that means we are making a positive impact throughout the world *together*. I won't forget that, and I hope you don't either.

Index

INDEX

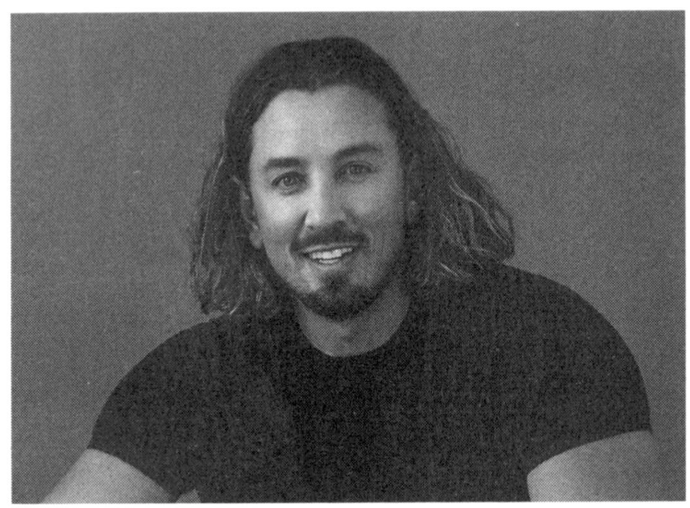

Simon Hill is the founder of the hugely popular *Plant Proof* podcast and blog of the same name, and a nutritionist and physiotherapist. On top of his formal education, Simon spends hours and hours deciphering scientific studies so he can break down how to fuel your body to promote longevity and reduce the chance of developing disease while simultaneously achieving whatever health and fitness goals you may have. He is the plant-based food contributor to Chris Hemsworth's fitness app, Centr, and in 2019 Simon opened a plant-based restaurant, Eden, in his Sydney neighbourhood of Bondi.

@plant_proof

@plant_proof

@plantproofnutrition

plantproof.com